The Beginnings of Modern Medicine in Iran

Willem Floor

MAGE PUBLISHERS

Mage Publishers Inc
www.mage.com

Library of Congress Cataloging-in-Publication Data
Available at the Library of Congress

First hardcover edition
ISBN: 978-1949445-23-7

Visit Mage online:
www.mage.com
eMAIL: as@mage.com

CONTENTS

II

The Beginning of Iran's Nursing schools

III

The Beginnings of Obstetrics in Iran

IV

American Missionary Hospitals: A Role Model

V

Qal`eh-ye Mehrab Khan: the First Leprosarium in Iran

Bibliography

TABLES

ILLUSTRATIONS

FOREWORD

In the field of the history of medicine in Iran, more has been written about the traditional medical system than about the introduction and spread of modern medicine. As a result, much of the early beginnings of modern medicine in Iran still remain unknown. Also, what has been written about that period alleges that French medicine and physicians had a major influence on the medical field in Iran. Therefore, the aim of this book is to correct this lacuna as well as to highlight the important and influential role of American physicians (as well as British physicians) in the development of medical care in Iran.

In chapter one the idea that the Dar ol-Fonun, established in 1851, was the first medical school in Iran is shown to be erroneous. Although medical training of Iranian students had already started by Dr. Holmes in 1876 in Urumiyeh, the first medical school was established by Dr. Cochran in 1885 in that same city, while two other medical training programs also existed at the American hospitals of Hamadan and Tehran. It was only after the American schools ceased their medical schools in 1914 that, in 1918, the government of Iran decided to separate the medical department from the Dar ol-Fonun and establish it as a separate medical school. However, it was only after 1934 that this school began operating as an all-round medical school, when it also taught the more practical side of medical science and its facilities were upgraded. The then *Daneshkadeh-ye Tebb* became a real medical school when it modernized its study program and dissections were allowed thus enabling Iranian students to really learn the anatomy of the human body. The establishment of the medical faculty of the newly created University of Tehran in 1938 signified that the teaching of medicine had achieved parity with medical schools elsewhere in the world.

Chapter two discusses the initiative taken by American physicians to address the total absence of nursing staff in Iran. Because nurses are an essential component of modern medical care, the American Hospital in Tabriz established the first formal nurses school in 1915, shortly thereafter followed by the American Hospital in Urumiyeh. After WW I, the other American Hospitals also started training nurses, an activity that was continuous, because as soon as the nurses were trained, they often married, or were lured away by government or other hospitals. In 1936, relying on assistance from American and British nurses the government of Iran launched its own schools of nursing, which only lasted until 1940. Thereafter, the American Hospitals continued with their own nurses' schools, an activity that was adopted by the newly established Iranian hospitals as of the 1950s.

Chapter three highlights the need for mother-and-child care in Iran, where mortality among both mothers and new-born babies was high. In the early 1930s, American Hospitals began a rigorous program of obstetrics, which soon thereafter was extended to include pre- and post-natal care. As a result, giving birth in a hospital became an acceptable option for a growing, albeit still a small number of women. Also, the American Hospitals began a program of Baby Clinics, in which they followed the British Christian Missionary Society (CMS) that had begun such a program in Yazd in 1932. It was only lack of funds that prevented the government of Iran from full-scale adoption of the same ob-gyn and pediatric approach. Nevertheless the first Iranian initiatives in this area were inspired by the example of the American Hospitals.

In chapter four some hardware and software issues for medical care are highlighted. To offer better care the American physicians introduced the X-ray machine, the hospital laboratory, and other technological instruments that enhance medical diagnosis and treatment. Furthermore, apart from surgical operations (also provided by British physicians) as well as new surgical techniques, they introduced new treatments for some endemic diseases (e.g. for favus and tuberculosis). Similarly, American physicians tried to establish a non-threatening environment, one of cooperation and collegiality, rather than one of competition with their Iranian colleagues through professional collaboration, seminars, and other forms of collegial exchange of information, including the creation of medical societies in Mashhad and Tehran.

In the last chapter, the targeted approach by the American Hospital in Mashhad to help leprosy patients is discussed. Little is known about the occurrence of leprosy in Iran throughout the centuries, even as late as the 1920s. Although segregated villages with lepers existed prior to 1926, it was only as of then that the Mehrab Khan village became the first true Iranian leprosarium, when regular institutional medical treatment was offered by American missionary physicians. The funding agencies, medical personal and treatment, the living environment of lepers and their number in Mehrab Khan are discussed as well as how its population size and status changed over time, and how it was transformed into a structural component of public medical care. Finally and briefly, the establishment and functioning of two other Iranian leprosaria is discussed as well as the slow but sure disappearance of the disease in Iran.[1]

American missionary physicians in Iran like their Iranian colleagues wanted to provide good medical care. However, in addition, they wanted to do something more than that. After all, unlike their Iranian colleagues they had not chosen their employment to make money. For American missionary doctors wanted above all to spread their religion and using the vehicle of medical care gave them a captive audience, either lying prone in a bed, in the consultation room, or in the waiting line at the dispensary. Therefore, they wanted to have good relations with the government, with their professional colleagues and with their patients. To that end, they provided any professional help to their colleagues and the government (technical assistance, lab, consultation, exchange of views, etc.). To improve those relations, they believed that the quality, success and non-competitiveness of their work would have that desired result. In doing so they certainly improved and saved

1. This chapter was earlier published as an article in *Iranian Studies* 53/1-2 (2020), pp. 9-41 and appears here with the permission of the editor-in-chief of that journal.

the lives of many patients, developed and improved medical training, medical care, and public health policy and facilities in Iran.

I wish to express my thanks to Dr. Mohammad Ali Azizi (Tehran) for making a scan of the *Rahnama-ye daneshkadeh-e pezeshki* available to me and Dr. Hormoz Ebrahimnejad for having read and commented on the text. Further, to the staff of the Presbyterian Historical Society (Philadelphia) for facilitating my research by their very helpful attitude. Finally, to my friend Keith Openshaw for being once again my guardian to see that I didn't botch the Queen's English too much.

I

THE FIRST MEDICAL SCHOOL IN MODERN IRAN

The Establishment of the Dar ol-Fonun

When Amir Kabir became grand vizier in 1848 he initiated a series of initiatives with the intention to make Iran a modern state. This meant that Iran needed to have a stronger and more capable military to defend its borders, a modern industry to reduce imports, and a class of officials trained in European sciences and languages that would strengthen the government's overall capabilities. One of these initiatives was the establishment of a modern school to train this new class of officials. In 1849, therefore, Amir Kabir instructed the British trained Mirza Reza *mohandes-bashi* to design a building for his new school that generally was called Dar ol-Fonun. Together with Mohammad Taqi Khan *me`mar-bashi* he built the school over the next two years. The location was part of the royal palace that previously had been used as barracks.[1]

Although teaching medicine was part of the school's curriculum, the main objective of the establishment of the Dar ol-Fonun in Tehran was to create a modern military and technical capacity in Iran. Medicine and other subjects were ancillary to this objective, because Amir Kabir wanted to meet the medical needs of the army.[2] This is clear from the school's curriculum, from the students' military uniform, as well as from the composition of the first group of European teachers, most of whom were military (Nemiro, Gumoëns, Kržiž, and Zatti). Although

1. Gurney and Nabavi 1993; Ardakani 1368, vol. 1, p. 255; Rahnama 1333, pp. 26, 28; Elgood 1951, p. 511; Dowlatabadi 1336, vol. 1, pp. 327-28.
2. Gurney and Nabavi 1993; Amanat 1997, p. 127; Ardakani 1368, vol. 1, p. 255; Adamiyat 1354, pp. 353-54.

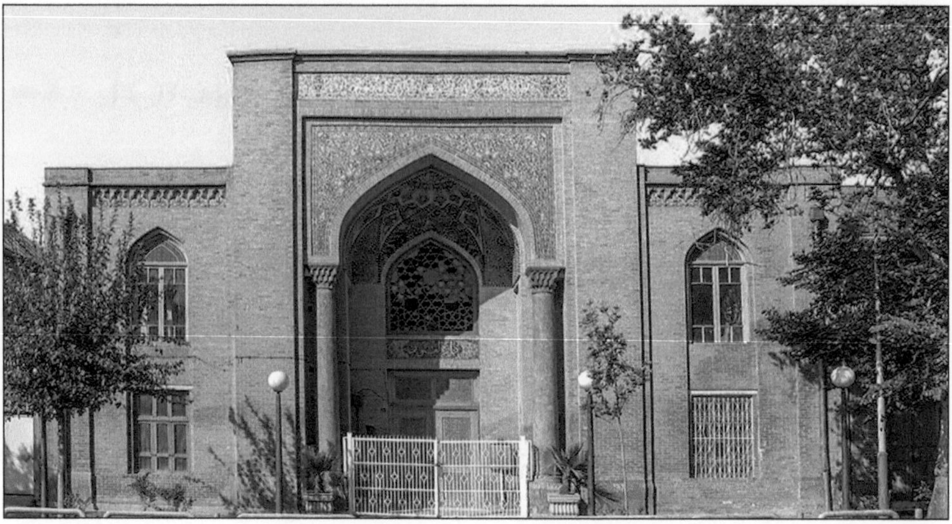

The main entrance of the Dar ol-Fonun in Tehran

the Dar ol-Fonun remained a military school until the beginning of the 20th century, Amir Kabir also wanted to create the beginnings of a class of physicians trained in modern medicine to sustain his policy concerning public health. For example, in 1851 he promulgated a law making it compulsory for all Iranian subjects to be vaccinated against smallpox.[3]

However, not everybody agreed with Amir Kabir's reforms, including the establishment of his school. Opposition against the new school came from the olama and conservative court circles, who felt that the new teachings would undermine the monarchy, Islamic values and the olama's monopoly on education. It also came from traditional physicians such as Mirza Baba Shirazi Malek al-Atteba, who was adamantly opposed to modern Western medicine. To torpedo any chance of Western medicine ever becoming accepted in Iran he wrote

---

3. *Vaqaye`-ye Ettefaqiyeh* 1373-74, vol. 1, p. 122 (no. 25, 25 Ramadan 1267/23 July 1851). UNESCO 1343, vol. 1, p. 735; Gurney and Nabavi 1993. Sometimes the school is explicitly referred to as *Madraseh-e mobarakeh-ye nezamiyeh-ye Iran mowsum be Dar al-Fonun*. (the blessed military school of Iran known as Dar al-Fonun). Hedayat 1338-39, vol. 10, p. 560.

the *Resaleh-ye Jowhariyeh*. Therefore, to placate the olama, theology and public prayer was made part of the curriculum, and, to appease the traditional healers, traditional medicine was taught at the school.[4]

To avoid British-Russian rivalry, Amir Kabir asked Austria, a neutral country without interest in Iranian affairs, to send teachers for the Dar ol-Fonun. Mirza Jan Davud Khan, first interpreter at the Ministry of Foreign Affairs, was sent to Vienna to hire competent teachers. He hired the following people:[5]

Lt. August Karl Kržiž	Artillery
Alfred Baron de Gumoëns	Infantry
Johann von Nemiro	Cavalry
Joseph Czarnotta	Mineralogy
Jacob Eduard Polak	Medical science
Capt. Guido Zatti	Mathematics & architecture

Fochetti,[6] an Italian, who taught physics and pharmacology, came somewhat later, in 1852, but it is not clear who had hired him.

Amir Kabir was dismissed as grand vizier on 20 November 1851, and on 24 November Jan (Jean) Davud Khan arrived with six Austrian teachers. Polak ascribed the appointment of Mirza Aqa Khan Nuri as the new grand vizier as part of the reason for the less successful achievement of the school, because he opposed any reform proposed by Amir Kabir. In fact, he wanted to pay the seven teachers an indemnity so that they might return home. Also, Col. Sheil, the British envoy did not favor the arrival of the Austrian teachers and preferred to use Italian

4. Gurney and Nabavi 1993; Ardakani 1368, vol. 1, p. 255; Rahnama 1333, vol. 1, pp. 26, 28; Elgood 1951, p. 511; Dowlatabadi 1336, vol. 1, pp. 327-28; Ebrahimnejad 2014, p. 89.

5. Rahnama 1333, p. 28; Polak 1865, vol. 1, p. 298; Gurney and Nabavi 1993; Slaby 1982, pp. 68-73.

6. Sani` al-Dowleh 1296, vol. 2, p. 84 says he was Italian. Also, he was not part of the group hired in Austria and apparently came separately, because, on arrival, Polak was prepared to teach pharmacology.

officers, who had been hired by the Iranian Legation in Istanbul.[7] The olama and traditional healers reiterated their objections to the school. However, Naser al-Din Shah supported the Dar ol-Fonun plan and, therefore, he disregarded the opponents to the school.[8] As long as Mirza Aqa Khan Nuri was grand vizier the Austrian teachers were treated poorly. According to Polak, they were denied the customary robes of honor as well as food and accommodations befitting their rank during the official reception by the Shah.[9] Because Austria had no diplomatic relationship with Iran and wanted to avoid any accusation that it wanted to meddle in Iran's internal affairs, like Russia and Great Britain did, it declined to support the Austrian teachers or even to be kept abreast of their situation. Austria considered them private citizens who had accepted employment in Iran not to represent their country, but to make money.[10]

THE FIRST CURRICULUM

On 30 November 1851, the Iranian and European teachers, interpreters and the 105 first year students were presented to Naser al-Din Shah, who officially opened the school on 29 December 1851.[11] Because the government had asked the 14-15 year-old sons of the country's governing and socio-economic elite (*a`yan* and *ashraf*) to be sent to the school, the first class of students consisted mostly of princes, sons of courtiers and other high government officials. In fact, the

7. These Italian army officers also taught at the Dar ol-Fonun, because by 1854 the Austrian group had been halved in number. On these Italian officers, see Piemontese 1984. Therefore, additional teachers were needed, see *Vaqaye`-ye Ettefaqiyeh* 1373-74, vol. 2, p. 856 (no. 137, 11 Dhu'l-Hijjah) (Gumoëns, who was a querulous man, was replaced by Fedor Karaczay and Zatti by the Frenchman Buhler); Rahnama 1333, vol. 1, p. 40; Slaby 1982, p. 74; Polak 1862, p. 235.

8. Polak 1865, vol. 1, p. 301; Dowlatabadi 1336, vol. 1, pp. 327-28.

9. Polak 1865, vol. 1, pp. 298, 302.

10. Polak 1865, vol. 1, p. 298; Slaby 1982, pp. 69-70.

11. Hedayat 1338-39, vol. 10, p. 523. According to Hazefi 1332, vol. 1, p. 28 there were 100 students at the Shah's opening of the school.

shah ordered all his governors to send their sons and other talented young men to the school. Later classes consisted in more socially and education diverse groups, be it that students still came from the upper and upper-middle class. The main reason was that, apart from traditional *maktab*s and theological seminars, there were no schools in Iran and thus, the supply of potential students was small.[12] Therefore, many of the medical students were sons of traditional physicians.[13]

Students were given two sets of uniforms (for summer and winter), food, books and a monthly or an annual stipend ranging from 12 to 100 *tuman*s per year. Each department (*kelas*) wore a uniform of a different color, and with the arrival of new classes, each new class had a uniform in a color that was peculiar to it. Also, the term class (*kelas*) here should be understood as denoting a separate department within the Dar ol-Fonun; the following 'classes' were known:

Military and music (*nezami va muzik*)
Literature (*adabiyat*)
Mining (*ma`dan-shenasi*)
Fine arts (*honarha-ye ziba*)
Mathematics and architecture (*riyazat va mohandesi*)
Medicine and pharmacology (*tebb va daru-sazi*).[14]

Mirza Mohammad `Ali Khan, Minister of Foreign Affairs, was the first director of the school, who reported personally to the shah about the school's activities. He died in February 1852 and his successors, all military officers, did not interfere with the school's operation. In fact, during 1852, it was the deputy-director, Rezaqoli Khan Hedayat,

---

12. *Vaqaye`-ye Ettefaqiyeh* 1373-74, p. 223 (no. 43, 3 Safar 1268/28 November 1851); Rahnama 1333, vol. 1, pp. 28, 30; Polak 1865, vol. 1, p. 303. For the problems in getting students with some level of education, see Ebrahimnejad 2014, pp. 90-91.
13. Ebrahimnejad 2014, p. 117; Rahnama 1333, vol. 1, p. 30.
14. *Vaqaye`-ye Ettefaqiyeh* 1373-74, vol. 1, p. 253 (no. 48, 9 Rabi` I 1268); Hedayat 1338-39, vol. 10, p. 522; Polak 1862, p. 236; Ardakani 1368, vol. 1, pp. 266, 268, 293; Yaghma'i 1349, p. 300; Rahnama 1333, vol. 1, p. 33.

and the European instructors, who shaped the school's curriculum and work program, which were based on their various specialties and work experience. At the beginning of the second school year a detailed program was established. The total duration of the study was supposed to last 12 years, divided into four grades (*martabeh*) of three years. Students could only advance to the next grade by passing an exam at the end of each 3-year period.[15] The 'upgrading' as well as the acceptance of each student, was subject to royal approval, because Naser al-Din Shah was very interested in the school's activities. He visited it regularly and handed out prizes and (copper, silver, gold-plated and gold) medals to deserving students after exams. Also, the head of the school regularly reported to the Shah about the school's activities and progress.[16]

The curriculum, which included prayer and listening to sermons in the school's mosque,[17] consisted in: military arts (cavalry, infantry, artillery, music); medicine and pharmacology; mathematics and technology; mineralogy, literature, art (mostly painting) and sports. Foreign languages, initially only French (in 3 classes), were taught, which were obligatory for students in medicine, technology and mineralogy.[18] Literature meant Persian and Arabic literature as well

15. Ardakani 1368, vol. 1, pp. 300-05; Yaghma'i 1349, pp. 303-05; Piemontese 1969, p. 431; Sani` al-Dowleh 1295-97, vol. 2, p. 90.

16. Mostawfi 1343, vol. 1, p. 124; Hedayat 1338-39, vol. 10, pp. 521-22; Rahnama 1333, vol. 1, pp. 29, 31-32, 37-39 ; Sani` al-Dowleh 1296, vol. 2, p. 281; Gurney and Nabavi 1993. According to Sani` al-Dowleh 1296, vol. 3, p. 12, the revenues of Malayer and Tuyserkan were allocated E`tezad al-Saltaneh to pay for the cost of the Dar ol-Fonun.

17. *Vaqaye`-ye Ettefaqiyeh* 1373-74, vol. 1, p. 253 (no. 48, 9 Rabi` I 1268); Polak 1862, p. 236.

18. Rahnama 1333, vol. 1, pp. 33-34; but later (1880s) also English, Russian and German (each only in one class); E'temad-al-Salṭaneh 1307, p. 92; Ehtesham al-Saltaneh 1366, pp. 26-27; Ardakani 1368, vol. 1, pp. 300-05; Yaghma'i 1349, pp. 302-06. See also Polak's remarks on the beginning of the discussions about the curriculum. Polak 1865, p. 1, pp. 302-03.

as theology and was taught by Sheikh Mohammad Saleh Esfahani and Rezaqoli Khan Hedayat.[19]

All students had to study reading, writing, Arabic, and philosophy. These were in particular important for medical students, because of the sources of Galenic medicine such as Ibn Sina and Razi were written in Arabic. This subject, as noted above, was part of the curriculum. Mirza Ahmad Tabib Kashani taught Galenic medicine, because most Iranians did not believe in Western medicine. He read the students from the *Qanun*, *Tebb-e Akbar* and *Sharh-e Asbab* and occasionally discussed the text with them. He taught this subject until 1870. He was not the only one, because Mirza Sayyed `Ali also taught traditional medicine, in addition to modern medicine, being a former student of Dr. Cloquet and Dr. Polak. He taught *Sharh-e Nafisi* by Ibn Nafis and *Qanuncheh* by Mohammad b. Mahmud Chaghmimi.[20] French was also a subject that was acquired during the study. To help students in these subjects, some Persian teachers (Armenians and Moslems) were hired.[21] The level of knowledge and commitment of the incoming students differed, of course. Therefore, some were able to complete their studies in six to seven years, while others took 10-12 years to do so. There also were some who failed to graduate.[22]

---

19. Hedayat 1338-39, vol. 10, p. 522.

20. *Vaqaye`-ye Ettefaqiyeh* 1373-74, vol. 1, p. 609 (no. 102, 3 Rabi` II 1269/14 January 1853). Others such as Mirza Hoseyn-e Doktor also taught Galenic medicine at the school. Ebrahimnejad 2014, p. 92.

21. *Vaqaye`-ye Ettefaqiyeh* 1373-74, vol. 4, p. 2290 (no. 456, 19 Jomadi I/14 December 1859); Rahnama 1333, vol. 1, pp. 28, 33. For a list of teachers and translators in 1268/1852, see *Vaqaye`-ye Ettefaqiyeh* 1373-74, vol. 1, p. 582 (no. 98, 5 Rabi` I 1269/17 December 1852).

22. Rahnama 1333, vol. 1, pp. 32-33, 35, 38; Sani` al-Dowleh 1296, vol. 2, p. 90; Gurney and Nabavi 1993. Polak made some negative remarks about the interest of many students in learning (Slaby 1982, pp. 80-81), although he was positive about those studying medicine. Polak 1865, vol. 1, p. 303.

THE FORMATIVE YEARS

DR. JACOB EDUARD POLAK

Dr. Polak was 31 years old when he started teaching. At that time, there were 14 medical students, according to Polak, but 20 according to the *Rahnama-ye Pezeshki*.[23] The latter source probably refers to a later date, because in May 1852 Polak wrote that there were 15 students, about whom he was satisfied, as they were better than he had expected.[24] He first taught in French, which was translated by Mohammad Hasan Khan Qajar, who had been sent to France to study during Mohammad Shah's reign. To be more effective, Polak learnt Persian and later taught in that language.[25] Each day, except Friday and Sunday, Polak taught for two hours. After six months he began teaching in Persian with the help of fingers, signs, drawings and specimen. From Europe he had taken a skeleton and specimens in alcohol. Later other aids were imported from Europe such as anatomical models and physiological instruments.[26]

The European teachers realized that their Persian students lacked the necessary knowledge, background, and time to become fully trained physicians. According to Schlimmer, the objective of the training of students in medical science was therefore the following:

> To better understand the reasons why in teaching my Oriental students I always have preferred the narrative genre that

23. Polak 1862, p. 235; Rahnama 1333, vol. 1, p. 29.
24. Polak 1852, p. 742.
25. Polak 1852, p. 742; Idem 1865, vol. 1, p. 304; Idem 1862, p. 235, where he remarks that he later found out that his translator was not translating his words, but told the students all kinds of things that Polak later had to try to erase from their minds what traditional Iranian medicine said about the substance discussed. These translators, who later also were teaching assistants, were called *khalifeh*. The teaching assistants were drawn from the ranks of the higher grades' students. Rahnama 1333, vol. 1, p. 34.
26. Polak 1862, p. 235.

> combines the useful and the fun, I have to say that these students are too little accustomed to serious study and that the only requirement for their admission as medical students is the knowledge of the Persian language (read and write fluently) and of Arabic, sufficient to understand the derivations and the grammatical roots. In general, they have no preliminary idea of science at all, and may, with much effort on their part and of that of their teachers, become what were Health Officers in Europe at the beginning of the [nineteenth] century. Nevertheless, let's not despair. It would be impracticable for the Persian government, with its limited means and the limited number of teachers of diverse nationalities that it found to be available at the moment of the creation of the School to dictate study plans such as are current in Europe. It was therefore, necessary to be content and train practical Persian physicians, who would know to diagnose diseases in an encyclopedic manner based pathognomic symptoms, which European science have established in an unequivocal manner, and to treat these maladies with remedies that have been accepted by the most famous professors. In all civilized countries one demands in addition that one makes the students recognize at the same time the different modifications that the nature of the country and the way of life of its inhabitants make necessary. As to surgeons, we require just enough knowledge of topographical anatomy that is required to generally perform non-invasive operations, dress wounds and the necessary routine capacities to be able to prepare themselves the required drugs in the field.[27]

Already in the first year Polak introduced medical practice in his teaching. He knew that he was unable to train his students to become full-fledged physicians, which was not his intention anyway, but also, he lacked the means to do so. However, he wanted his students to have a good idea of what medicine and natural sciences entailed and thus, to induce them to continue their studies in Iran, or go to Europe

27. Schlimmer 1970, pp. 228-29.

for additional education.[28] According to a progress report published in the government newspaper *Vaqaye`-ye Ettefaqiyeh*:

> Dr. Polak has twenty students who are progressing well. His students completed the study of anatomy, a course which normally takes a year, in three months. His students also study pharmacology and the diagnosis of ailments. At the moment, they have made such remarkable progress that Dr. Polak is planning to take them along to the hospital, so that they can gain some practical experience. He has assured his students that at least two of them can accompany him at each surgery session to observe surgical procedures up-close.[29]

As of the end of December 1852, Dr. Polak worked at the *Dowlat* or State Hospital,[30] where he was assisted by his students. They also assisted him in his city dispensary. Because he was a surgeon (he operated on wealthy Iranians in his private practice) Dr. Polak also wanted his students to have knowledge of that part of medicine. Thus, the idea was to provide the students with a good basis of medical science that would allow them to deal with the most common diseases and to do simple surgery as well as to continue their studies abroad after graduation and then become real physicians.

> I would like to teach my students how to perform small operations. Then, they would be able to come with me to visit patients and assist me in important operations. After some time, I will allow them to perform amputations independently.[31]

Dr. Polak was indeed partly successful in this regard. In March 1854 he wrote that already some of his students were able to make a

28. Polak 1865, vol. 1, pp. 305-06.
29. *Vaqaye`-ye Ettefaqiyeh* 1373-74, vol. 1, p. 582 (no. 98, 5 Rabi` al-Avval 1269/17 December 1852).
30. Polak 1853, p. 221.
31. Polak 1865, vol. 1, p. 305.

useful diagnosis and some he allowed to do small operations under his supervision, which later they were able to do independently.[32]

In 1854, Dr. Polak wanted to establish a 20-bed military hospital outside the city. Although Iranian military physicians opposed his plan, he was able to realize it. However, the Iranian military physician in charge of the hospital managed it in such a way that Dr. Polak resigned from his job working in that hospital, because it was useless, according to him. However, his students continued to work there for some time and thus, learnt the practice of hospital care, including the writing of case histories.[33] He also had the shah order the military physicians to come to the Dar ol-Fonun in the mornings to learn about the basics of modern medicine and in particular about the diseases from which soldiers suffered and died mostly, i.e. malaria, dysentery, typhus and frostbite. Dr. Polak also wrote a treatise on these four diseases, which the military physicians had to study. The treatise was sent to the provinces so that military and other physicians might benefit from the information. To make the text comprehensible, Dr. Polak had phrased the instructions in paragraphs. Various officers told Dr. Polak that these instructions had been very useful in remote places like Shush and Dezful and had reduced mortality among soldiers significantly.[34] However, the attendance of military physicians fell into abeyance, for the order was repeated in 1868.[35]

Dr. Polak was a strong believer in on-the-job training, exposing his students to medicine in practice. This again is clear from a report in the newspaper *Vaqaye`-ye Ettefaqiyeh* in 1854.

---

32. Polak 1853, p. 219; Idem 1854, p. 396; Idem 1862, pp. 249-50.

33. Polak 1854, p. 396; Idem 1862, p. 249. For the critical reaction of the military physicians to Polak's hospital plans, see Ebrahimnejad 2004. For the appalling conditions in the military hospital, see Polak 1865, vol. 1, pp. 307-11; Floor 2004, pp. 190-91.

34. Polak 1865, vol. 1, p. 300; Idem 1862, p. 251; Rahnama 1333, vol. 1, p. 41.

35. *Ruznameh* 1370-72 (no. 6349/11/1868, vol. 2, p. 1168).

> In 1852, under the instruction of Dr. Polak, at the time of the cholera epidemic, the students took measures to administer treatment. Each time Dr. Polak made a house visit three of his students accompanied him. Sometimes, Dar ol-Fonun medical students were sent to the provinces on special assignments.[36]

Apart from teaching, Dr. Polak also ensured that students had access to a number of books that explained several subjects of modern medicine in Persian.

> Books and treatises written by the teaching staff at the school were often translated by the students and printed by the Dar ol-Fonun Press. This press is operated by the students, thus facilitating the rapid printing of books. The first medical book to be printed by the Dar ol-Fonun Press was the Anatomy of the Human body by Dr. Polak.[37]

This book on anatomy was indeed Dr. Polak's first publication, which was translated by his student Mirza Mohammad Hoseyn Afshar. This first effort was incomplete and rudimentary, because as Polak admitted, he lacked sufficient knowledge of the language and because he did not want to make it too complicated. In this way, Dr. Polak and his student-translators contributed to medical terminology.[38] Prior to the publication of his book on anatomy (*Tashrih*) in 1852,[39] Persian physicians only had `Ali b. al-`Abbas `Ala al-Din al-Majusi's *Kamel*

---

36. *Vaqaye`-ye Ettefaqiyeh* 1373-74, vol. 2, p. 997 (no. 157, 4 Jomadi I 1270/2 February 1854).
37. *Vaqaye`-ye Ettefaqiyeh* 1373-74, vol. 2, p. 997 (no. 157, 4 Jomadi I 1270/2 February 1854); Yaghma'i 1349, p. 361; Rahnama 1333, vol. 1, p. 34 (on the printing press).
38. Hedayat 1338-39, vol. 10, p. 522; Polak 1852, pp. 78-90; Polak 1854, p. 396; Rahnama 1333, vol. 1, p. 44.
39. Polak's *Tashrih-e Badan* (Anatomy of the [Human] Body) was printed at the Dar ol-Fonun Press and was offered for sale at a price of 6,000 dinars. *Vaqaye`-ye Ettefaqiyeh* 1373-74, vol. 2, pp. 1115 (no. 173, 7 Sha`ban 1270/25 May, 1854).

al-Sena`at (from 994 CE) and Avicenna's *Qanun fi'l-Tebb* (from 1037 CE) to guide them in matters of anatomy. There also was an earlier European-type study on anatomy, published in Arabic by the Abu Zabel School. Mullah Mohammad Qobuli published a Persian translation in lithographic form around 1854. However, according to Dr. Schlimmer, this Persian translation was filled with mistakes and mysterious formulations, which he ascribed to the ignorance of the translator. Finally, this book's main function was to serve as packing material for the druggists.[40] In addition, there was the treatise that Mirza Mohammad *Hakim-bashi-ye koll* had written. It was a study on medicine entitled *Anvar-e Naseriyyeh* in three volumes. The first volume was on anatomy with 56 plates and an index. The second volume was on surgery, and the third volume on general medicine.[41]

The anatomical knowledge of Iranian physicians remained, however, still very theoretical, despite their improved sources of information. Dissection was forbidden (*haram*) and thus, anatomy was a subject learned from a book. The only case of a dissection that ever occurred was an autopsy done by Dr. Polak on the corpse of his compatriot Zatti to determine whether foul play had been involved in his death.[42] This allowed his students a view into the inside of a human body.[43] When in 1852, he was allowed to use the corpses of executed

---

40. Schlimmer 1970, pp. 38-39; *Vaqaye`-ye Ettefaqiyeh* 1373-74, vol. 2, pp. 1105 (Polak's anatomy), 1115 (Polak's anatomy), 1121 (Polak's anatomy in Persian, 6,000 dinars).

41. *Vaqaye`-ye Ettefaqiyeh* 1373-74, vol. 2, p. 1988 (no. 305, 4 Rabi` II 1273/2 December, 1856). Not having seen this treatise it is not possible to form an opinion about its value added.

42. Schlimmer 1970, p. 69 (q.v. autopsy or *fath*); *Vaqaye`-ye Ettefaqiyeh* 1373-74, vol. 2, (no. 138, Dhu'l-Hijjah 1269/September-October 1853); Polak 1865, vol. 1, p. 313 wrote that Zatti died of coal dust suffocation, but Slaby 1982, p. 73 reported that he had been strangled by an infuriated Persian officer. However, autopsy continued to be considered a ghoulish and un-Islamic activity. Clarke 1837, p. 708 ("A man to be seen dissecting would be taken for a ghoul, and he would be shunned as a degraded being").

43. Schlimmer 1970, p. 69 (autopsie); Rahnama 1333, vol. 1, p. 32.

Babi members for teaching purposes, Polak refused, because he did not want to be a tool of the government and out of fear for the hatred on members of the sect.[44] Although European teachers, of course, wanted their students to be proficient in doing dissections as well, no Iranian at that time was really willing to learn or to do so, because of Islamic and culture prejudice. Even, as late as 1926, Dr. Neligan noted that, "Persian practice is largely medical. There are very few surgeons."[45] The same also held true for those Iranians who had studied medicine in Europe (mostly in France), such as Mirza Sheikh Jalal, who, despite their medical studies in Paris, still remained tradition-bound doctors.[46] The best one could hope for was that Dr. Polak helped his students to overcome their initial fear to touch bones, which they considered to be *najes* or impure. To that end, Polak also had his students handle real skeletons. After initial reluctance to perform such a ritually unclean act, they soon overcame this attitude. Thereafter, they made haste to get skulls from gravesites to be used as study objects.[47]

Dr. Polak's second book was on surgery, which was a translation of the work by Chelius, to which he added some sections on typical Middle Eastern diseases, such as Aleppo boils, guinea worm, leprosy, etc. as well as on eye diseases. His courses were written down and partly published on subjects such as pathology, materia medica, etc. He further wrote a medical dictionary (Persian, Latin, Arabic) as well as a 'Compendium on Physiology.'[48]

Dr. Polak's teaching had some encouraging success. By 1858, 18 students, who had majored in medicine graduated. Of the first class he taught, five succeeded quite well after they had completed their studies in France: Mirza Hoseyn b. Mirza Ahmad Tabib; Mirza

---

44. Polak 1865, vol. 1, p. 306.
45. Neligan 1926, part III, p. 742.
46. Lycklama 1875, vol. 2, p. 166; `Eyn al-Saltaneh 1345, vol. 1, p. 795 (Dr. Ehya al-Molk Sheykh Morad had studied in Paris); Polak 1865, vol. 1, p. 311 (Dr. Mirza Hoseyn, Dr. Mirza Reza b. Moqim and Dr. Mirza `Ali Naqi); in general see Ebrahimnejad 2002, pp. 100-07.
47. Polak 1865, vol. 1, p. 304.
48. Rahnama 1333, vol. 1, p. 44; Polak 1854, p. 396.

Hoseyn b. Mirza Bozorg hakim-bashi, Mirza Reza b. Mirza Moghim Mostowfi; Nosrat `Ali Mirza d. Seyfollah Mirza, and Mirza `Ali Naqi b. Hajj Aqa Esma`il.[49] Another of Polak's students, Mirza `Abdol `Ali, settled in Tabriz and performed operations such as lithotomy and others.[50] Given the success of Polak's students in France, in 1859 it was decided to send some 18 students (in three waves) to study medicine and four students to study pharmacology (*davasazi*), half of whom were students of the Dar ol-Fonun.[51] This study abroad program was strongly supported by E`tezad al-Dowleh, the new school director since 1857, a grand-uncle of the shah, with whom he was on good terms.[52] E`tezad al-Saltaneh also reduced the study time for certain subjects, restructured the various courses, and saw to it that the student body became socially more diverse and did not remain limited to upper-class students. Therefore, the selection of these students was purely based on merit.[53]

Dr. Johan Schlimmer

Before Dr. Polak's departure, the Dutch physician Dr. Johan Schlimmer had started teaching at the school. According to Najmabadi, Schlimmer started teaching at the Dar ol-Fonun in 1860, when Polak left.[54] However, in January 1851/Rabi` I 1267, Schlimmer was already chosen to teach at the Dar ol-Fonun.[55] It seems that Schlimmer continued to serve as military physician until April 1856, when he was appointed

---

49. Rahnama 1333, vol. 1, pp. 35-37.
50. Hedayat 1338-39, vol. 10, p. 522. The title Doctor was only allowed to physicians who had studied in Europe; those who had done so in Iran used the title of 'doctor' after there name, thus, Mirza Reza Doktor. Rahnama 1333, vol. 1, p. 32.
51. Ardakani 1368, vol. 1, p. 303; Rahnama 1333, vol. 1, p. 35. For an overview of the graduates and their careers see Ekhtiar 1994, pp. 178-82, 184-85, 188-91, 195-99.
52. For a biography of this prince, see Amanat 1999.
53. Gurney and Nabavi 1993; Ardakani 1368, vol. 1, pp. 320-55.
54. Najmabadi 1349, p. 575.
55. Adamiyat 1348, p. 356.

Polak's deputy to teach the students at the government hospital and on that occasion Naser al-Din Shah bestowed a *termeh* shawl on him.[56] In June 1857, Dr. Schlimmer is mentioned as being the Shah's personal physician (*hakim-bashi*) and engaged in teaching at Dar ol-Fonun.[57] In 1866, Dr. Schlimmer resigned and was succeeded by Dr. Mirza Reza Tehrani. Why Dr. Schlimmer stopped teaching is unknown, although he remained in government service.[58] During his period at the Dar ol-Fonun, Dr. Schlimmer also engaged in private practice.[59]

Dr. Schlimmer had a good reputation in Iran, not only because he treated poor patients free of charge, but also because patients generally felt that he was effective. For that reason, he was still well-known among people of the older generation of Rasht in the 1950s, according to Najmabadi.[60] Iranian physicians also respected Dr. Schlimmer, because he in turn respected them and their methods,[61] although he criticized these when he thought they did not make sense.[62] When these methods were useful, however, he even argued for their adoption in Europe. For example, traditional Persian physicians prescribed patients not only a remedy, but also gave them a written prescription, which were kept by the patient for later reference. Therefore, any physician, in case of a future consultation, would be able to study all

---

56. *Vaqaye`-ye Ettefaqiyeh* 1373-74, vol. 3, p. 1738 (no. 271, 4 Sha`ban 1272/ 10 April 1856).

57. *Vaqaye`-ye Ettefaqiyeh* 1373-74, vol. 3, p. 2185 (no. 332, 8 Shavval 1273/1 June 1857). According to Elgood 1951, p. 512, Schlimmer began teaching "on 9 May 1858 on leprosy … he spoke Persian fluently." For a list of some of Schlimmer's students, see Ardakani 1368, vol. 1, p. 303.

58. Najmabadi 1349, pp. 577-78; Schlimmer 1970, frontispiece.

59. *Ruznameh* 1370-72, vol. 2, p. 657 (25 Sha`ban 1280/4 February 1864).

60. Najmabadi 1349, p. 575.

61. Najmabadi 1349, p. 579.

62. Schlimmer 1970, pp. 32 (q.v. *amaigrissement*), 305 (q.v. *graisse de la bosse*).

previous prescriptions and thus form an opinion about the medical history of the patient.[63]

Dr. Schlimmer's most important contribution was in helping to shape the teaching of medical science in Iran. The European teachers at the Dar ol-Fonun realized that their Iranian students lacked the necessary background and time to become fully trained physicians. According to Schlimmer, the objective of the training of students was to provide them with a good basis of medical science that would allow them to deal with the most common diseases and to do simple surgery as well as to continue their studies abroad after graduation and then become a real physician.

> At present we need to train physicians who are able to make correct diagnoses after gaining a basic knowledge of symptoms and to prescribe the appropriate drugs when necessary. With regard to surgery, they must know enough about anatomy so that they are able to perform surgery safely. After a few medical students have graduated from the Dar ol-Fonun, many major cities will have access to young Iranian physicians, who are aware of the advances of modern medicine. Medical students will accompany doctors on visits to hospital so that they grow familiar with medical terminology and procedures. Occasionally, less complicated cases will be sent to the Dar ol-Fonun for treatment. The school has been supplied with basic medical diagrams and skeletons imported from Europe.[64]

Apart from exposing the students of the Dar ol-Fonun to Western medical science and its latest developments, mainly through oral teaching, some of the professors, as mentioned above, wrote textbooks for the school, most of which remained in manuscript form. Apart from the fact that there were no textbooks on Western medicine in Persian, the European professors realized the need for the creation of a body of medical knowledge in Persian to modernize Iranian medical

---

63. Schlimmer 1970, p. 482 (*recette*).

64. *Vaqaye`-ye Ettefaqiyeh* 1373-74, vol. 1, p. 582 (no. 98, 5 Rabi` I 1269/17 December 1852).

practice as well as to facilitate the transition from Islamic-Galenic to Western medical methods. Dr. Schlimmer wrote: "In the beginning of the teaching the absence of a scientific nomenclature in Persian was a great handicap."[65]

Between 1854 and 1875, four professors wrote most of the available books and manuscripts for use as teaching material at the Dar ol-Fonun. Dr. Schlimmer wrote the largest number of manuscripts (14) on various subjects, such as pharmacology, pathology, ophthalmology, and pediatrics.[66] Some of these texts were printed by the Dar ol-Fonun Press,[67] and some were printed at the author's expense, such as the *Serr al-Hekmat* (the Secret of Medicine), a book about human anatomy (1863) and the *Zeynat al-Abdan* (On skin diseases), a book dealing with the effects of venereal diseases.[68] However, most of the medical texts written remained in manuscript form. These manuscript courses passed from hand to hand and were kept by students for future reference.[69] The students were also encouraged to distribute their lecture notes on cholera among doctors and laymen alike to be used in the case of an outbreak of cholera.[70]

Table 1: List of medical books written by Schlimmer

	Titles	Pub. Date
1*	Serr al-Hekmat (the Secret of medicine).	1279/1862
2*	Zeynat al-Abdan (the Ornament of Bodies; on skin diseases).	1279/1862
3*	Shafā'iyeh (On remedies).	1284/1867

65. Schlimmer 1970, p. 229.

66. Arjah 1371, index; Elgood 1951, p. 502.

67. *Vaqaye`-ye Ettefaqiyeh* 1373-74, p. 630 (no. 105, 4 Jomadi al-Avval 1269/December 17, 1852).

68. *Ruznameh* 1370-72, vol. 1, pp. 509 (17 Rajab 1279/8 January 1863), 511 (24 Rajab 1279/15 January 1863). See Shteglova 1975, vol. 1, pp. 307-08 (*Ketab-e Serr al-Hekmat* in 1862; *Ketab-e Zeynat al-Abdan* in 1862).

69. Najmabadi 1439, p. 577.

70. Ebrahimnejad 2000, p. 173.

	Titles	Pub. Date
4	Loghatnameh (Persian French dictionary)	1291/1874
5*	Qavā'ed al-Amrāz (Pathology).	1292/1875
6	Asbab al-Tadviyeh (Pharmacology)	? 1292/1875
7	Meftah al-Khavass (On the use of medications)	? 1277/1860
8	Jala' al-`Oyun (Ophthalmology)	? 1277/1860
9	Adviyeh va noskhehha (Drugs and prescriptions)	?
10	Amraz al-Sebyan (Children diseases)	?
11	Patuluzhi (Pathology)	?
12	Tohfeh-ye Naseri (Naseri's Gift)	?
13	Tashrih-e madeh-ye `asabi (Anatomy of the nervous system)	1294/1877
14	Qarabadeyn (Pharmacopoeia)	1292/1895
15	Montakhab al-shafa'iyeh (Selected treatments)	1305/1888

Source: Arjah 1371, Index; Najmabadi 1349, p. 579.

* Means published in lithograph.

In 1874, Dr. Schlimmer published his most important work entitled: *Terminologie Medico-Pharmaceutique*.[71] It had started as a small dictionary of Persian equivalents for common French medical terms, but had grown into a major pharmacopoeia. According to Elgood, "it was indeed a gigantic attempt to make the transition from Avicenna to Harvey least abrupt, to fit the old nomenclature to the new ideas, and to standardize the technical terms of the new university."[72] In this way, these pioneering teachers and translators, and in particular Schlimmer, created and codified much of the medical terminology used in Iran for many decades. Being a public health official, Schlimmer

71. Its impending publication was announced in *The Athenaeum* 1874, p. 528. Schlimmer's contemporary, Hedayat 1344, p. 58 considered it to be a very valuable book that deserved to be republished. It was only in 1970 that the first reprint was published to be followed by a third reprint in 2001.

72. Elgood 1951, p. 502. For an analysis of these treatises written by the European teachers of the Dar ol-Fonun see Najmabadi 1354 and Ibid. 1364.

was probably also the first to define the concept of public health in Persian, viz. *hefz-e sehhat* (health protection) and *jelow-e maraz gereftan* (preventing disease).[73] Schlimmer further published in Persian a treatise on animal chemistry, a treatise on skins diseases, and a first edition, without notes, of the *Terminologie*.

> My course on pathology and special therapy together with a large pharmacopeia of about 700 pages remains in manuscript and half done on lithographic stone due to lack of funds; my Treatise of medical ophthalmology with illustrations after Beer and others is ready to be lithographed. I also have dictated a *Treatise of Pharmacodynamics*, and another medical primer, a course on pathology and general therapy, and a course on semiotics, all of them in manuscript with my students, and even some traditional doctors have hastened to obtain copies of them.[74]

DR. JOSEPH DÉSIRÉ THOLOZAN.

When, in 1858, Polak was planning to return to Vienna,[75] the Shah asked his ambassador in France to find a French physician to replace him. The government of France proposed Dr. Tholozan. Already in 1857, the Iranian government had asked France to send a large group of mainly military instructors to teach at the Dar ol-Fonun. Although a much smaller group of French teachers came at the end of 1858, it included, Tholozan, who was appointed *hakim-bashi*, i.e. one of the Shah's personal physicians as well as teacher at the Dar ol-Fonun.[76] The French teachers were not only supposed to teach, but also to improve the curriculum and emphasize the core function of the school. Therefore, the school's new director as of 1860, E`tezad al-Saltaneh, the Shah's great-uncle, wanted to have a student body based on merit

73. Schlimmer 1970, p. 473 (q.v. *preservation*).
74. Schlimmer 1970, p. 230; see also Hedayat 1344, p. 58.
75. According to Polak 1859, p. 765, in 1858 he had enough of French intrigues against him and decided to return home.
76. Floor 2018, p. 157.

rather than on privilege, and a curriculum that emphasized actual practice of the subjects taught. Students were to receive a stipend, free lunches and a uniform, the length of the studies were reduced to five years. To better prepare students for the unfamiliar subjects they had to study, the first 2-3 years were aimed at giving them a solid foundation in essential subjects, so as to enable them to more effectively engage in more specialized studies thereafter (5-6 years).[77]

In the 1860s, Dr. Tholozan gave lessons concerning descriptive and microscopic anatomy of the nervous system as well as a special course on the dissection of the sanguinary system using sheep as subjects. The course was followed with great interest by the students and even by some practicing traditional doctors, who had never studied at the school.[78] Tholozan further introduced aegophonia or auscultation (*sowt-e bozi*) in the Dar ol-Fonun. However, the availability of medical textbooks remained one of the constraints for students to acquire the necessary knowledge and therefore, Tholozan wrote the *Badaye` al-Hikmat-e Naseri*, a treatise on auscultation, percussion and palpitation that clearly demonstrated its workings in the lithographed version. It was translated by his assistant Mostafa b. Aghil al-Alavi al-Esfahani and published in March 1861 in Tehran. In his preface to the book, Tholozan writes that he meant the book to a sort of guide how to diagnose illnesses of the chest and belly with the most simple and practical methods.[79] He further wrote a *Quinology* in Persian, dealing with pharmacological and therapeutical applications as well as describing the most recent European developments in the field. Finally, Tholozan wrote a textbook, *Badaye` al-Hekmat*, which was published in lithographed version in Tehran in 1277/1861. Some of the interpreters of the European professors at the school translated various medical texts into Persian. Tholozan also wrote other books

77. *Vaqaye`-ye Ettefaqiyeh* 1373-74, p. 2998 (no. 458, 19 Jomada II 1276/13 January 1860).
78. Schlimmer 1970, p. 229.
79. Schlimmer 1970, p. 45.

relevant for teaching at the Dar ol-Fonun, some of which were dictated to his students.[80]

These various publications by European physicians and by Mirza Reza Doktor, Mirza `Ali Doktor, and Abu'l-Qasem Hakim-bashi as well as articles in government newspapers helped to popularize Western medicine and to allay existing prejudice against it. European medicine also influenced Islamic-Galenic medicine, because its terminology and concepts were gradually adopted by traditional Persian physicians in their treatises. As discussed above, to facilitate the transmission of European medical science many of the textbooks developed for teaching at the Dar ol-Fonun were also translated into Persian. These were used by students as well as by opponents to Western medicine and thus influenced their theoretical framework in which they carried on their discussion.[81]

THE SCHOOL'S DECLINE

This early period of relative success was followed by decades of neglect. It began in October 1861, when Naser al-Din Shah upset by the presence of the so-called *faramush-khaneh* in the school, to which many students and staff belonged, banned this activity and exiled its instigator, Malkom Khan, a translator and teacher at the school. The Shah suspected the adherents to this new and secret society of having subversive intentions to overthrow the monarchy.[82] Although the Shah's actions had no further immediate negative impact on the school's mission or performance it was, nevertheless, the beginning of the Shah's loss of interest in his educational experiment. Because E`tezad al-Saltaneh continued as director, while the administration remained in the hands of the Hedayat family (first Rezaqoli Khan

80. Schlimmer 1970, pp. 17, 229; Arjah 1371, p. xi. See also Tholozan's biography for his public health activities and his list of publications in Floor, 2018, pp. 156-67.

81. Ebrahimnejad 2000, p. 176; Ibid. 2002, pp. 104-05.

82. Algar 1969, p. 49; Dowlatabadi 1336, vol. 1, p. 327.

Hedayat and then his younger son Ja'farqoli Khan Nayyer-al-Molk), who all enjoyed the Shah's confidence, the school was able to continue its activities. The Hedayats had been instrumental in establishing the administrative procedures and rules during the last decade, and thus, the school was able to continue to follow the old rules and routine. However, by 1870, gone were the days of enthusiasm, dedication and commitment, while mediocrity among teachers and students prevailed. The main reason was that Naser al-Din Shah had lost interest in educational reforms. His original intention to open schools similar to the Dar ol-Fonun in other in other provinces was shelved, sending a clear signal to education and other reformers.[83] Therefore, neither the directors of the school nor its teachers made an effort to make the school a success by motivating students to learn. Instead, everybody, including the students, went through the motions of attending and teaching, but the spirit was gone. It may be said that after 1870, the Dar ol-Fonun languished for many decades.

Another reason was that despite the continued prominence given to the teaching of Western medicine at the Dar ol-Fonun and the study program in France this did not mean that this subject enjoyed much popular support. In January 1860, the opposition against European medicine was sufficiently strong for the government to once again inform the public that the teaching of traditional medicine was an integral part of the Dar ol-Fonun's curriculum. It did so by having E`tezad al-Saltaneh, the school's director, announce in the government newspaper *Vaqaye`-ye Ettefaqiyeh*: "Since some of the people of Iran are not yet convinced of European medical practice, in order to inform medical students of the prevailing Iranian medical practice, Mirza Mohammad Hakimbashi Kashani, who, both in terms of practice and knowledge is the best of the Iranian doctors, was assigned to teach Iranian medicine in the blessed school."[84] The policy that manifested

---

83. *Vaqaye`-ye Ettefaqiyeh* 1373-74, p. 2998 (no. 458, 19 Jomada II 1276/13 January 1860); also cited in Ardakani 1368, vol. 1, pp. 311-14.

84. *Vaqaye`-ye Ettefaqiyeh* 1373-74, vol. 4, p. 2998 (no. 548 19 Jomadi 1276/January 13, 1860).

itself in this statement was reinforced by a report on the nature of medical teaching and practice at the Dar ol-Fonun.

> As the medical students of the Dar ol-Fonun are knowledgeable about Iranian as well as European medicine, many people consult them and often their treatments have been effective. However, since some of them have not perfected their skills enough, E`tezad al-Saltaneh strictly forbids them to treat people unless they are examined and their skills approved by Dr. Tholozan in Western medicine and by Mirza Ahmad Hakim-bashi-ye Kashan in Iranian medicine. Once their capacity to treat patients is approved, Dr. Tholozan and Mirza Ahmad will provide them with a license to practice; otherwise they must not receive any patients. After exams, the names of those who have received such a license will be published in the journal.[85]

After the late 1860s, most of the teaching was done by Iranian physicians, who were graduates of the Dar ol-Fonun and of French universities. They were, Mirza Sayyed `Ali (Persian, *i.e.*, Islamic-Galenic medicine), Mirza Ahmad Tabib Kashani (Islamic-Galenic medicine; until 1870), Mirza Taqi Khan Ansari (Western medicine), Mirza Reza (Western medicine), Mirza Kazem Mahallati (chemistry), Mirza Abu'l-Qasem Hakim-bashi (Islamic-Galenic medicine; as of 1877), Mirza `Ali Doktor Mo`tamed al-Atebba (Western medicine; as of 1877), Mirza Hoseyn Doktor (Western medicine; as of 1864), Dr. Abu'l-Hasan Khan Bahrami (Western medicine to second year students; as of 1879), and Mirza Mohammad Doktor Kermanshahi (Western medicine; as of 1881). Although there was a drop in the quality of the teaching this was not due to the use of Iranian teachers. More importantly, was the total lack of interest that Naser al-Din Shah showed in the school in particular and modernization in general.[86]

---

85. Ebrahimnejad 2014, p. 93, translation of *Ruznameh 1370-72,* vol. 1, p. 550 (no. 541,17/04/1863). For a facsimile of an report of examiners of medical students, see Ebrahimnejad 2014, p. 69.

86. Rahnama 1333, vol. 1, pp. 50-53 (with short bios of Mirza Reza Doktor, Mirza `Ali Doktor and Dr. Khalil Khan A`lam al-Dowleh

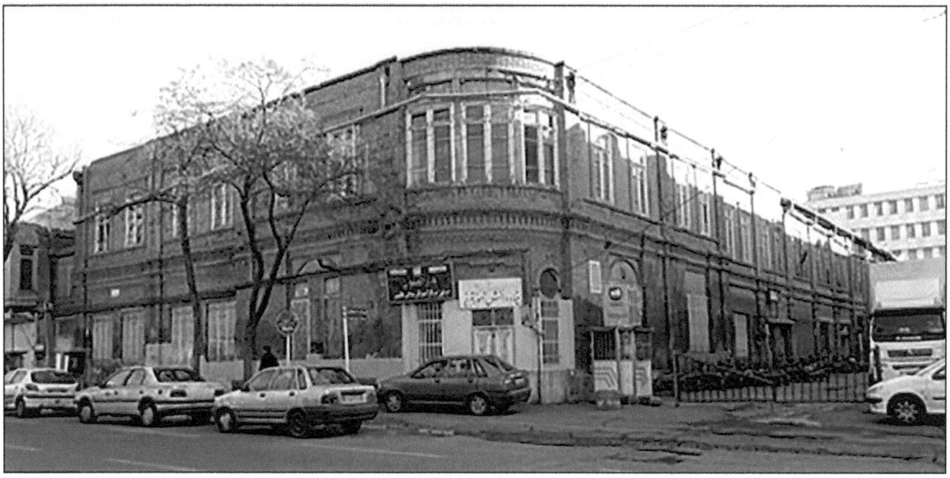

The former Mozaffar School or the Dar ol-Fonun in Tabriz

Despite the Shah's flagging interest in modern education, in 1876, Mozaffar, a government school was opened in Tabriz that was modeled on the Tehran Dar ol-Fonun. Like in Tehran, students were trained for public and military service and about half received financial support from the government. Its medical department employed teachers, who had graduated from the Dar ol-Fonun of Tehran. In 1896, after 20 years, he Tabriz school was closed down. Nothing is known about the curriculum of students who studied medicine, their number and how long their study lasted. Although at least one of the school's graduates (Dr. Jalil Saburi Naser al-Hokama) later became a well-known physician in Tabriz, we don't know whether his medical training was limited to that school. According to Wilson, "The graduates in medicine are for the most part given appointments in the army."[87]

When Mirza Hoseyn Khan, Naser al-Din Shah's reform-minded grand-vizier visited the school in 1875, he wrote with dismay that

Thaqafi); Ekhtiar 1994, pp. 171-74 (Persian teachers), 205-10 (changing shah's attitude). For a bio of Dr. Mohammad Kermanshahi, see Mahdavi 2009.

87. Sardari-Niya 1382; Wilson 1895, p. 188.

the only European teacher was M. Richard, the other teachers were former students. Of the supposedly 150 students only 79 were found, including the teacher and their assistants.[88] However, this visit provided not even a temporary upsurge in the school's activities and the school remained in a status of total irrelevance, if we may believe Ehtesham al-Dowleh, who was a student of the school at that time:

> It is not clear why the Dar ol-Fonun was thus called and what kind of plan and program the founder and instigator had in mind, because at that time we [i.e. he and his two brothers] were sent to that school to be educated, for many years prior and after that time it was nothing more than a *maktab-khaneh* at the level of an elementary school. [...] The result and outcome of my eight years at this school was so little and scant that I am certain that during that long period I gained less knowledge than a person who was taught [at another school] in six months. The reasons were that there was no supervision, nobody asked anything, there was no program and from neither the student nor the teacher a responsible attitude was demanded. Of course, the children had no interest in learning and being taught. [...] After eight years of studying French, if somebody would say two words of French to me, I was unable to answer. In short, the years that I spent at the Dar ol-Fonun, which were the best years and the best opportunity in life for learning, I am very sorry to say, were wasted.[89]

Ehtesham al-Dowleh opined that the worst misdeed was the school's total lack of care for and interest in the students. He went even so far to state that, "the bad state of affairs and the cause of

88. Ekhtiar 1994, p. 209. About the teaching qualities of Richard and others, see Ehtesham al-Saltaneh 1366, pp. 26-27.

89. Ehtesham al-Saltaneh 1366, pp. 25, 28. As to the quality of teaching English, see Eyn al-Saltaneh 1376, vol. 1, pp. 330 (English), 577-78 (comparison with the quality of teaching at the American missionary school in Hamadan).

backwardness of Iran, in my opinion, may only be sought in the Dar ol-Fonun."[90]

The diminishing interest shown by Naser al-Din Shah in the Dar ol-Fonun translated itself in 1873 in a cessation of the flow of government-sponsored students to Europe to receive further medical training and education.[91] It also was shown in the quality of teaching at the Dar ol-Fonun that left much to be desired after about 1870, according to both European and Iranian observers. For Ehtesham al-Dowleh was not the only one to criticize the quality of education at the Dar ol-Fonun. `Eyn al-Saltaneh qualified the school in 1892 as useless, where students learnt nothing, while Dr. Neligan, looking back at the results obtained towards the end of the Qajar era, opined that, "Medical education in Persia, in spite of years of experience and expense, is, it must be candidly stated, of a very low standard."[92] Dr. Hakim A`zam wrote about the medical students of the Dar ol-Fonun at that time:

> They are those who only by making some notes with the professors and are present at their consulting room (*mahkameh*) consider themselves a physician, although called 'doctor' they engage in the exercise of medicine without any official testimony. The author, as he did not consider the teaching at the Dar ol-Fonun and the consulting rooms [practice] sufficient, went to Europe and after ten years of study returned.[93]

The lack of royal interest in the school and its subsequent deterioration as an educational institution was also reflected in the rather

90. Ehtesham al-Saltaneh 1366, p. 29.

91. Although Naser al-Din Shah reportedly continued to visit the Dar ol-Fonun this custom was not continued by his successors. Rahnama 1333, vol. 1, p. 31; Sani` al-Dowleh 1300, vol. 3, p. 376.

92. Government of Great Britain 1945, pp. 408-09; `Eyn al-Saltaneh 1376, vol. 1, pp. 330 (not one good student graduated from that school), 577 (1893: apart from music and gymnastics students knew nothing), 849 (lying, useless students); Rahnama 1333, vol. 1, p. 54.

93. Rahnama 1333, vol. 1, p. 54.

low number of students who graduated. In 1882 it was reported that since 1853 only 237 students had graduated, who were employed by the government.[94] Despite the lackluster if not negligent performance of the school, members of the elite continued to send their children to get an education there. This had nothing to do with the quality of education, or lack thereof, but rather that, apart from the fact that it was the only modern school in town, it was expected to send your sons to the Dar ol-Fonun. The Shah may not have had much interest in the school any longer, but it had become a well-known institution, it had an acquired certain cachet, it was the only institute of modern education in Tehran, and, therefore, everybody who was anybody still sent their sons there. Despite all the negative aspects of the school, some of the leading 20th century political and educational reformers attended it in the 1890s.[95]

This situation did not fundamentally change in 1882, after Mokhber al-Dowleh, Minister of Education had visited Germany. On his return he brought three teachers with him, among whom was Dr. Albo. They were to teach at the Dar ol-Fonun. Dr. Albo, however, spent much of his time working in the state hospital.[96] Dr. Albo taught internal medicine, and normal and pathological physiology about which he wrote a book. Because he was mainly hired to work in the hospital he used his patients as teaching prop. In 1890 he returned to Europe.[97] There was still a need for additional medical text books. Therefore, Dr. Albo produced six manuscripts, mostly on surgery, physiology and general medicine, while Abu'l-Hasan Khan wrote a text on therapeutics and `Ali Ra'is al-Atebba on anatomy.[98] Dr. Khalil Khan

94. Ebrahimnejad 2014, p. 91.

95. Ekhtiar 1994, p. 210.

96. This hospital, known as *Marizkhaneh-ye Dowlati* or State Hospital (later Ebn Sina), was built at Naser al-Din Shah's orders after his return from his first visit to Europe, see Floor 2012, p. 50.

97. Rahnama 1333, vol. 1, pp. 34, 51-52; Elgood 1951, p. 502.

98. Arjah 1371 (index); Elgood 1951, p. 502. Two of Schlimmer's texts were published. Shteglova 1975, vol. 1, pp. 307-08 (*Ketab-e Serr al-Hekmat* in 1862; *Ketab-e Zeynat al-Abdan* in 1862). Tholozan's

A`lam al-Dowleh Thaqafi,[99] son of E`tezad al-Atteba worked as Dr. Albo's assistant and taught the first two classes of the school. He also taught first aid and vaccination in the military school and was one of Naser al-Din Shah's physicians. Dr. Albo was replaced by Dr. Basil, a British-trained Armenian, who taught at the Dar ol-Fonun until 1914.[100] Mirza Ahmad Tabib Kashani, who taught traditional medicine until 1870, was succeeded by Mirza `Abdol-Vahhab (1870-77), one of the shah's physicians. In 1877, he was replaced by Mirza Abu'l-Qasem Na'ini Soltan al-Hokama. He taught this subject (about which he published a number of books) for 26 years until his death in 1913.[101]

In 1851, the school had 100 students; in 1861 this number had hardly changed being only 107, while in 1866 there were still only 123 students. In 1883, there were 185 regular students plus 50 who only studied languages, while in 1890 there were less than 250 students.[102] Because of the establishment of the Military College (*Madraseh-ye nezami*), in 1885, and in 1899 of the College of Political Sciences (*Madraseh-ye `olum-e siyasi*); the latter within the Ministry of Foreign Affairs, the body of students at the Dar ol-Fonun grew less than it

---

book on the plague was printed in Tehran in 1876, see Ibid., vol. 1. p. 309 (*Resaleh dar keyfiyat-e marz-e ta`un*). Therefore, it is highly questionable whether Tholozan initiated the *réforme litéraire*, as Ebrahimnejad 2000, p. 171 has it.

99. He began his studies at the Dar ol-Fonun in 1876 and during his 4-year study he also was interpreter for a French geography teacher. He was the first Dar ol-Fonun student to get the title doctor without having studied abroad. In 1894 he was sent to Paris at Tholozan's recommendation. After Naser al-Din Shah's death he returned to Iran and became Mozaffar al-Din's physician and was influential in having the Shah agree to the Constitution. Rahnama 1333, vol. 1, p. 52; Elgood 1951, p. 564.

100. Rahnama 1333, vol. 1, p. 52.

101. Rahnama 1333, vol. 1, pp. 33, 42, 67; Ebrahimnejad 2014, p. 92.

102. Ebrahimnejad 2014, p. 91. By November 1871, there allegedly were about 200 (for names of ninety-eight students and the subjects studied, see Yaghma'i 1349, pp. 303-06). In 1889, Curzon 1892, vol. 1, p. 494 mentioned 255 students, while Ehtesham al-Saltaneh 1366, p. 26 gave the number as 250.

might have.[103] In fact, the number of medical students at the Dar ol-Fonun dropped, because following leading Iranian physicians, who had been trained in Europe, offered an attractive (shorter, and perhaps also cheaper) educational alternative in their practice (see below).[104]

ATTEMPTS TO IMPROVE DAR OL-FONUN'S QUALITY

Dr. Schneider, who became the shah's personal physician in 1893, was instrumental in establishing a new medical curriculum within the Dar ol-Fonun. However, without active government support for and interest in the school this did not change the general situation of almost irrelevancy of the school. In 1323/1905 of the 312 students only 40 were enrolled in the medical class.[105] Even the arrival of a group of French teachers in 1905 brought no improvement. In that year, `Ala ol-Molk, the Minister of Education, hired a number of European teachers. Those teaching medical-related subjects were: Dr. George (internal), Dr. Gualet (surgery, descriptive anatomy), M. Dantan (biology), and M. Olmer (chemistry, physics). The physicians were all military men, who had taught at the Army Medical College of Lyon. Dr. Gualet was an excellent draughtsman, which helped student better understand human anatomy. In addition, in 1908, there were the following Iranian assistant-teachers (*khalifeh*): `Ali Asghar Khan Mo'addab al-Dowleh Nafisi (anatomy), Nasrollah Khan (surgery,

103. Gurney and Nabavi 1993; `Eyn al-Saltaneh 1376, vol. 1, p. 505 qualified the military college in 1892 as a buffoonery (*luti-bazi*); Rahnama 1333, vol. 1, p. 54.

104. Rahnama 1333, vol. 1, p. 61 (see below). Ehtesham al-Saltaneh 1366, p. 26 mentions that his father had to pay 40,000 *tuman*s per year for his education of the Dar ol-Fonun, which means that school attendance may not have been financed by the State any longer.

105. Rahnama 1333, vol. 1, p. 58 (at that time the school's staff consisted of Rezaqoli Khan Nayyer al-Molk II, Adib al-Dowleh,director, Dr. Basil, Mr. Maulion – Soltan al-Hokama had died one year earlier; sometimes Dr. Luf (sic; Loew?) of the *Dowlat* Hospital also taught).

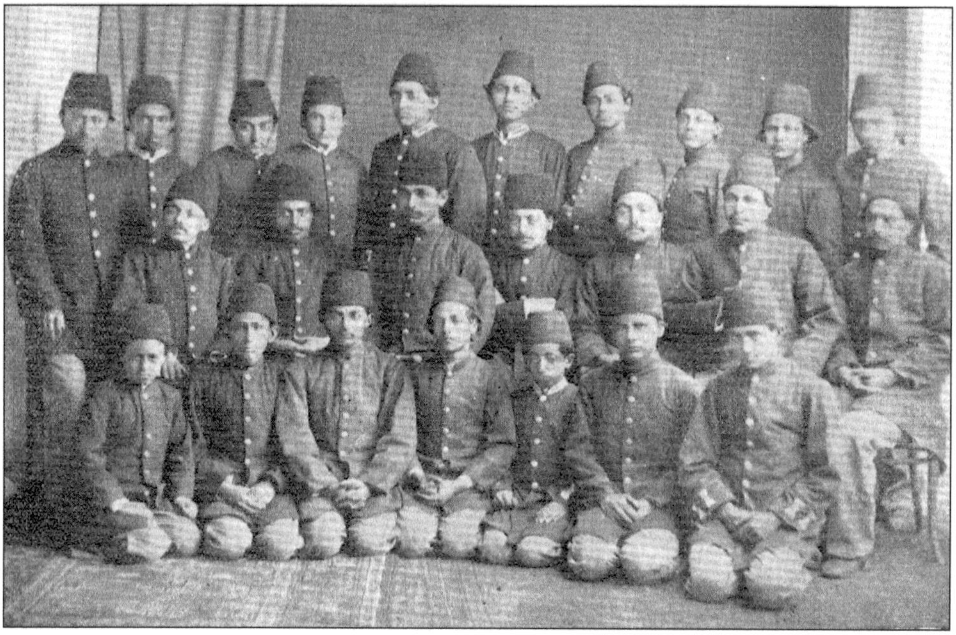

Students of the Dar ol-Fonun in their official uniforms

external) Mahmud Khan Shimi, son of Mirza Kazem Shimi (asst. biology), who also worked as translators.[106]

The objective of the hiring of European professors had been to upgrade the quality of teaching that had suffered in the preceding period. Despite the fact that the Dar ol-Fonun had existed 50 years, there still were no entry requirements or a compulsory study plan for students. Therefore, in September 1906/30 Sha`ban 1324 such entrance requirements and a study plan (*ketabcheh-ye sharayet-e qabul-e shagerdan va perogram-e darsha-ye madraseh*) were published by the Ministry of Education. Henceforth, the study would last seven years and there was an entrance exam equivalent to grade one of a high school. Two years of preparatory education in natural science

106. Rahnama 1333, vol. 1, pp. 59-60, 63 (here also details about the problems between the French teachers and the government). Mo'addab al-Dowleh Nafisi left the school after a disagreement with Gualet and began teaching students in his father's practice. Dr. Amir A`alam, who just had finished his studies in Europe replaced him.

and languages subjects were followed by one year of biology, medical chemistry and physics. After these three years, and after having passed the examination, the medical study lasted another four years. The school year lasted from 15 September to 15 June and at the end of each year an exam had to be taken. Students who finished the entire study were given a diploma by the Ministry of Education that gave them the right to treat patients, but they were not allowed to call themselves doctor. It was from this moment onwards that the European practice of issuing of so-called four-tiered (*chahar khanehha*) diplomas became and remained current in Iran. The broad study plan for medical students looked as follows:

> Year 1: descriptive (*tashrih-e tafsili va tarsimi*) anatomy; physics, natural chemistry, parasitology
>
> Year 2-4: anatomy, physiology, general pathology, internal and external pathology, surgery and therapeutics.

Because the Dar ol-Fonun didn't have its own hospital, students had to examine patients in the school itself under the supervision of their teachers.[107]

In 1906, there were only 22 medical students. Therefore, to attract more students, it was made known that those studying with private physicians would be accepted and only had to study for three years. During year I, students had classes the whole day (medicine only in the morning) and in Years II and III received half-day instruction. This had some success as in 1908 there were 60 medical students. By the third year about half dropped out, because they did not know a foreign language and/or had difficulty understanding the substance taught. Therefore, the drop-outs preferred to learn medicine the traditional way, in the service of a *hakim*; the remaining 30 students graduated after three years. In 1909, there were only 12 regular students, who graduated after seven years of study. At that time, two students remained who graduated in 1914. "In that year the auditoria of the

---

107. Rahnama 1333, vol. 1, pp. 61-62.

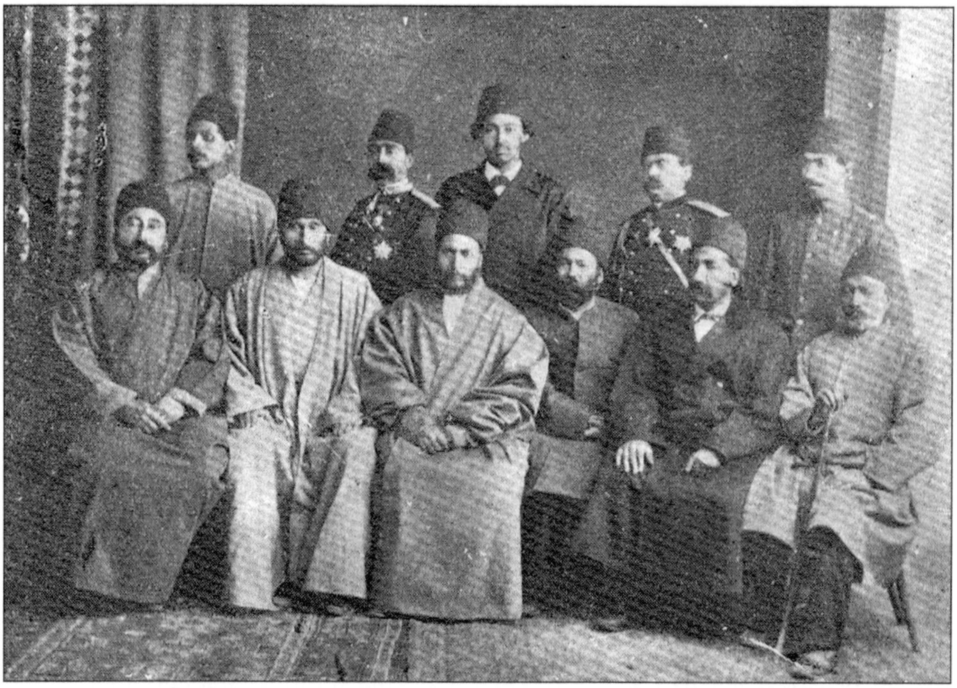

Teachers of the Dar ol-Fonun ca. 1890. From left to right: Yahya Khan, translator Artillery department; Martyrs Khan, Russian teacher; Mokhber al-Saltaneh, translator Infantry department; Mozayyan al-Dowleh, French translator and painter; Amanollah Khan, teacher and translator Medical department. Seated: Baqer Khan, mineralogy teacher; Dr. Mohammad Khan Kermanshahi; Mirza Kazem Khan Shimi; Mirza `Ali Ra'is al-Atteba; Mirza Abu'l-Qasem Na'ini Soltan al-Hokama; Mirza `Ali Khan Qajar.

Dar ol-Fonun remained empty and nobody wanted to study there," wrote Dr. `Ali Partow.[108]

Because of lack of medical students, seven years of medical study were felt to be too long, because training by private physicians was much shorter. Therefore, in 1912, the Minister of Education announced that 3-years of study were also possible, be it that graduates were not allowed to call themselves doctor. As a result, about 60 students came. After three years a few asked to be allowed to study an additional year to receive the school's diploma. In 1912, the French

108. Rahnama 1333, vol. 1, p. 63 (with the names of the graduates).

teachers returned to France at the end of their contract, because of differences of opinion between them and the Ministry of Education concerning working conditions and other issues. They were replaced by Drs. Gachet (internal medicine), Duchense (external medicine and surgery), Lattes (physics and chemistry), Combel and Le Blanc (biology). However, in 1914 they all left Iran after the outbreak of WW I. Of the Iranian teachers Nafisi had already left in 1906, he was replaced by Dr. Amir A`lam, teaching descriptive anatomy. In 1908, Dr. `Ali Partow Hakim A`zam (1877-1938) returned from Europe and taught hygiene, physiology and forensic medicine, and later also internal medicine.[109]

Although Dr. Polak and Dr. Schlimmer both had written a text on eye diseases the subject was not formally taught at the Dar ol-Fonun. It was only in 1892, after Dr. Hatulde had established the ophthalmic department at the Imperial Hospital that he gave some lectures at the Dar ol-Fonun, but that ceased after two years. It was only in 1915 that it became a regular subject at the Dar ol-Fonun at the insistence of Dr. Yahya Mirza Shams Lesan al-Hokama, a former student of Dr. Albo and Dr. Hatulde. From 1898-1905 he had studied and practiced ophthalmology in Paris. He taught this subject until the end of his life in 1945.[110]

In 1917, the medical department of the Dar ol-Fonun was known as the *kelas-e tebbi*, where the following physicians taught: Amir A`lam (therapeutics, special anatomy, external disease, pediatrics); `Ali Partow (hygiene, forensic medicine, physiology, internal medicine); Gholam Hoseyn Khan A`lam (minor surgery); Yahya Mirza Shams (ophthalmology); Ehya al-Molk and Malekzadeh (anatomy); Loqman

109. Rahnama 1333, vol. 1, p. 60 (here also details about the problems between the French teachers and the government). On 29 Sha`ban 1329, the Majles approved the renewal by three years of Dr. Lattes contract, as well the hiring of a teacher of natural history to replace Dr. Kambu (Combel?), and a French physician, who had to have the academic rank of *agregée*, to teach medicine. Majmu`eh-ye qavanin, p. 446.

110. Rahnama 1333, vol. 1, pp. 51, 66 (with the names of the students who took and graduated from this course).

al-Molk (urology); Hoseyn Khan Mo`tamed (medical physics and chemistry); and `Abdollah Khan Ahmadiyeh (biology).[111]

Another Attempt at Regulation

The Ministry of Education with the help of Dr. Lattes had developed a plan to improve the quality of the Dar ol-Fonun so that over time a medical faculty might be established within the school that would train students to the level of a bachelor diploma. Such a diploma would give these students access to medical schools in Europe. However, the necessary funds to implement the changes were not there and thus, the plan was shelved. However, the exercise was not without effect, because the Majles, urged by several of its members who were well-known physicians, decided to discuss when somebody was allowed to practice medicine.[112]

The choice of becoming a 'modern doctor' was not necessarily a good one from an economic point of view. The modern trained physicians were in competition with the traditional *hakim*s and most people preferred the latter, unless surgery was required, when the 'modern' doctors had the advantage.[113] Therefore, it was important both for the protection of the patients and the new modern physicians that standards were formulated that established what a 'physician' was. This was also but the logical result of the curriculum that was used at the Dar ol-Fonun and other medical educational institutions. On 2 June 1911, the Majles passed a new law, which required that physicians had to receive a license to practice or work for the government in a medical capacity from the Minister of Education, which had to be registered with the Ministry of the Interior. To qualify for a license the physician had to have a diploma from [Iranian] medical

111. Rahnama 1333, vol. 1, pp. 66-67 (with their salaries).

112. Rahnama 1333, vol. 1, p. 65. Already in the 1870s a board was established to examine physicians, however, nothing is known about its composition, how it functioned and how long it lasted. E'temad-al-Saltaneh 1307, p. 114; Yaghma'i 1349, p. 234.

113. Rahnama 1333, vol. 1, p. 64; Mostowfi 1343, vol. 1, p. 713.

state schools (*madares-e tebbi-y dowlat*), which did not yet exist, or a medical diploma issued by foreign governments (articles 1, 2 and 11). This meant that training by private physicians (see below) should be less attractive than studying at the Dar ol-Fonun. Those without a diploma, but who had been practicing medicine in Tehran for less than five years would not be given license to practice (art. 4). Those without a diploma, but having practiced medicine in Tehran for more than five and less than 10 years were entitled to receive a license to practice, if, within three years, they would pass an examination by a special commission. (art. 5) The examination commission was composed of one of the medical teachers of the Dar ol-Fonun, one of the physicians of the American hospital, one well-known Iranian physician, and two representatives of the Ministry of Education, one of whom was the president of the commission. (art. 7). An exception would be made for the following categories, if, within four months, they would submit a diploma issued by a well-known established physician, or by physicians of the state or American hospitals (art. 5). Those having practiced for more than 10 years in Tehran qualified for a license to practice (art. 6). In accordance with art. 5, candidates had to pass an exam given by a commission that would sit twice per year (in spring and fall) during the next three years. The commission was composed of medical teachers of the Dar ol-Fonun, four well-known Iranian physicians, and one representative of the Ministry of Education, who was president of the commission (art. 8). At all events, those wishing to practice medicine or dentistry had to get a license to do so within one year. Those failing to do so would be banned from medical practice (art. 9). Those practicing without a license would first get a warning and the second time would be given 4-month imprisonment (art. 10).[114]

---

114. Government of Iran n.d. B, pp. 393-96 (*Qanun-e Tebb 3 Jomadi II* 1329). This law was to a great extent a copy of the substance of an earlier draft regulation proposed by the Sanitary Council in 1907, which had among its responsibilities the task if examination of practitioners and the appointment of traditional and modern physicians. Ebrahimnejad 2014, pp. 140, 155.

The implementation of this law tentatively was resumed as of 1917/18, after the end of WW I, because of the unsettled political situation in Iran during 1911-1918.[115] From the diplomas given, whether in 1899 or 1917, it is clear that many candidates had first studied traditional medicine and then modern medicine and surgery.[116] In 1919, a new superintendent of education in Rasht- a Cambridge man- tried to enforce the laws requiring licenses of all physicians. He asked Dr. Frame of the American Missionary Hospital to examine a number of doctors, who had been practicing without a license to give them a temporary one, as the permanent one had to come from Tehran. Dr. Frame asked that Dr. Tashchiyan, an Iranian colleague working in Rasht, be associated with him. They examined six men, one quit, three passed and two were recommended for temporary permits to be re-examined after one year.[117]

The Madraseh-ye `Ali-ye Tebb (1918-34)

Given the need for more modern physicians there was a great need to develop and improve Iran's national capacity to train those physicians. The more so, because many a European physician, such as Dr. Neligan, the physician of the British Legation and member of the Sanitary Board, was not much impressed with the quality of medical teaching at the Dar ol-Fonun. In 1919, he wrote:

> For perhaps 30 years the Iranian government maintained a medical school with a faculty of Iranian and French teachers. In 1914, at the Dar ol-Fonun, there were two French professors (both military officers), who did part of the teaching. They gave three lectures each week, for the rest they were engaged in private practice. It was reported that they would be replaced. The other teachers were young Iranians, several of whom had a French medical diploma. The teaching was

115. For an exception to this statement, see Ebrahimnejad 2014, p. 155, reporting a failed attempt to apply the law in Hamadan in 1913.

116. Ebrahimnejad 2014, p. 93.

117. RG 91-19-9, Report Medical Work 1919-20.

> entirely theory, there was no clinical teaching, although its students presented themselves in an irregular fashion at different local hospitals and clinics. There was no practical teaching in pathology or bacteriology, while the school's gold medalists could not say what a well-stained preparation of blood under the microscope was. I once gave a series of lectures on tropical diseases occurring in Iran with illustrations and microscopic demonstrations. They were well attended, but he was never asked again, although the students asked him to do so. […] The different missionary hospitals [give] a good practical training with very little theoretical work.[118]

However, the American missionaries for a variety of reasons had ceased to train medical doctors (see below) and thus, something had to be done to address the lackluster performance of the Dar ol-Fonun. It would seem that the Iranian government also leaned that way, because in October 1918, at the Shah's orders, Dr. Mohammad Hasan Khan Adham Loqman al-Dowleh became head of the medical part of the Dar ol-Fonun, which thereafter was called *Madraseh-ye Tebb*. Until that time, the director of the Dar ol-Fonun was also the head of the medical department (*kelas-e tebbi*), which now became a separate

---

118. FO 248/1291. Memo Dr. Neligan to Minister, Tehran, 28 January 1920; Elgood 1951, p. 535 ("In the [British] mission hospitals in a far humbler manner young Persians were receiving a grounding in anatomy and physiology"); see also, IOR/L/MIL/17/15/23, Military report on Tehran and adjacent Provinces of North-West Persia (including the Caspian Littoral), p. 204 ("A graduate of the Dar ol-Fonun school has attained a standard of education equivalent to that of an Indian Secondary School. There are some 400 pupils of about 13 to 18 years of age. Admittance is by entrance examination, and no fees are charged except perhaps a ' douceur ' for the examiners. The Faculties of Law and Medicine have a 5 years' course. Each is attended by some 60 students who have graduated from the school. Students undergo a five years' course of purely theoretical instruction, there is no dissection, histology, bacteriology, or regular classes of clinical medicine. In short, at the end of his 5 years' study, the student has no practical knowledge or experience. Add to this the lectures in Law and Medicine are all in French, and only partly intelligible to the audience.").

institution. Therefore, part of the Dar ol-Fonun (the *hayat-e nezam*) was allocated to the *Madraseh-ye Tebb*. The Ministry of Education also made a change in the curriculum. The new curriculum for the first year was called P.C.N. (i.e., physics, chemistry, and natural science). A medical museum, a museum of natural history, and a chemistry and microbiology laboratory were planned to be added to the school, although these investments were either not made or poorly executed (see below). Instead of seven years the study henceforth lasted five years, of which the first year was reserved for physics, chemistry and biology. Also, a chemistry, physics, and bacteriological laboratory were supposed to be added to the school. Moreover, Dr. Hoseyn Mo`tamed, Dr. Yahya Mirza Shams and Dr. Loqman al-Dowleh had to teach surgery, ophthalmology and medicine four days per week in the Imperial Hospital to students of years three to five. Traditional Galenic medicine, which had been omitted from the curriculum since 1913, was taught again. Dr. Sehhat al-Dowleh was charged with this subject. Dr. Yunes Afrukhteh had to teach midwifery, which until then had not been part of the school's curriculum. Finally, it was decided that the professors would meet once a month to discuss progress made in education and to resolve problems. The new independent medical school started with a group of 34 students.[119]

However well-intentioned, the establishment of a separate and independent *madraseh-ye tebb* did not change the reality that the quality of education at the school still left much to be desired. According to Dr. Neligan, Iran badly needed a modern and well-equipped medical school. Therefore, he supported Col. Hince's plan to establish a modern medical school in Iran. However, where should this school be located? In the South (Kerman), as Col. Hince proposed, or in the center, such as Isfahan, where, according to Neligan, the best hospital in the country, was to be found; this was operated and staffed by the CMS. Or should there be two schools, one in the North and the other in the South? Neligan opined that one well-equipped medical school sufficed for a poor country with 10 million inhabitants. Meanwhile, once Great

---

119. Rahnama 1333, vol. 1, p. 67 (the plans for the separate medical school had already been planned in 1906).

Britain had taken over the management of the Imperial hospital,[120] Neligan induced the school authorities to insist that students came there for clinical teaching and pass through the hospital's different departments. Because shortly, the Imperial hospital was expected to reach its limits of 60-70 beds, the Iranian government promised to build a new hospital large enough to meet the city's needs. Neligan was in favor of establishing a medical school in connection with this new hospital. He further argued that Great Britain should take charge of that hospital and the medical school. However, there were two difficulties. One was the presence of the French professors, the other the use of French, which was the most widely spoken foreign language in Tehran. However, English was gaining ground and, if there were English teachers and with additional supportive activities, the use of English would make great strides, he argued. Neligan did not favor teaching in Persian, although he was often forced to do so. He insisted that students needed to know a foreign language otherwise they would be cut off from the medical literature. Also, Persian was deficient in scientific terms.[121]

On 25 October 1920, Lt. Col. Fortescue of the British Legation called on Alim al-Soltan, director of secondary education of the *Vezarat-e Ma`aref*. The latter informed Fortescue that he had made a plan for the attachment of a hospital to the Dar ol-Fonun in which the two French professors, Dr. Pourac and Dr. Wilhelm,[122] were to have wards and give lectures. He admitted this was done after much pressure by the French Minister on the Iranian government. Apparently, Firuz Mirza, when engaging the two French doctors in Paris, had signed a contract with them that they would be given hospital wards and a laboratorium, and the French Minister insisted that this contractual

120. This was at the request of the government of Iran within the context of the proposed 1919 Perso-British Agreement with Vothuq al-Dowleh, see Floor, *History of Hospitals* (forthcoming).

121. FO 248/1291, Memo Dr. Neligan to Minister, Tehran, 28 January 1920.

122. The original text mistakenly calls these physicians Polak and Willem.

obligation be honored. Fortescue wanted the British Legation to take strong action against the realization of any such plan given that two British doctors and two British nurses were working in the Imperial hospital and that this hospital was 2,000 *tuman*s in debt. As a result, no member of the staff of the Imperial Hospital had received any pay for the last two months. The hospital, which could accommodate 100 patients, was unable to admit urgent cases as there were no funds to feed them. Also, there was a great shortage of drugs and dressings. Almost 500 syphilis patients attended the out-patient department and there was no salvaran to treat them. Therefore, Lt. Col. Fortescue concluded, that to spend 1,200 *tuman*s/month on a new institution "for purely political reasons is a scandal."[123] However, the British pressure was to no avail. In 1921, the Sheikh Hadi hospital was resuscitated and turned over to the French professors in the medical school, to satisfy the French Minister's demand.[124]

The Madraseh-ye `Ali-ye Tebb Plods Onwards

Because of the changes and the hiring of new French teachers the American doctors of the missionary hospital in Tehran were somewhat encouraged. They commented that indeed after1918 there had been attempts to bring the Dar ol-Fonun more up-to-date. The course had been lengthened to seven years and exams had to be passed before graduation, as a result the graduates were better than before. The latest improvement, in 1921, was the establishment of the Pasteur Institute under a French professor. Its objective was to supply the country with vaccines and serum.[125] But in spite of all these changes they were still considered to be insufficient.

> The Tehran medical college had a couple of French teachers, also a few Iranians who had studied in France. Most lectures were given in French, in the afternoon only, so students

---

123. FO 248/1291, Lt. Col. Fortescue to Minister, Tehran 26/10/1920.
124. RG 91-19-11-1, Notes on medical work of Teheran station Jan. 1922
125. RG 91-19-11-1, Notes on medical work of Teheran station Jan. 1922

> might serve as apprentices to doctors. Anatomy was taught from charts and a skeleton only. There was no dissection, no laboratories, no nursing profession, no surgery.[126]

The American doctors were of the opinion that this situation had to change. Whereas, the practice of medicine in Tehran approximated that of Europe and the US,[127] there were only about 200 to 250 doctors trained in Western medicine in the whole country. Therefore, there was a great need for physicians trained in modern medical methods. In 1927, because the Tehran missionary hospital was unable to provide that necessary training, the US Presbyterian Iran Mission recommended "that a pre-medical course be provided in the Tehran College for men and that the proper medical course be pursued either at the Imperial Polytechnic School at Tehran [i.e. the *madraseh-ye tebb*], or preferably in the Beirut Medical School."[128] Although nothing came of this plan, it would seem that all the good efforts spent to improve the *madraseh-ye tebb* also proved to be in vain. According to Dr. Neligan, the medical school at Tehran in the early 1920s was "very poorly equipped and the teaching is largely theoretical. No fees are charged. There is a long list of so-called professors, two (the lecturers on surgery and bacteriology) are French, the others are Persian, some of whom have French diplomas. The two Europeans have no say in the management of the school. The religious law does not permit dissection. Hospital attendance is not compulsory."[129] Unfortunately, the British officials were correct, because the French physicians were unable to make a difference, which was the reason why they had been hired, and, as a result, medical education did not improve measurably.

Although Dr. Neligan implies that the French teachers were not star performers, the lack of improvement in the quality of teaching cannot have been because the French physicians were technically

---

126. RG 231-1-6, Hoffman, *Pioneering in Meshed*, pp. 28-29

127. RG 91-19-11-1, Notes on medical work of Teheran station Jan. 1922

128. Presbyterian Church 1928 b, pp. 188, 190. Although the American missionary hospitals had ceased training Iranian physicians, they offered internships to medical students, in particular in Tehran.

129. Government of Great Britain 1945, pp. 408-09.

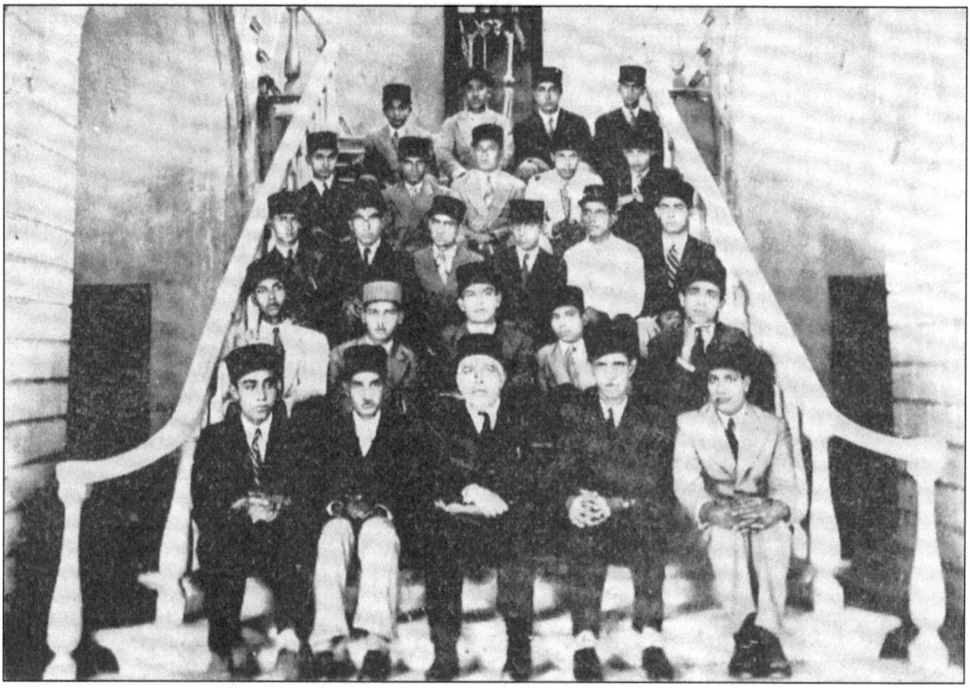

Professors and students of the *Madraseh-ye `Ali-ye Tebb*

incompetent. After all, as of 1918, foreign teachers, who were vetted as to their qualifications, only could be hired with the approval of parliament. However, most of the French teachers did not stay very long, which, of course, must have had a negative impact on the students. For example, in 1920, Dr. Pourac had been hired to teach internal medicine until 24 April 1923, but he left already in 1921. After Dr. Pourac's return to Europe, Dr. A`lam al-Molk was hired for three years to teach internal medicine, and one year later to teach general medicine and pediatrics. He also had to work one day/week in the Vaziri hospital to teach students clinical care (*balini*). In 1303/1924, Dr. Roland was hired to replace Dr. Pourac to teach internal medicine, but he did not stay long either. M. Odigiet (?) was hired for three years on 18 April 1923 as was Mr. Monet, who had to teach botany for a period of three years. On 26 December 1922, Dr. Wilhelm, a French surgeon was hired to teach surgery and work in the Vaziri Hospital. In addition, a few other Frenchmen worked at the *madraseh-ye `ali-ye tebb* between 1922-25, all for short periods, to wit: Messrs. Corandel:

microbiology; André: biology; Bonville: biology. On 15 January 1925, the Turkish Armenian Dr. Paparian was hired to teach pharmacology, although he mostly taught at the school of pharmacology. After Mirza Abu'l-Qasem Na'ini Soltan al-Hokama's death in 1913, the subject of traditional medicine was not taught for five years, until it was included again in 1918 and taught by Sehhat al-Dowleh. He was not a physician of the old school and thus, his teaching was mostly of a comparative nature. The subject was known as *Qarabadin-e Irani*, i.e. traditional Iranian drugs. It continued to be taught (in the last few years by E`tezad al-Hokama) until 1934. The subject was replaced by the history of medicine.[130] On 4 Jadi 1301/26 December 1922, Dr. Wilhelm was hired for 3 years as of 23 April 1923 to teach surgery at the *madraseh-ye tebb* and to be responsible for lessons of manual procedures (*a`mal-e yadi*) at the Vaziri hospital.[131]

Table 2: Teachers and teaching program of the medical school in the early 1920s

Name instructor	Subject	Time / week
Dr. Amir A`lam	Descriptive anatomy; therapeutics	3 hours
Dr. Hakim A`zam	Internal medicine, physiology, forensic medicine	Idem
Dr. Gholam Hoseyn A`lam	Pediatrics; minor surgery	Idem
Dr. Abdollah Khan	Parasitology; history of medicine	Five days
Dr. Loqman al-Molk	External medicine, urology	Idem
Dr. Sehhat al-Dowleh	Iranian traditional medicine	One day

130. Rahnama 1333, vol. 1, pp. 67-68. Ebrahimnejad 2014, p. 196, n. 49 mentions a text from 1868 called *Qarabadin-e Salehi*, a book on compound drugs.

131. *Majmu`eh-ye qavanin*, p. 678.

Name instructor	Subject	Time / week
Dr. Hoseyn Khan Mo`tamed	Medical physics and chemistry; VD; scientific medicine	Six days [67]
Dr. Ehya al-Molk	Public health	One day
Dr. Mehdi Malekzadeh	Anatomy	Five days
Dr. Yunes Khan	Midwifery and bacteriology	Two days
Dr. Lesan al-Hokama	Ophthalmology	Idem
Dr. Loqman al-Dowleh	General medicine	One day
Dr. Abu'l-Qasem Khan Bahrami	Biology; zoology	Two days

Source: Rahnama 1333, vol. 1, pp. 67–68.

Dr. Neligan was correct as to the poor equipment available at the *Madraseh-ye Tebb*, which, given its limited annual budget, is no surprise. In 1298/1919-20, the budget for the school amounted to 9,720 *tuman*s and in 1299/1920-21 it was 12,300 *tuman*s. During 1322-24/1923-35, the budget was about 16,500 *tuman*s. If we realize that the annual salary of, e.g., Dr. Wilhelm was 5,000 *tuman*s and we add the cost of the salaries of the other European teachers, one may question the wisdom of hiring European teachers.[132] In the short-term, moreover, there was no change in the poor housing and equipment of the *madraseh-ye `ali-ye tebb*. It remained in the same *hayat-e nezam* until 1923. In 1922, the government bought the *Emarat-e Mas`udiyeh*, which, after repairs, became the seat of the Ministry of Education and the *madraseh-ye tebb*. A few years later the school moved temporarily to a location in the Khiyaban-e Laleh Zar-e Now, but, soon thereafter, it moved to the Mo`tamed Hospital. This hospital had been founded

132. Rahnama 1333, vol. 1, pp. 67-68.

by Hoseyn Mo`tamed one of the school's professors. It was only in 1316/1937 that the school moved to new premises (see below).[133]

For a number of years, there was no major change in the school's situation. Until 1928, the professors remained those listed in Table 2; any changes were mostly in the rotation of French professors, who served only for short periods (see above). In 1928, Dr. Valiollah Khan Nasr became the new head of the *Madraseh-ye Tebb* and Dr. Ali Farahmandi his deputy. Together they laid the foundation of the new medical curriculum for the school and of the later medical faculty of the new University of Tehran. They also hired a new team of teachers (see Table 3) that had to implement the new and revamped study program.

Table 3: Names of teachers of the *Madraseh-ye `Ali-ye Tebb* during 1928-34/1307-13

Name instructor	Subject
Dr. Valiollah Khan Nasr	Director of the school
Dr. Sa`id Khan Malek	Teacher
Dr. Dr. `Ali Khan Partow A`zam	Idem
Dr. Amir A`zam	Idem
Dr. Moh. Hoseyn Khan Loqman Adham	Idem
Dr. `Abbas Khan Adham	Idem
Dr. Hoseyn Khan Mo`tamad	Idem
Dr. `Ali Farahmandi	Teacher and deputy director
Dr. Moh. Hoseyn Khan Pezeshkpur	Teacher
Dr. Mohsen Sayyah	Idem

133. Rahnama 1333, vol. 1, p. 84.

Name instructor	Subject
Dr. Sayyed Mostafa Bani Hashemi	Teacher and budget officer
Dr. A`lam`ali Khan Mina	Teacher
Dr. Yahya Sokut [?]	Idem
Dr. Mo'taman`	Idem
Dr. Parviz Khan Sadiq	Chief of the laboratory
Dr. Andre	Natural sciences teacher
Dr. Grandel	Microbiology teacher
Dr. Jean Azma	Chemistry teacher
Dr. Paparian	Teacher at the school of pharmacology
Dr. Paul Bonville	Natural sciences teacher

Source: Rahnama 1332, vol. 1, p. 69

The new teaching program was approved in September 1928 and was based on a five-year study. It started with 1-year of physics, chemistry and biology. Further: medical chemistry: 2 hours/week with practice; medical physics: 3 hours; descriptive anatomy: 3 hours; physiology: 3 hours; histology and embryology: 1 hour. Other courses: 30 hours. Also, more attention was paid to the practical side of medicine (See Table 4), so that students also had to aquire clinical experience. Nevertheless, much of the teaching remained theoretical and essential facilities, such as a laboratory were lacking. For example,

> Pathology was taught in theory with no slide presentations, gross or microscopic examinations, or medical laboratory. The teachers used handwritten books or copies of previous textbooks. Extant are reports of tissue examination from the American Hospital, the British Oil Company Hospital, or from

employees of foreign embassies which were sent abroad. Tissue examination facilities were not available for ordinary patients.[134]

Table 4: Curriculum of the *Madraseh-ye `Ali-ye Tebb* as of 1928

Theoretical classes	Time per week	Practical lessons
Medical chemistry	2 hours	Laboratory
Medical physics	3 hours	Idem
Descriptive anatomy	Idem	-
Physiology	Idem	Laboratory
Histology and embryology	1 hour	Idem
Theoretical anatomy	2 hours	-
Forensic medicine and public health	Idem	-
Midwifery	Idem	-

134. Bahadori 2015, p. 14 is mistaken that no tissue examinations were done of ordinary Iranian patients. Apart from the fact the American hospital served mainly (99.9%) Iranian patients and that the NIOC hospitals also had a majority of Iranian patients, both institutions, as well as the American Hospital in Mashhad, sent pathology specimens either to the American Hospital in Beirut (see below p. 254 in this book) or, in case of the NIOC, did the testing themselves. The hospitals in the oilfields had a pathologist with a pathology lab. The British physicians did extensive research in, e.g., sulfur dioxide exposure about which oil workers complained, see Floor 2018, p. 128; Williamson 1927, pp. 128-132; Gilmour 1924, p. 39, IOR/L/MIL/17/15/24, 'Military Report on The Anglo-Iranian Oil Company's (South Iranian) Oilfield Area', p. 49. Also, when the Dowlat hospital was still under British management (1921-23) it employed a pathologist. RG 91-19-11-1, Notes on medical work of Teheran station Jan. 1922. The CMS hospital in Kerman also employed a pathologist at times. Administration Report 1935, p. 38.

Theoretical classes	Time per week	Practical lessons
Physicians' duties – discussion	Idem	-
Parasitology	3 hours	Laboratory
Pathology	2 hours	-
Bacteriology	1 hour	Laboratory
External diseases	3 hours	-
Internal and tropical diseases	Idem	-
Pharmacology and simple drugs	1 hour	Laboratory
Mouth and teeth diseases	2 hours	-
General medicine and diagnostics	Idem	-
Principles of therapy	Idem	-
Practical medicine	1 hour	-
Minor surgery	Idem	Operations
Ancient Iranian medicine	Idem	-

Rahnama 1332, vol. 1, pp. 69-70

In addition to class room and practical instruction, students also had to follow clinical lessons, as follows:

1. Clinic of internal diseases: each morning in the hospital.
2. Clinic of external diseases: idem
3. Urology and gynecology: 3 hours/week in the hospital.
4. Ophthalmology clinic: 2 hours

5. Clinic of dermatology and venereal diseases:
   4 hours/week in the hospital.
6. Mouth and teeth diseases: 2 hours/week in the hospital.
7. Ear, throat, nose clinic: 2 hours/week in the hospital.
8. Radiology: 2 hours/week in the hospital.
9. Midwifery: 2 hours/week in the morning in the hospital.

The clinical lessons took place either in the Dowlati or the Vaziri hospital. In 1309/1930, the ear-nose-throat and obstetric clinical lessons took place in the American hospital. Students had to pass an exam in each of the subjects taught at the end of the year.[135]

Despite all these improvements Dr. Garrison of the Johns Hopkins School, perhaps influenced by Dr. Elgood, whose help he acknowledged, wrote:

> The only medical school is that of Tehran, but the teaching is unsatisfactory by reason of faulty training in physics and chemistry, neglect of dissecting, which is forbidden by Mohammedan law, total indifference to diseases of women, and the lack of a lying-in hospital manageable by men. The Medical School is staffed by 12 Persian physicians, most of whom hold a French diploma. Teaching is entirely along French lines.[136]

Regulating the Medical Profession

To upgrade and improve the quality of physicians and their number, the government took two important steps. One was to establish the qualifications of the physicians, who wanted to practice medicine, and the other was to send a large number of students to Europe and the USA to study medicine and thus increase the country's medical capacity and quality. In 1290/1911, as discussed above, the *Majles* had passed a law that required a physician to have a valid diploma from a domestic or foreign medical school to practice.[137] However, due to the

135. For details, see Rahnama 1333, vol. 1, pp. 70-71.
136. Garrison 1933, p. 152.
137. Rahnama 1333, vol. 1, p. 71.

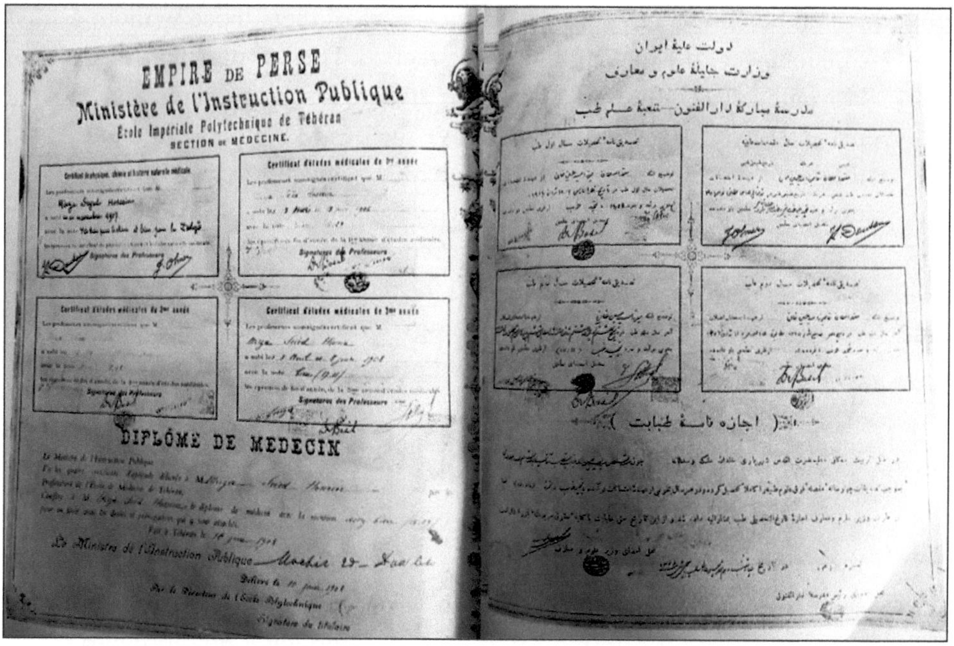

So-called four-tiered (*chahar-khaneh*) medical diploma and license to practice

uncertain and unstable political times as well as the outbreak of WW I this law remained a dead letter. After WW I there was the sporadic attempt to apply the law, such as in 1919, in Rasht. There, `Isa Sadeq, a new superintendent of education- a Cambridge man- tried to enforce the laws requiring licenses of all physicians. However, he was accused of acting as if he still was in the past period of absolutism and doctors and others started a media campaign (in the papers, rumor mongering, calls to politicians) to make Sadeq stop his unwanted interference. However, he persevered and succeeded in applying the law.[138]

To make the physician's licensing law effective the *Majles* passed a new law in Shahrivar 1306/August 1927 stating that those medical practitioners who did not yet have a permit to practice, but had practiced for 10 years might pass an exam in the provincial capital in the presence of group of physicians who had a permit, and, if successful,

138. Sadeq 1340, vol. 1, pp. 202-03; RG 91-19-9, Resht Medical Report 1924-25.

would be allowed to practice. However, as of then, those without a diploma were no longer allowed to practice. The law of Adhar 1306/ November 1927 allowed a period of 2 years for these exams to take place. However, the law did not have the desired effect either, and, therefore, on 25 Esfand 1308/16 March 1930 the *Majles* passed a law extending the 1306/1927 law by three years, although the exam could only be taken once per year in Mehr (Sept–Oct). On 10 Mordad 1309/1 August 1930, the *Majles* established the requirements for the medical exam to be taken: anatomy, physiology, internal medicine, external medicine (ophthalmology; gynecology and midwifery were part of the exam concerning external medicine), causes and symptoms and diagnosis and prescription as to internal and external diseases, and essentials of therapy. In this way, the medical profession, had acquired a legal foundation and in theory provided reliability for patients as to the physicians' qualifications. It also made clear who had the right to the title of 'doctor' and who did not.[139]

The reason for opting for a gradual, although a revolutionary, approach was that Persia just did not have enough Western trained doctors. The reality was that most doctors were those trained in the Islamic-Galenic system and it was not realistic to forbid them to practice. The law, therefore, provided a grandfather clause. If you had practiced outside Tehran for more than 10 years and thus had shown that your treatments had not been harmful, you were allowed to continue to practice. Traditional doctors who had practiced in Tehran for more than five but less than 10 years were required to pass a government examination within a period of three years. Some *Majles* deputies had argued that the law should apply to the country as a whole, because otherwise quacks that were not allowed to operate in Tehran would "go to the provinces and there engage in murder." But the view that there should be an immediate cut with the past throughout the country did not win out. It was also argued that in Tehran more specialists would practice who needed modern drugs, which, if used improperly, might be harmful.[140]

139. Rahnama 1333, vol. 1, pp. 71-72.

140. Government of Iran n.d A., vol. 3, pp. 1576-80.

Among the provincial groups of licensed physicians foreign ones, who happened to work there, often American missionary physicians were asked to become a member. McDowell of the American Hospital of Tehran served some years on the National Board of Medical Examiners. In 1935 he spent several days examining graduates of the medical college.[141] In Mashhad, governor Pakravan asked Dr. Hoffman to be one of the three doctors of the commission, who checked the qualifications of applicants for medical licenses. "'Doctors' were licensed by a Board in Tehran but there was a class called 'tabeebs' who were not permitted to do surgery."[142] This type of service was not limited to the American Hospital in Tehran. Also, in Hamadan, for example, mission doctors were often called to sit on examining boards or called to confer on various matters helping to raise the standards set for Iranian doctors.[143] In 1936, the department of health asked the American doctors to sit in on exams of applicants for licenses to practice medicine. These applicants were no graduates from any school, but

> are those who practiced a number of years without licenses, either on their own with picked-up or studied knowledge, or an assistant or student under some practitioner. These ranged from 30 to 70 years of age and were examined on the whole range of medicine. We were given to understand that the government did not expect us to ask difficult questions, but in spite of our leniency, not more than half of the thirty some applicants passed. It is of interest to note that all four of the examiners, together with the head of the health department who superintended, were all Christian doctors."[144]

---

141. RG 91-19-11-1, Tehran Medical Report 1935-1936; Idem, Report of Medical Work Teheran 1937-1938; RG 231-1-2, Hoffman to N.N., no date (probably 1938).

142. RG 231-1-6, Hoffman, Pioneering in Meshed, p. 119; RG 91-20-2, Mashad Medical Report 1929-1930 (Dr. Hoffman sat on the Board of Medical Examiners for the past 2 years.).

143. Presbyterian Church 1932, p. 169.

144. RG 91-19-27, Healing in the Home of Avicenna June 30, 1936

The concern was that despite these legal requirements the majority of Iranians still did not have access to medical care from a licensed physician and, therefore, traditional practitioners and quacks still treated more patients than physicians trained in modern scientific medicine. By 1924, a total of 905 doctors were licensed to practice in Persia. Of these, 253 had a diploma (this number includes European and American doctors residing in Iran), the remaining 652 had been authorized to practice as a result of the 1911 law. Of these, very few had any notion of modern Western medicine, although some enjoyed a good reputation. This number of official doctors translated into one doctor per 11,000 inhabitants. However, of the 905 doctors, a total of 323 practiced in Tehran, so that, excluding Tehran, in 1924, there was one doctor per 16,800 inhabitants. The corresponding figure for Tehran was one per 680 inhabitants. Given the worrisome public health situation in Iran, it is clear that these doctors did not serve the population at large. Also, at the same time there was a much larger number of unregulated practitioners of folk medicine operating in Persia, who served the bulk of the population. It would seem that in line with the focus of traditional medicine few of the trained Persian physicians took surgery as a specialty.[145]

THE DANESHKADEH-YE `ALI-YE TEBB

In 1309/1930-31, Dr. `Ali Khan Farhmandi was appointed director of the *madraseh-ye `ali-ye tebb* and of the school of pharmacology.[146] He remained director of the schools until 1312/1933-34, when he was replaced by Dr. Loqman al-Dowleh, who was joined in 1313/1934 by Dr. Abu'l-Qasem Bakhtiyar as his deputy. The latter resigned one year

145. Gilmour 1924, pp. 33-36 (including the text of the law). In Kermanshah there were 20 doctors, five of whom had diplomas, the remaining 15 did not. Soltani 1370, vol. 1, p. 535. In fact, in Maragheh none of the traditional doctors were licensed to practice. Some them, therefore, opted for training to be able to pass the state exam, see Good 1981, pp. 68, 71-72. By 1920, only one or two Iranian women had taken up Western medicine as a profession. Rice 1923, pp. 252-53.

146. Rahnama 1333, vol. 1, p. 69.

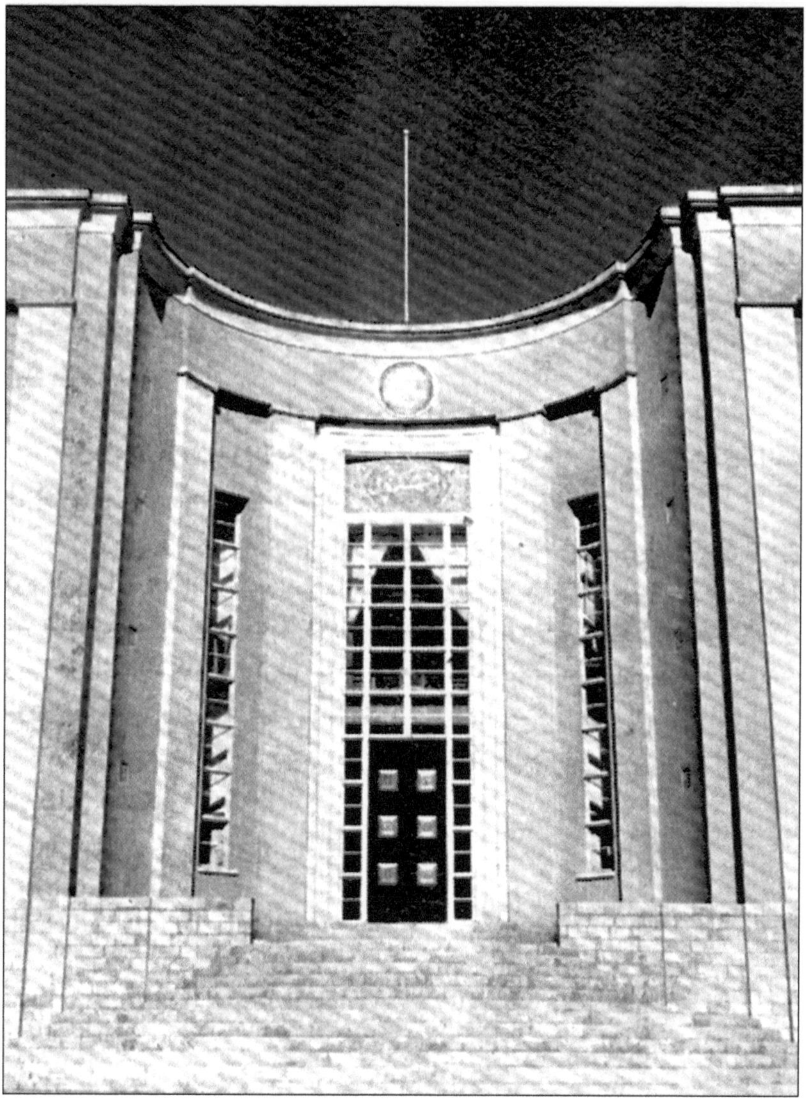

Southern portico of the Medical School of the University of Tehran. The master plan of the campus buildings was drawn up by French architects Roland Dubrulle and Maxime Siroux, Swiss architect Alexandre Moser, as well as Andre Godard, Nicolai Markov and Mohsen Foroughi.

later and was replaced by Dr. Javad Shetiyani [?]. On 30 May 1934 Parliament passed a law (5 Khordad 1313/26 May 1934) establishing that the various *madrasehha-ye `ali* became *daneshkadeh*s. Until then, the *Madraseh-ye `Ali-ye Tebb* was housed in rented facilities. Therefore, a large piece of land was bought (200,000 sq. m) for 90,000 *tumans* to build a new university, which was designed by M. Markov. The first stone was laid on 3 Tir 1313/24 June 1934 and the official opening in the presence of Reza Shah took place on 15 Bahman 1314/5 February 1936.[147]

Not only a new institution was created and a new building erected, but at the same time the government saw to it that the study program of medical students was updated, which was built on the one established in 1928 (see above). In 1313/1934 a new law required that graduates write a thesis to get the title of 'doctor,' while the study period remained fixed at five years. The curriculum that emphasized increased practical experience was re-organized as follows:

> Year 1: practical anatomy 384 hours; theoretical anatomy and diseases of the nervous system 576 hours; psychiatry and dermatology 192 hours.
> Year 2: practical descriptive anatomy 144 hours; theoretical descriptive anatomy 120 hours; theoretical physiology 96 hours; practice 48 hours; medical chemistry and physics 192 hours; practice 48 hours.[148]
> Year 3: topical anatomy 3 hours/week; physiology 3 hours/week, including 3 hours of practical lessons during summer; clinical anatomy 3 hours/week plus one-hour practice/week during winter; practical surgery; parasitology; natural birth; minor surgery each one hour/week.

---

147. The law of 2 Bahman 1312/22 February 1934 also changed the rules governing appointment and dismissal of staff, which until that time was at the discretion of the Minister of Education. The new law established a council that was composed of government officials and university staff to deal with those administrative rules and issues. Rahnama 1333, vol. 1, p. 74-75.

148. In year 1, the study lasted 144 weeks (8-hour day) and in year 2, 81 weeks/year. I assume that other subjects were taught in the remaining weeks.

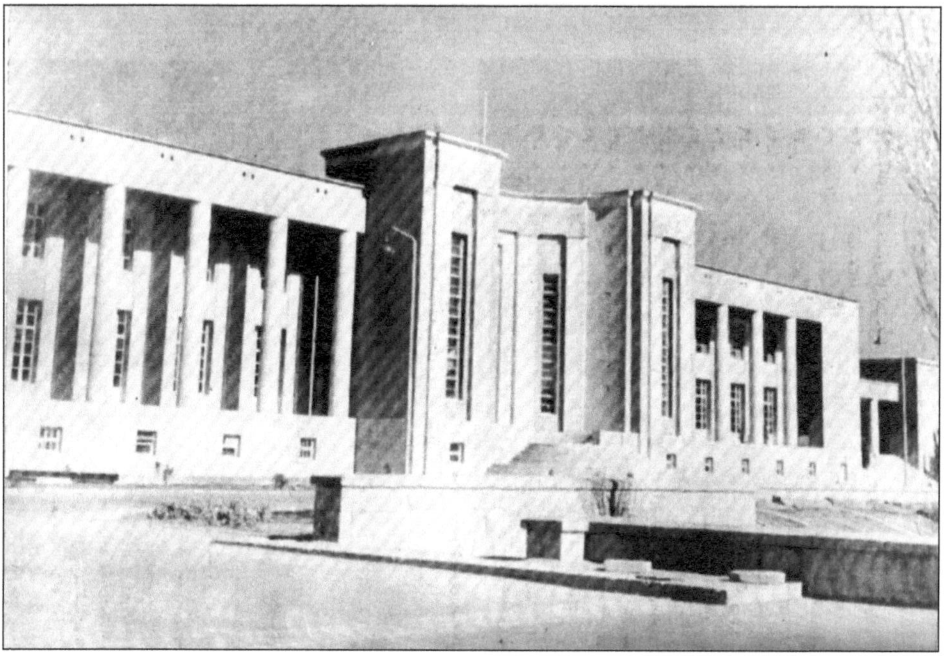

A view of the Medical School of the University of Tehran

Year 4: urological diseases; microbiology (3 hours/week); parasitology, pathological anatomy, difficult birth,[149] venereal diseases; principles of therapy (2 hours/week); elements of medicine; pharmacology (1 hour/week).
Year 5: principles of therapeutics; forensic medicine; ophthalmology; radiology; throat-ear-and nose diseases; mouth and teeth diseases (2 hours/week); male and female urological diseases; public health (2 hours/ week) history of medicine (1 hour/week).
Clinics: medical clinic, surgery, venereal (zahravi) and skin; urology; midwifery and gynecology; ophthalmology; ear-throat-nose; teeth and mouth; radiology; brain diseases.

149. The term used, *qabeligi-ye gheyr tabi`i*, or 'unnatural delivery', refers to difficult delivery cases which may need Cesarean section, forceps delivery etc. (in contrast to normal vaginal delivery).

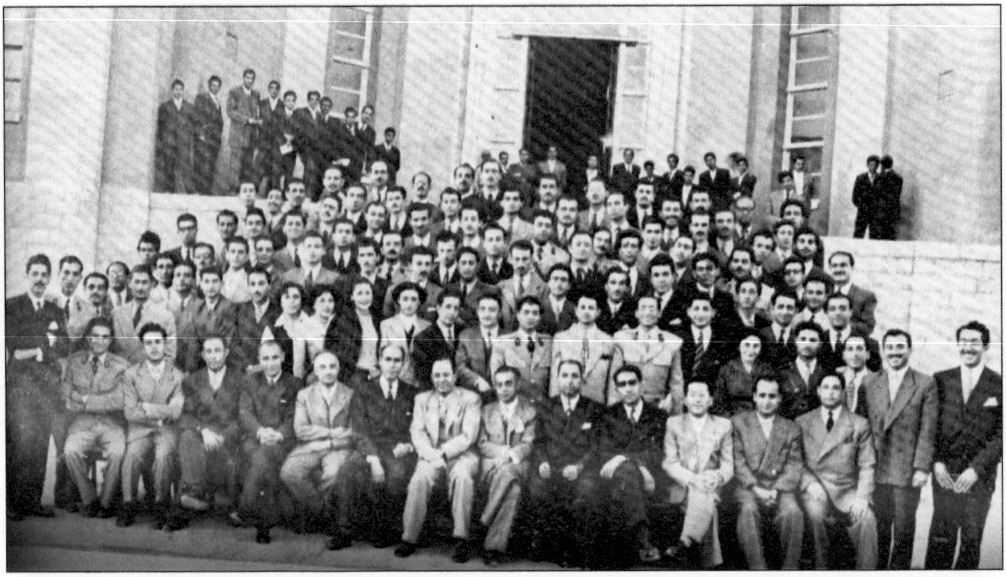

Medical teachers and graduates of 1951-1952, Tehran School of Medicine

As of 1314-15, minor changes were made to this teaching program:

> Year 1: practical and theoretical anatomy; psychiatry; dermatology; medical physics and chemistry.
> Year 2: physiology; medical chemistry and physics; minor surgery; internal and external diseases; midwifery; urology; general diseases; theoretical and practical parasitology.
> Year 3: pathological anatomy; clinical anatomy of diseases; internal and external diseases; obstetrics; urology; general diseases; practical and theoretical parasitology.
> Year 4: urology; microbiology; pathological anatomy; female diseases; pharmacology; internal and external medicine; practical medicine.
> Year 5: principles of medical treatment; public health; forensic medicine; ophthalmology; radiology; ear-nose-throat diseases; history of medicine; mouth and teeth diseases; mental diseases; essential surgery.[150]

150. Rahnama 1333, vol. 1, p. 75. "Pathology, together with histology and embryology, were taught in a small room at Dr. Motamed Hospital where the only Iranian 'Madraseh-Teb' was located. […] microscopic slides [were shown] to students" by Dr. Mostafa Habibi. Bahadori 2015, p. 15.

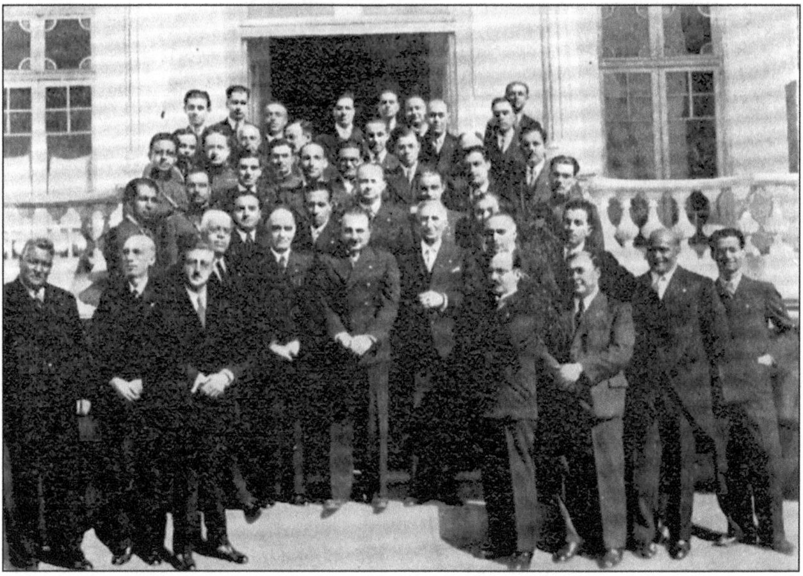

The faculty and medical students, Motamed Hospital, academic year 1935-1936

In 1937, the *daneshkadeh-ye `ali-ye tebb* moved to the new university buildings. From 1940 it was called *daneshkadeh-ye pezeshki*. In Dey 1318/December 1939, the government created 34 professorial chairs for the teaching of medicine at the new university, to wit: 23 for medicine, 8 for pharmacology and 3 for dentistry. Practical teaching took place in the Dowlat, Razi, Vaziri and Nesvan hospitals.[151] In 1939, medical students followed a six-year course "with practical work in the Tehran civil hospitals, before obtaining their diplomas. The course of study in pharmacy lasts four years and dental surgery three years. The present numbers of students are reported to be as under :

Medical	456
Pharmacy	146
Dentistry	27."[152]

151. Rahnama 1333, vol. 1, p. 80. For the names of the professors and the subjects they taught, see Rahnama 1333, vol. 1, pp. 80-81. For information on these hospitals, see Floor 2012.

152. IOR/L/PS/12/3503, Intelligence Summary no. 3 for the period ending February 11, 1939, p. 1.

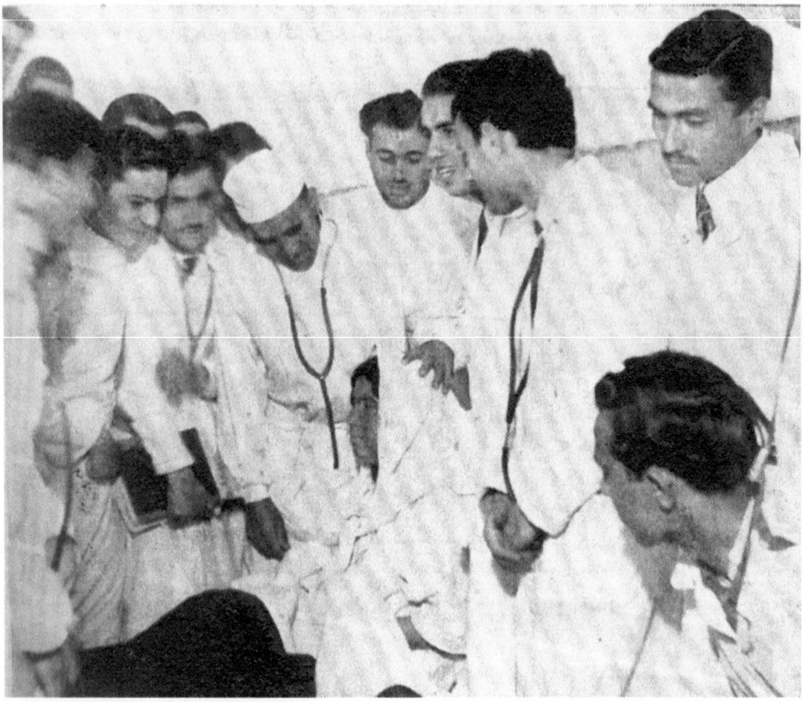

Professor Mehdi Azar, internists and medical students, examining a patient, Vaziri Hospital, Tehran

The American missionary doctors, with some exceptions, did not teach at the government medical school, but some of its students were an important part of the Tehran American hospital's personnel. At least one medical student was permanently on its staff the whole year. Three other students volunteered, and four to five picked up clinical instruction regularly, when they were free from classes.[153] It was only in the field of anatomy that Dr. Blair of the American Hospital provided his services to the anatomical institute, a.k.a. the Ibn Sina Institute, which was the first medical institute that opened on 5 February 1935. Dr. Edward Blair of the American Christian Hospital was hired to teach anatomy. Because dissection henceforth was officially allowed, he taught the subject using cadavers as well as how to make specimens from them. The first formal autopsy was

153. RG 91-19-11-1, Annual Report of Teheran Hospital, June 30, 1933

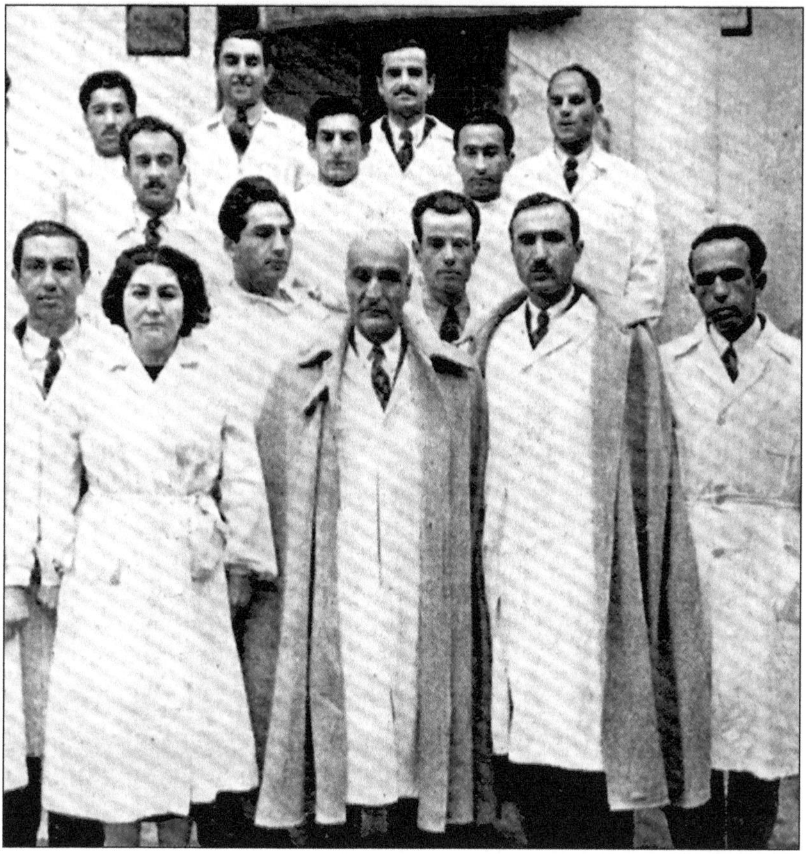

Razi Hospital, Department of dermatology and venereal diseases

performed by Dr. Hashem Hanjan at the *Daneshkadeh* in 1937.[154] Although officially allowed, dissection was still an anathema to the olama. Therefore, initially, Dr. Abu'l-Qasem Bakhtiyar, professor of obstetrics smuggled a number of bodies from the public hospitals to the anatomy laboratory in his own car.[155] Dr. Blair's Gross Anatomy course was much appreciated. Both Iranian laymen and doctors praised his work. Dr. Blair continued teaching in the Anatomy Department

154. Bahadori 2014, p. 146.
155. Karamati 1999.

at the Medical School until his departure in 1938, which the School very much regretted. [156]

In 1939, with the appointment of Dr. Pierre Oberlin as head of the medical faculty, a new chapter in the teaching of modern medicine began.[157] The new generation of Iranian doctors, whether trained in Tehran or abroad signaled a sea change for the future of Iran's public health, in more than one sense. The once skeptical American missionary doctors were pleased with this development. For example, Dr. Lichtwardt (Hamadan hospital) commented that "the new University [in Tehran] is turning out well-equipped [medical] young men."[158] From Mashhad, Dr. Hoffman opined: "Its 'med school' has improved, has a building of its own to house its class rooms; it trains young men as doctor's assistants or village doctors to meet great demand."[159]

---

156. RG 91-19-11-1, Annual Report, June 30, 1936; Idem, Report of Medical Work-Teheran Station 1937-1938; RG 231-1-2, Hoffman to NN, no date.

157. How the medical faculty developed after that date, see Rahnama 1333 and Karamati 1999. For a short biography of Dr. Oberling, see Azizi 2014 a.

158. RG 91-19-27, Healing in the Home of Avicenna June 30, 1936.

159. RG 91-20-2, Mashad Medical Report, 1945-1946.

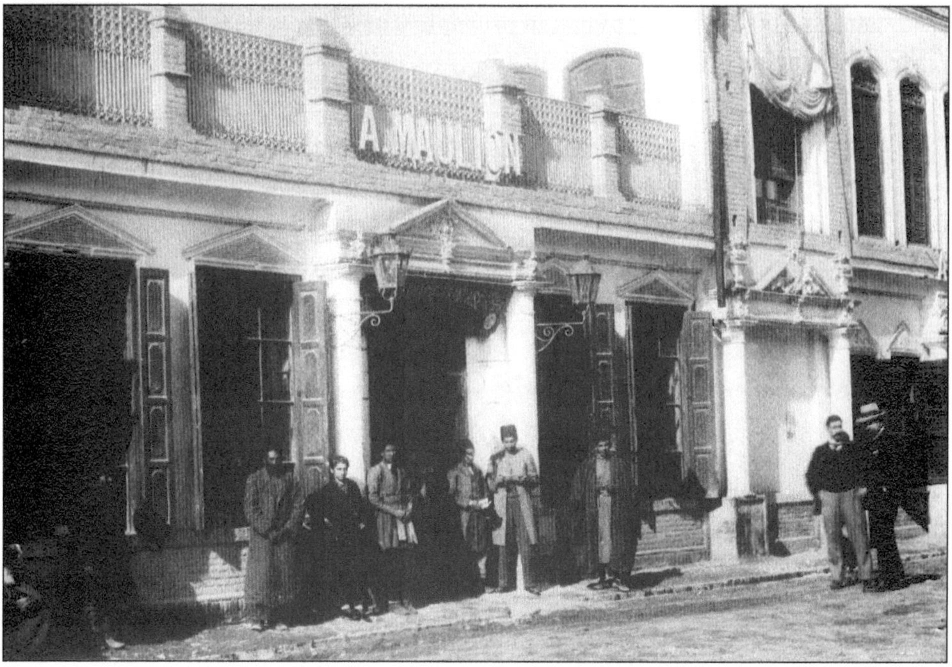

The Maulion Pharmacy in Tehran

The School of Pharmacology

When in 1918 the *madraseh-ye `ali-ye tebb* separated from the Dar ol-Fonun, a separate school of pharmacology (*daru-sazi*) was established to train pharmacists. Pharmacology had been a subject taught from the very beginning of the Dar ol-Fonun. Fochetti, who was among the first group of foreign teachers who arrived in Tehran in December 1851, taught pharmacology and sciences at the Dar ol-Fonun, where he had seven students. In 1852, two of these received honorary awards for making much needed drugs. One of them was Mirza Kazem Mahallati a.k.a. Mirza Kazemi.[160] Fochetti taught in French, which was translated by Mirza Reza Kashani. In 1857, Fochetti went to Europe to buy equipment for a laboratory that he wanted to establish inside the Dar ol-Fonun. It was ready in 1858, and it was the first pharmaceutical and chemical lab in Iran, where he conducted

160. *Vaqaye`-ye Ettefaqiyeh* 1373-74, p. 852 (no. 98, 5 Rabi I 1269/1852).

analyses of traditional Persian drugs. In 1859 it was decided to send four students to study pharmacology (*davasazi*), half of whom were students of the Dar ol-Fonun.[161]

To support the work and needs of the laboratory, Dr. Schlimmer made an effort to introduce the manufacturing of glassware at the school to produce instruments for medical use. However, his effort produced no lasting result, except for the following poetic outburst by a local wit:

Ey Shlimer yek zaman dar kar-e khod andisheh kon
Agar namigardad bolur in kureh anra shisheh kon.

O Schlimmer why don't you think for a moment about your class
If this kiln does not produce crystal then have it produce glass.[162]

Although the lab was able to produce a number of drugs and allegedly in large amounts, the school still required local drugs.[163] Fochetti left Iran in 1861 and was replaced by one of his students, Mirza Kazem Shimi, who had gone to France to complete his studies. He taught pharmacology, chemistry and sciences till his death in 1896 and was also head of the pharmacology department. After his death, Mirza Kazem Shimi was replaced by M. Rocquebrun, who served from 1898-1901. He was succeeded by a German, Dr. Schwerin, and after some time, another Frenchman replaced him, M. Maulion or Mauléon.[164] He was assisted by Dr. Mahmud Khan Shimi, the son of Mirza Kazem Shimi, who had studied in France. He also acted as interpreters for these three European teachers. Other pharmacology

---

161. Ardakani 1368, vol. 1, p. 303; Hazefi 1332, vol. 1, p. 35. For an overview of the graduates and their careers, see Ekhtiar 1994, pp. 178-82, 184-85, 188-91, 195-99.

162. Hedayat 1344, p. 58.

163. Ebrahimnejad 2014, pp. 92-93.

164. Rahnama 1333, vol. 1, p. 43. Each of these foreign teachers opened a modern pharmacy retail shop in Tehran. Rahnama 1333, vol. 1, p. 81; E'temad-al-Salṭaneh 1307, p. 92.

teachers mentioned include Banati [?] (France) and Petrosian, but it is not precisely known when they taught at the school.[165]

I do not know whether any of the Dar ol-Fonun graduates opened a modern public pharmacy, but Schwerin, the German teacher of pharmacology, opened a retail pharmacy on Kh. Naseriyeh, despite violent public opposition. Another professor of pharmacology at the Dar ol-Fonun, Maulion, also opened a chemist shop, and later a number of Armenian doctors (Petrosiyan, Papaziyan, and Garnik), who had been trained in Beirut and Switzerland, did the same. Petrosian also taught at the Dar ol-Fonun.[166] Many Iranian and foreign entrepreneurs also opened modern pharmacies, both in Tehran and in other Iranian cities. However, the traditional herbalists remained the main suppliers of medicine to the population at large.[167]

In 1903, the Persian government hired two French pharmacologists. One of whom was Gustave Lecomte, a French army officer, who was hired to head the royal pharmacological laboratory and pharmacy. He set up a laboratory in the government theater (*Takiyeh-e ye Dowlat*) where the two Frenchmen taught their courses. Lecomte also conducted research concerning mineral water and wine. He published the result of his research in 1906 in Paris. In his laboratory he taught many pharmacists, and Abbasqoli Qarib translated for him.[168] Nothing is known about the teaching of pharmacology until 1918, when the school of pharmacology was separated from the *madraseh-ye `ali-ye tebb* and became an independent institution. However, this soon was considered to be an unworkable situation. Therefore, in 1301/1922, the school of pharmacology was merged again with the *madraseh-ye `ali-ye*

---

165. Rahnama 1333, vol. 1, p. 81.

166. Hasanbegi 1377, p. 205; *Tarbiyat* 1377, index q.v. *Muliyun*, *Davakhaneh*, and *Davasazi*. For other modern pharmacies, see Floor 2004, pp. 218; Anonymous 1911; Aubin 1908, p. 46; Sepehr 1368, p. 194; Grothe 1911, p. 132 (German pharmacies in Rasht, Barforush, Tehran, Tabriz, Hamadan, Senneh, Kermanshah).

167. Shahri 1368, vol. 4, pp. 327-28.

168. Neligan 1926, part III, p. 742; Government of France 1914, p. 40; Rahnama 1333, vol. 1, p. 82.

tebb. In 1924, Dr. Gilmour qualified it as a poorly equipped school of pharmacology. The study period at the school of pharmacology was initially three years, but later five. Students studying medicine also followed courses there. Pharmacology students needed to have a state certificate showing they had an elementary school education as well as two years of having worked in a pharmacy. During their study, which included botany, herbal pharmacology, chemistry and physics, they also needed to be employed in a state-certified pharmacy.[169]

Initially, Dr. Paparian, who had been hired in 1925, was the only teacher for pharmacology. The other teachers were Ali ol-Molk (physics); Mahmud Khan Shimi (chemistry); Hakim al-Saltanat (pharmacy).[170] Dr. Namdar was the first head of the school of pharmacology. During 1310-19/1931-40, pharmacology was taught by Dr. Moqaddam. In 1928, Dr. Heinrich Streng, head of the German technical school, was appointed for practical teaching (pharmacology, chemistry, biology) at the pharmacological school. Therefore, students did their practical work in the laboratory of the German technical school. Gradually the direction of the school came into the hands of Iranians trained in Europe. In 1311-12, the teachers at the school were Dr. Streng, Dr. Moqaddam, Dr. Fathollah A`lam, Dr. Paparian, and Dr. Namdar. Compulsory subjects not covered by these teachers were taught by teachers of the medical school.[171]

In 1317–18/1938–39, the school employed the following teachers: Dr. Namdar (botany), Dr. Sharqi (physics, chemistry, biology), Dr. Fathollah A`lam (toxicology, mineral chemistry), Dr. Gagig [?] (descriptive chemistry, theory and practice), Dr. Moqaddam (microbiology, hygiene, earth and water science, Galenic medicine), Dr. Mozaffari

169. Gilmour 1924, pp. 16; Rahnama 1333, vol. 1, pp. 68, 82.

170. Rahnama 1333, vol. 1, pp. 68-69. Dr. Paparian, a Turkish subject, was hired by law 24 Dey 1304/25 December 1925 for 2 years and 3 months with a salary of 75 *tumans*/month. His contract was renewed as of 1306/1927 for 2 years and 9 months.

171. Rahnama 1333, vol. 1, p. 82. Dr. Streng was hired by law of 7 Jadi 1304/28 December 1925.

(organic chemistry, chemical drugs) and Dr. Mohammad Sadri (pharma-codology ?).[172]

The teaching of pharmacology was only one aspect that needed to be developed to provide better health care for the people of Iran. A related subject was that of standards for the qualifications of pharmacists and the products they made and sold.[173] Prior to the establishment of modern pharmacies, the shop of the druggist (*`attar*) was the closest thing to the institution of a modern pharmacy, which did not yet exist in Iran. The only ones of that kind were those managed by European physicians and were private in nature. Even after the opening of modern pharmacies as of the 1880s, the *`attar*s remained the main source of supply for medicines to the majority of the population. This was not a minor issue, because the quality of the products sold by druggists (*`attar*) was not guaranteed. In fact, one Iranian author accused them of "selling rotten and corrupt medications."[174] This was, for example, the case in Bandar `Abbas where in 1910, the British medical quarantine officer had to get supplies from the British consulate, because the stocks of the druggists in the bazaar were rotten or too old to be used.[175] It also happened that they gave the patient the wrong product instead of that which the doctor had prescribed.[176] Moreover, there was also a rise in pharmacy shops, which were not regulated either. In 1926, Dr. Neligan, concerning the situation in Tehran, wrote, "Chemists' shops are numerous."[177] For example, in 1929 there were no less than 148 of such shops in Tehran. In 1926, there were 19 chemist shops in Kermanshah.[178] Already, in 1906, the

---

172. Rahnama 1333, vol. 1, pp. 83.

173. On the profession of the herbalist or *`attar*, see Floor 2004, pp. 130-36.

174. Ebrahimnejad 2002, p. 171.

175. Sadid al-Saltaneh 1342, p. 169.

176. *Vaqaye`-ye Ettefaqiyeh* 1373-74, vol. 1, p. 237 (no. 45, 17 Safar 1268/12 December, 1851).

177. Neligan 1926, part III, p. 742; Government of France 1914, p. 40.

178. Baladiyyeh-ye Tehran 1310, pp. 78-79; Soltani 1370, vol. 1, pp. 535-36.

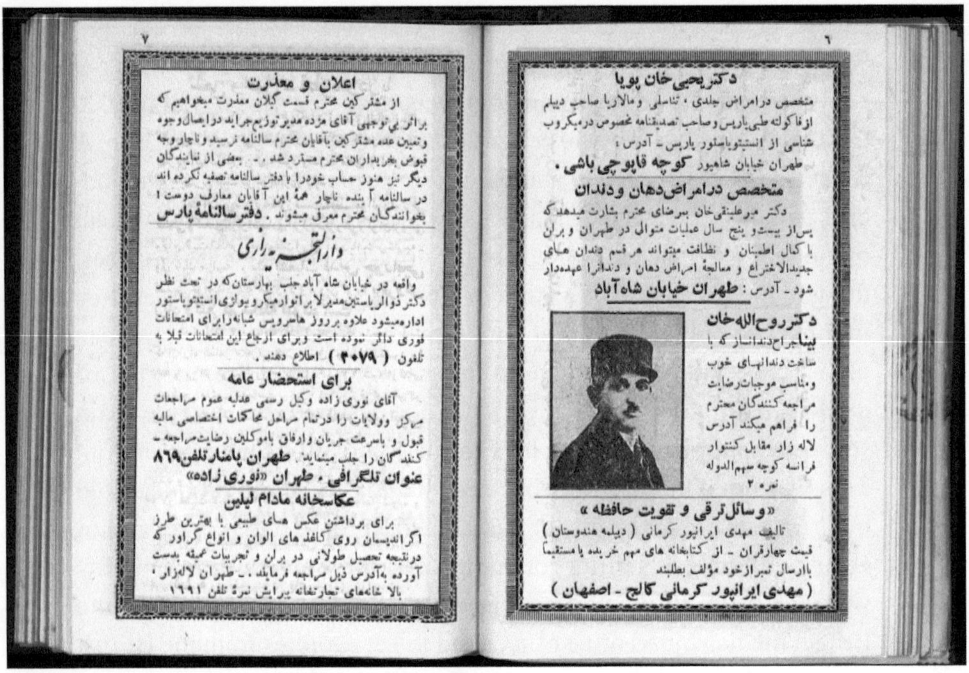

Ad for Dr. Yahya Khan Puya, dentist, 1936

Majles had announced the intention to regulate pharmacies.[179] To deal with this unsatisfactory situation, in October 1919, the government issued a rule regulating the business of the sale of drugs (*`attari*). Only those who had been licensed by the Ministry of Public Education were allowed to engage in this business. To qualify for a license, you had to (i) have a diploma in pharmacology issued by a university in Europe or by the Dar ol-Fonun, or (ii) have worked for at least five years in a recognized pharmacy shop, or (iii) pass an examination of practical pharmacology. Only those who held European university diplomas were allowed to be chemists in Tehran. Outside the capital the examinations were still applied.[180] These exams indeed took place. In 1924, Dr. Frame of the American Missionary Hospital in Rasht

179. *Tarbiyat*, vol. 3, p. 2266.

180. Gilmour 1924, pp. 36-38 (with the text of the law); Rahnama 1333, vol. 1, p. 81.

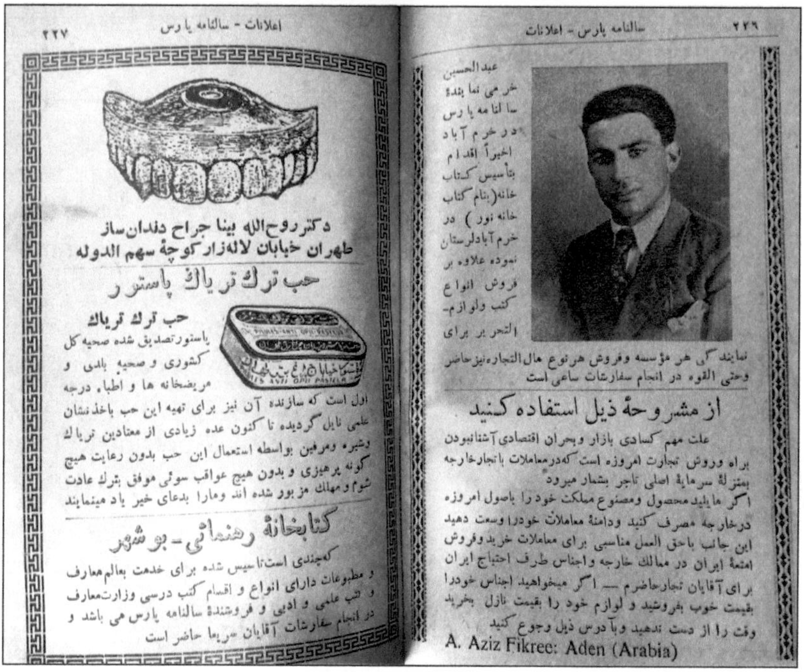

Ad for Dr. Ruhollah Bina, orthodontist, 1936

was asked to become a member of the Pharmaceutical Examining Board and a Public Health Advisory Committee of the Municipality.[181] However, the application of the law outside Tehran was incidental. The traditional pharmacists like traditional doctors severely criticized such actions, but the government refused to give in.[182]

To address this lack of success, the government issued a new order on 13 Khordad 1306/4 June 1927 that those pharmacists who had worked as such for more than 5 years were given the opportunity to pass an exam, and if they passed, the Ministry would give them a license to practice. In June 1927, a law was passed that pharmacists with 5 years of experience were allowed to take an exam to obtain a permit. Within the context of the application of the law licensing physicians of 10 Mordad 1309/1 August 1930, after that date requests for exams by

181. RG 91-19-9, Resht Medical Report 1924-25 [img0973-82]
182. Sadeq 1340, vol. 1, pp. 202-03.

pharmacists and dentists and midwives were disallowed. Candidates had to get training at the relevant schools. However, according to the law of 20 Tir 1310/12 July 1921 and the regulations concerning examinations of dentists and pharmacists it was allowed that those with five years of consecutive experience in these professions were allowed to take the exam and had time to submit their candidature until Mehr 1311/23 September 1932. However, the examination commission only convened in Tehran and thus, applicants from outside the city had to incur travel and lodging cost. The examination committee had to consist of three licensed pharmacists and two licensed physicians. The exam covered the following subjects: general chemistry, organic chemistry, general physics, botany, zoology, pharmacology, public health, writing and filling prescriptions (*noskheh-khvani* and *noskheh-pichi*).[183]

This "modernization' of a branch of the medical infrastructure that traditionally also dispensed medical advice in addition to medicines meant that slowly, but certainly this aspect of their work was brought to an end. The increased use of chemical instead of herbal medicines also reduced the role of the traditional herbalists (*`attar*), while promoting that of the modern chemist shops.[184]

THE SCHOOL OF DENTISTRY

Until recent times, the barber (*salmani*, *dallak*) enjoyed the monopoly of dentistry. He used no anesthetics, and the pulling of teeth was done with the simplest tools such as forceps and pincers (*kalbateyn*; *gazon-bor*).[185] There were no modern dentists in Persia until Naser al-Din Shah brought a dentist back from Europe, whom he employed as the royal dentist.[186] Most members of the elite initially did not make use

183. Rahnama 1333, vol. 1, pp. 81-82.

184. Good 1981, p. 73. Of course, just like elsewhere in the world, traditional or alternative drugs and medicines remain used and even popular, also in Iran. See, e.g., Jozani 1994.

185. Floor 20074, pp. 154-55.

186. `Eyn al-Saltaneh 1376, vol. 1, p. 904; vol. 2, p. 1323; E`temad

of this European dentist, according to Mostowfi.[187] Nevertheless, by the end of the Qajar period, in addition to the royal dentist (then Dr. Stamp), there were some locally trained dentists in Tehran, who only had to pass a simple examination.[188]

In 1906, the newspaper *Tarbiyat* published a number of articles on the importance of dentistry and dental hygiene.[189] *Majles* deputies deemed the subject of sufficient importance to include dentistry in the physicians' licensing law of 1911. This law considered dentists to be physicians, who needed a diploma and a license to practice from the Ministry of Education for which request a time of one year was given (see above).[190] In 1922, Dr. Stamp, the long-time sole European dentist in Persia wrote an article in which he lamented the sorry state of dental health and of the dentist profession in Persia.[191]

The situation in Mashhad, where the Presbyterians had established a modern hospital, was rather typical for the rest of the country. In 1929, there was no dentist in Mashhad and not only the local population, but also the US missionary phycisians needed dental care.[192] Therefore, at the hospital many dental extractions were done. The

---

al-Saltaneh 1345, pp. 109 (M. Le Mormuz [?], *yakanchi-bashi*), 200, 237, 548, 600, 614, 618, 757, 998; Wishard 1908, p. 266 ("For many years, M. Hybennet, dentist to the Court, was the only one in Tehran"); E`temad al-Saltaneh 1345, p. 26 (*chahar-shanbeh* 28).

187. Mostowfi 1343, vol. 1, p. 529; E`temad al-Saltaneh 1345, pp. 84, 663.

188. Neligan 1926, part III, p. 742; Wishard 1908, p. 266.

189. "Mohsenat-e dandan az asli va `ariyeh," in the newspaper *Tarbiyat* 1377, vol. 3, pp. 2058-59 (year 6, no. 693, 15 Dhu'l-Qa`deh, 1323/11 January, 1906), see also "Ahammiyat-e kar-e dandan va dandansazi," Idem, vol. 3, pp. 2145-46 (year 6, no. 404, 12 Jomadi I, 1324/5 July, 1906).

190. Government of Iran n.d. B, pp. 393-96 (Persian text of the *Qanun-e Tebabat* dated 3 Jomadi II 1329/11 June, 1911). For the French text, see Gilmour 1924, pp. 34-36.

191. Stamp 1922.

192. RG 91-20-2, Mashhad Medical Report 1928-1929. "One of our Persian Christians has set up a dental shop in Nishapur." RG 231-1-2, Hoffman to parents, 25/07/1920.

traditional method was to ask a barber to do so, who used forceps. Patients told the American doctors that, "I didn't know it would be so easy; the barbers hurt us so much, we prefer the toothache." The Iranian assistants to the American physicians had been trained in doing simple extractions. Armenian nurses helped them operating.[193] The Christian hospital not only was engaged in dentistry, because the barbers were so bad at it, but also because bad teeth were a leading cause of morbidity. As a result, by 1936, dental extraction was by far their most common operation; sometimes they did >100/month. Those patients who had been able to afford a modern dentist, were not always treated well either. Dr. Hoffman observed that: "The dentists still love to put on gold caps, which are popular but often conceal masses of putrefaction."[194] The example of the missionary hospitals was adopted by other hospitals. For example, in some of the larger hospitals of the Trans-Iranian Railway there was a fully equipped dentistry unit.[195]

To address this situation of bad dentists and dentistry, the law of 1309/1930 gave those practicing dentistry no choice; they had to have completed their studies at the national school of dentistry to be allowed to practice. According to the law of 20 *Tir* 1310 (12/07/1931) and its regulations of 23 *Shahrivar* 1310 (15/09/1931), dentists who had practiced for at least five consecutive years were allowed to take an exam until 15 *Mehr* 1311 (07/10/1932), which only could be done in Tehran. The examination board consisted of four certified dentists and one physician. The exam had to be taken in the following subjects (both theory and practice): general anatomy of head and neck, special

---

193. RG 231-1-6, Hoffman, Pioneering in Meshed, pp. 78-80.

194. RG 91-20-2, Mashhad Medical Report 1935-1936; IOR/L/PS/10/209, Meshed Consular Diary no. 7 for the week ending the 17th February, p. 1 (The Rev. Esselstyn told the British Consul-General that it was possible an American dentist would establish himself in Mashhad).

195. Government of Iran 1317, p. 144. Some private hospitals, such as the *Mo`tamed* in Tehran, also offered dentistry services. *Salnameh-ye Pars* 1311. Large military hospitals also had a dentistry service, certainly as of the 1940s. Ettela`at 1329, p. 116.

anatomy of the teeth, diseases of the teeth, general and special therapy concerning the teeth, the drawing and filling of the teeth and diseases of the mouth. The practical part included the making of teeth from rubber and gold.[196]

Although dentistry was taught at the Dar ol-Fonun by Dr. Stamp, who came to Iran in 1912/13 as dentist to the Shah,[197] as yet, there did not exist a school of dentistry in Iran. In the summer of 1928, the *Madraseh-ye `ali-e tebb* was required to include courses on mouth and dental diseases in its curriculum.[198] On 12 Dey 1308/3 December 1929, a law was approved hiring Dr. Melczarski, a Polish dentist, to head the newly established dentistry department of the *madraseh-ye `ali-ye tebb*. By law of 23 September 1932/1 *Mehr* 1311 he was hired for three years. In 1930, a school of dentistry (*Madraseh-ye `ali-e dandan-pezeshki*) was attached to the medical college, offering a five-year diploma course; the first class included fifteen candidates. Dr. Melczarski was the first director and Dr. Mohsen Sayyaḥ his deputy. In October 1934, Dr. Sayyah succeeded him.[199] In the late 1950s, as a result of the establishment of the dental faculty, there were 1,050 dentists in Iran.[200]

---

196. Rahnama 1333, vol. 1, p. 83.

197. Elgood 1951, p. 537. In 1910, an Austrian dentist, trained in the USA, named Röhrlich or Roelich worked in Tehran. In March 1913, Dr. Stamp sent him to Mashhad, whence, in 1918, he was deported to India. IOR/L/PS/10/209, Meshed Consular the week ending 5th March 1913; IOR/L/PS/10/613, Telegram No. 166-C., dated the 20th August 1918. Consul-General, Meshed, to-The Foreign Secretary to the Government of India, Simla, Persian correspondence. (1917-18); IOR/L/PS/10/210, Meshed Diary no. 11, for the week ending March 13, 1915, p. 1.

198. Ardakani 1368, vol. 1, p. 262.

199. Rahnama 1333, vol. 1, p. 83. In 1921, Dr. Mohsen Sayyah, apparently the first fully qualified Persian dentist, returned to the country and, together with a Dr. Stepanian, trained in the United States, was licensed by the Ministry of Education to initiate classes to train dental technicians. Together these men laid the foundations of scientific dental education in Persia. Sajjadi 1994.

200. US Army 1963 p. 153.

OTHER OPPORTUNITIES FOR MODERN MEDICAL TRAINING

PRIVATE MODERN IRANIAN PHYSICIANS

The drop in the number of medical students at the Dar ol-Fonun was not an indication that there was less interest in the study of medicine. One of the reasons was the bad reputation that this school had acquired over the decades, while another was the availability of alternative possibilities to get training as a physician. In addition to the Dar ol-Fonun, a few Iranian physicians educated in Western medicine provided training in their private practice. This option for medical training followed the traditional model, i.e. on-the-job training as an assistant to a practicing physician. Nothing is known about what kind of teaching was given, how long the training lasted and whether there was any kind of formal examination, which seems unlikely. Among the physicians who offered such training the most important were:

> (i) Mirza Zeyn al-`Abedin Mo'tamen al-Atteba, who had been trained by Dr. Schlimmer and Dr. Tholozan. After having worked as a physician for the governor of Kermanshah he became one of the shah's physicians. After Tholozan's death he replaced him and in his private practice, which was mainly surgical in nature, he trained students until his death in 1908. His students mainly worked thereafter as surgeons in Tehran's hospitals that were established later.[201]
>
> (ii) Dr. Abu'l-Hasan Khan Bahrami (1844-1912) began his studies at the Dar ol-Fonun in 1863 under Mirza Reza Doktor and graduated in 1873/74. From 1874 to 1880 he taught therapeutics at the Dar ol-Fonun. In 1884 he went to Paris, where he studied medicine. In 1886 he returned and replaced Dr. Mohammad Kofri as director of the State Hospital. When in 1894, Dr. Luf [Loew?] took over as director of that hospital, Dr. Bahrami established a medical teaching school, where

201. Rahnama 1333, vol. 1, pp. 37, 49, 54-55.

he trained students such as Dr. Bozorgmehr, Dr. Mozayyan, Dr. Nejat Bina and Dr. Sarraj, who all became well-known physicians. He published a number of teaching books about anatomy, physiology, pathology, therapeutic and hygiene.[202]

(iii) Mirza `Ali Akbar Khan Nafisi Nazem al-Atteba. In the 1890s he had a private practice where he trained students, for whom he wrote study books, among other things a book on anatomy (1887) and *Pezeshki-nameh* (1889), which were used at the Dar ol-Fonun. As of 1909 he focused exclusively on his practice and his students until his death in 1924.[203]

American Medical Schools

The only other opportunity to study and practice modern medicine in Iran was at a small number of American missionary hospitals, in particular the one at Urumiyeh. Originally, teaching modern medicine and training young Iranians in this field had not been part of the missionaries' objectives. However, as one-man or one-woman missionary hospitals the demand and pressure on their time was such that these missionary doctors had to train staff to function better. For example, in Kermanshah, after Dr. Packhard's departure, Dr. Bussdicker was working alone and he found the workload overwhelming. He had to be administrator, surgeon, physician, intern, lab and X-ray technician, instructor for nurses, treasurer and accountant. The US nurse was not only instructor and nursing supervisor, but also anesthesist, floor nurse, and supply nurse. In short, everybody was overworked.[204] The oldest hospital, in Urumiyeh, was the first that started training Iranian students and soon established a formal medical school, where graduating students had to pass the same exam as aspiring physicians in

202. Elgood 1951, p. 502; Rahnama 1333, vol. 1, p. 55.

203. Rahnama 1333, vol. 1, pp. 56-57. Mira Sa`id Hoseyn Khan Nezam al-Hokama also trained students in his practice. Rahnama 1333, vol. 1, pp. 45, 57-58.

204. RG 91-19-28, Annual Report Westminster Hospital Kermanshah 1944-45.

the USA. What was also different in the missionary medical schools, which themselves also employed female teachers, was that women were accepted as students, who actually graduated as physicians.

URUMIYEH

In the fall of 1876, Dr. Holmes began a medical class of eight young men. Only one of them was Moslem, "whose family lives 150 miles away, he came to get a medical education." One year later the class had only seven students.[205] In 1883, a class of eight students, first taught by Dr. Holmes and then by Dr. Cochran, finished their medical course as prescribed by the best medical institutions in the USA and passed their exam before a panel of Moslem, Armenian, and Nestorian representatives.[206] In 1885, two medical students were being trained. Apart from medical studies they also had to study English with Ms Emma Cochran, who also helped them understand the English text books. After one year, the students were able to assist in the dispensary.[207] In 1896, Dr. Cochran, in addition to his regular medical duties, gave two lessons for students each day.[208]

Because he worked alone as of 1885, and, therefore, needed more medical staff, Dr. Cochran, formalizing Dr. Holmes' training method, established a medical training school, a first for Iran. To that end he built a wooden building, which contained lecture rooms and a laboratory. This building still exists. Although he had to train the Iranian physicians himself, Dr. Cochran's clinical and teaching task was eased when Dr. Emma Müller arrived in 1892. General courses consisted

205. Presbyterian Church 1876, p. 42; Idem 1877, p. 42. Ms Cochran's "knowledge of medicine, her thorough acquaintance with people, were humanly speaking all that saved Mr. S[tocking] from being buried by the side of his wife." Wells 1878, p. 26.

206. Presbyterian Church 1883, pp. 62-63 (One year later, Mirza Shimoil received a certificate that was equal to a MD degree. Another of Holmes' former students had become regimental surgeon in the Iranian army). Presbyterian Church 1884, p. 66.

207. Presbyterian Church 1886, p. 82.

208. Presbyterian Church 1897, p. 163.

in English, Persian, medical law and ethics. Basic medical sciences covered were physiology, anatomy, biochemistry and physics, and clinical sciences were pathology, contagious diseases and gynecology, while students also had to be knowledgeable about pharmacology. Students were required to attend the medical college for 9-10 months per year. However, the college was open around the clock. Students would study several hours each day and spend the rest of their time working in the hospital.[209]

In 1888, a new class of four medical students was started, because the demand for native educated doctors was increasing. Dr. Cochran sent Hakim Oshana to Edinburgh to take supplementary courses, which trip was paid by private individuals there.[210] Hakim Yohannan, another native graduate was sent to his people in Kurdistan.[211] In 1890, there was the graduation of another medical class of three men, who had studied four years. A new class of six medical students was begun in that year.[212] In 1893, seven young men graduated. Of those graduated earlier two were in practice in Urumiyeh, two in other cities, one in Mosul, one in the USA and one was assistant-physician in the American Urumiyeh hospital. A class of six medical students was expected to graduate next summer. Besides studying, they assisted in the drug room, in operations and dressing wounds.[213] In 1894, five men completed their four years' of course study in June and after examination received diplomas. They all started a private practice. A new group of eight medical students began.[214] In 1896, there was a medical class of five Nestorians; in the fall a Moslem student joined.[215] In 1901, there was a medical class of seven students, of which one was a Moslem.[216] The

---

209. Wilson 1896, pp. 74, 259; UNESCO 1343, vol. 2, p. 1449; Presbyterian Church 1920, p. 237.
210. Presbyterian Church 1887, p. 78.
211. Presbyterian Church 1889, p. 82.
212. Presbyterian Church 1891, p. 172.
213. Presbyterian Church 1894, p. 188.
214. Presbyterian Church 1895, p. 156.
215. Presbyterian Church 1897, p. 163.
216. Presbyterian Church 1902, p. 232.

third year class of four closed in June 1903 (one Moslem) - during the summer one was employed by a druggist, the other three practiced in a small way in Urumiyeh's environs.[217] In 1904, the four-year study of the medical class was ended; four students graduated; one Moslem and three Christians. All of them had a good knowledge of medicine and surgery.[218] When Dr. Cochran died in 1905, a total of 26 medical students had graduated by that time.[219]

In 1911, a new medical class was received, who had quarters in the hospital.[220] Fortunately, at the end of 1911, Dr. Ellis and his wife came, who shared in medical teaching until the completion of their 3-months course; five men received their diploma. All of them went into medical practice in the province, while two took service with the Red Cross.[221] It is of interest to see that the governor of Urumiyeh established a board of health to which practicing doctors had to present their diplomas, thus formalizing the recognition of the quality of the medical school graduates. Likewise, the local Russian physician also accepted the Urumiyeh medical school diplomas.[222] Because of the closure of the hospital in 1918, the difficulty in reopening it, and its final closure in 1934, there was no medical school activity after 1918.

The teaching situation in Hamadan and Tehran was different from that in Urumiyeh, where training was given in both medical theory and practice. The enabling circumstances (local modern schools, large number of graduates) that existed in Urumiyeh were not present in Hamadan and Tehran. Therefore, as Dr. Neligan rightly remarked,

---

217. Presbyterian Church 1904, pp. 255-56.

218. Presbyterian Church 1905, p. 292.

219. Wilson 1896, pp. 74, 259; UNESCO 1343, vol. 2, p. 1449; Presbyterian Church 1920, p. 237. On the training of Iranian physicians see Daniel 1901, pp. 207-209.

220. Presbyterian Church 1912, p. 363.

221. Presbyterian Church 1912, p. 363. In 1913 there were six boarding Assyrian students for the medical school. Presbyterian Church 1914, p. 341; Idem 1917, pp. 306-07.

222. Presbyterian Church 1915, p. 326.

training in the last two hospitals was more of a practical nature with less emphasis on theory.

Hamadan

In 1887, Dr. Alexander was assisted by a Mr. Terrill and Mirza Sa`id, who were his first medical students.[223] One year later Mirza Sa`id and Mirza Ya`qub are mentioned as his students.[224] They did much practical work and often worked full-time in the dispensary. In 1891, much dispensary work was done by Mirza Sa`id and Mirza Ya`qub, the Iranian assistant-doctors trained by Dr. Alexander.[225] Dr. Jessie C. Wilson, who arrived in the fall of 1891, was temporarily in charge of the dispensary. Here she was assisted by Mirza Sa`id and Mirza Ya`qub. The latter two looked after the male patients and Dr. Jessie Wilson after the female ones.[226] Mirza Sa`id, later served as chief physician to the governor of Hamadan.[227] In 1903, two medical students, Mirza Meyer and Mirza Tatevos, took care of the male patients, while Mirza Meyer also did 14 major operations.[228] Dr. Mary Allen was assisted by Dr. Khachatur, an Armenian graduate of the missionary medical school, who had assisted before.[229]

---

223. Presbyterian Church 1888, pp. 91-92. On Mirza Sa`id and his decision to study medicine and Dr. Alexander agreeing to this, see Rasooli and Allen 1958, p. 60.

224. Presbyterian Church 1890, pp. 182-84.

225. Presbyterian Church 1892, p. 198.

226. Presbyterian Church 1893, pp. 164-65. In April 1893, Mirza Sa`id's "period of contract having ended, he wished to terminate his service with the Mission and so tendered his resignation. He had served faithfully for twelve years as language teacher, doctor's assistant, and then physician." Rasooli and Allen 1958, p. 70.

227. Presbyterian Church 1901, p. 242. Mirza Sa`id served `Eyn al-Dowleh for one year as his physician and that of his retinue, see Rasooli and Allen 1958, p. 88.

228. Presbyterian Church 1904, p. 245.

229. Presbyterian Church 1914, pp. 329-30; RG 280-1-10, Report of the Women's Medical Work. Hamadan, July, 1914.

As of 1889, to enable to do his work better as well as to transfer know-how, Dr. Alexander had started a medical class of six students.[230] Dr. Holmes also trained many traditional Jewish merchants in the principles of modern medicine.[231] In the spring of 1896 the Senior medical class of two students graduated.[232] In 1897, the two first medical graduates returned from Tehran and opened dispensaries in Hamadan, which was an indication that there was a growing demand for physicians educated in modern medical science and practice. Mirza Sa`id, who had studied with Dr. Alexander, and later for a short period in the UK, had a full practice. He caught the eye of `Eyn al-Dowleh, who took him to Tehran and was urged to remain there.[233]

After Dr. Alexander had left, it was Dr. Holmes and Dr. Jessie Wilson who did the teaching of medical students.[234] The remaining medical students continued to make good progress.[235] They were an eager bunch of young men. In 1901, Dr. Blanche Wilson wrote that "shortly after my arrival the young doctors who had studied under Dr. Holmes and Dr. Jessie Wilson asked for a special course in diseases and treatment of the eye. I agreed provided they prepared lectures on the subject and deliver them to the class. They did so very well and one of them, Dr. Ossatur offered to give one day in the week for village work. In January 1901, four students began medical study. Dr. Meyer heard the recitation, while Dr. Blanche Wilson gave an exam once a month in each subject studied."[236] In 1906, there were two medical classes – two seniors and four juniors.[237] In May 1909,

230. Presbyterian Church 1890, pp. 182-84 (Dr. and Mrs. Alexander also made visits to Bahar, Kurzara and Soltanabad; his assistant made medical tours in the villages around Hamadan); Presbyterian Church 1891, pp. 161-62.

231. DCR 3189, p. 40.

232. Presbyterian Church 1897, pp. 158-59.

233. Presbyterian Church 1898, p. 182.

234. Presbyterian Church 1898, pp. 181-82.

235. Presbyterian Church 1899, pp. 192.

236. Presbyterian Church 1902, pp. 224, 231.

237. Presbyterian Church 1907, pp. 299, 313.

four students in medicine were given diplomas, having spent six years to complete their studies.[238] In March 1910, two more students graduated.[239] In 1912, two students received instruction, one a young woman whom Dr. Field had as her assistant, the other a young man.[240] "During the first half of the year [i.e. second half of 1913] regular classes were taught, part of the time every day, part of the time every other day, while during dispensary hours some preliminary teaching has been done better to prepare the girl above mentioned [in the dispensary section] to enter the medical school."[241] On 19 June 1914, three students who had been studying during the last 5-6 years graduated, one of which an Armenian woman, probably Anna Hoseph, the first Iranian woman to receive a diploma in medicine and become a physician![242] In 1918, the Medical Class continued as usual, but was reduced to four students, due to the marriage of a young woman.[243] This was perhaps a graduate of the missionaries' Girls' School, who had wanted to study at the medical school, and in 1914 assisted in the dispensary.[244] In 1919, the medical class of four continued their studies until Dr. Funk's departure in 1920, when they all graduated and were given their MD certificate. The government of Iran issued them all a license to practice as physicians.[245]

The people of Hamadan were pleased with the men trained by the American physicians and by 1910, all previous graduates, had become very successful practitioners. Some of them, after having received their diploma, did well in American missionary dispensaries

---

238. Presbyterian Church 1910, p. 327.
239. Presbyterian Church 1909, p. 343.
240. Presbyterian Church 1913, p. 317.
241. RG 280-1-10, Report of the Women's Medical Work. Hamadan, July, 1914.
242. Presbyterian Church 1915, pp. 316-17; Idem 1909, p. 343 (Anna Hoseph was an assistant and student of Dr. Smith).
243. Presbyterian Church 1919, p. 263.
244. Presbyterian Church 1914, pp. 329-30; RG 280-1-10, Report of the Women's Medical Work. Hamadan, July, 1914.
245. Presbyterian Church 1920, p. 313; Idem 1921, p. 332.

and hospitals, and they were making a good name for themselves. All, but 2-3 remained in Hamadan, although the missionaries had hoped they would become nuclei for their work elsewhere. In Hamadan itself, the doctors trained by the American physicians had largely supplanted the local traditional practitioners, and "are attracting patients that normally would have come to us. As a result, the Lily Reid Holt hospital for men had comparatively few in-patients this year."[246]

TEHRAN

In Tehran medical training must have started in 1893, for, in 1895, two students were in their third year of medical study,[247] while, in 1898, a new medical class of three students was started.[248] In 1904, three young men were given their diploma after six years of study. These diplomas were countersigned by several European doctors and by the Minister of Education.[249] In 1905, two students having completed the Hospital Medical Course were granted diplomas.[250] In 1904 a medical class was started and in 1910 the first class graduated. Thereafter, the lack of a male physician put an end to this activity.[251]

The last graduates were Mirza Qavam al-Din, Mirza Mozaffar Khan and Mirza Amir Khan. Their diploma, issued by the American Hospital in December 1909, stated that "they have studied anatomy, physiology, pharmacology, practiced medicine, surgery and the use of antiseptics, ophthalmology and midwifery for six years; they have always been present in the medical and surgical clinic at this hospital." The Ministry of Education issued their license to practice in January 1910, or two weeks later.[252]

---

246. Presbyterian Church 1911, pp. 318; Idem 1912, p. 355.
247. Presbyterian Church 1896, p. 184.
248. Presbyterian Church 1899, pp. 187-88.
249. Presbyterian Church 1905, pp. 274-75.
250. Presbyterian Church 1906, pp. 289-90.
251. RG 91-19-11-1, Historical Sketch of Teheran Medical Work
252. Ebrahimnejad 2014, p. 148.

Medical Study Abroad

Realizing that Iran lacked the institutional capacities and facilities to train physicians, the medical teachers at the Dar ol-Fonun convinced the government of Iran to send a number of the most promising students abroad for study. Under Fath Ali Shah and Mohammad Shah also students had been sent to Europe. However, under Naser al-Din Shah the dispatch of students were so to speak the natural follow-up to their preparatory study in Tehran. Whereas students before Naser al-Din Shah had been mostly sent to the Great Britain, the students of the Dar ol-Fonun went to France for further study, partly for linguistic reasons, and partly, if not mostly, to avoid being categorized either as an Anglophile or a Russophile. However, those sent and sponsored by the government to study medicine were only eight in number or almost 10% of the total number of students sent.

Table 5: Number of students sent to Europe for further study (1811-1911)

Year	Total no. of students	No. of medical students	Country
1811	2	1	England
1815	4	1	England
1845	5	1	France
1859	42	5	France
1911	30	-	France
Total	83	8	-

Source: Azizi and Azizi 2010, p. 356.

In 1858, the following five students, who had been trained by Dr. Polak, were sent to France: Mirza Hoseyn b. Mirza Ahmad Tabib; Mirza Hoseyn b. Mirza Bozorg hakim-bashi, Mirza Reza b. Mirza Moghim Mostowfi; Nosrat `Ali Mirza d. Seyfollah Mirza; and Mirza `Ali Naqi b. Hajj Aqa Esma`il. Tholozan also supported the study program in France, and thus, he helped the careers of some of its graduates, who were sent to France to get a (partial) medical degree, such as Loqman al-Mamalek, Mirza Zeyn al-`Abedin, A`lam al-Dowleh as well as Mo`in al-`Atebba and Khalil Khan Thaqafi; the latter two, both became physicians to Mozaffar al-Din Shah.[253]

In 1873, Naser al-Din Shah decided to stop sending students for study in Europe, because they had become too political and reformist-minded. The government-supported program was only restarted after the establishment of a constitutional government in 1907. In 1911, the *Majles* decided to send 30 students to Europe none of whom studied medicine. This was the last time that government-financed students were sent to Europe for study during the Qajar period. However, the number of students who studied in Europe was much larger than those financed by the government. There were students who went to Europe at their own expense. Between 1805 and 1920 some 1,000 students studied in Europe, of whom 55 pursued a medical degree.[254]

Many of these medical students did not complete their studies and asked the authorities of their University, via the Iranian ambassador in Paris, to be allowed to only take a major and a final exam, skipping the other subjects. While the French government and university authorities granted these requests for political reasons, Dr. Schneider, the physician of the French Legation in Tehran, was concerned about the quality of the diplomas given to these students and thus, the quality of medical knowledge and care in Iran. He expressed his concern not only for professional reasons, but also because his British colleague in Tehran publicly criticized the quality of a French medical diploma, because of the ease of obtaining one.[255]

In 1928, because of a shortage of modern physicians and insufficient capacity and facilities in Tehran to train physicians, the government of Iran again decided to send student abroad to get medical training.

---

253. Rahnama 1333, vol. 1, p. 52-53; Bamdad 1356, vol. 1, pp. 487-89; vol. 3, pp. 282-83.

254. Azizi and Azizi 2010, p. 355, n. 35.

255. Ebrahimnejad 2014, pp. 127-28 (e.g., Mirza Mohammad Khan and Mo`in al-Atebba).

On 1 Khordad 1307/22 May 1928 a law was passed enabling the government to send students abroad to obtain a higher education. A budget of 100,000 *tumans* was allocated for that purpose and until 1312/1933 each year the same amount would be added. Those students who were accepted for training abroad had to commit themselves to serve the government for a period that was double that of their study. The government from its side had to employ the returning students. The number of students sent abroad between 1307/1928 and 1312/1933 amounted to 640. In 1307/1928, 20 medical students went to France and two to Great Britain. In 1308/1929, 21 students were sent to France for medical study. Thus, in total more than 125 medical students were sent abroad for training. After their return, some worked in the *Madraseh-ye Tebb* as teachers.[256]

Table 6: Number of medical students abroad and their destinations 1307-12/1928-1933

Year	France	UK	Switzerland	Germany	USA	Belgium
1307	20	2	-	-	-	-
1308	21	1	1	1	-	1
1309	18	1	-	1	-	1
1310	16	1	-	1	-	-
1311	15	1	-	1	-	-
1312	17	1	-	-	1	-

Source: Rahnama 1333, vol. 1, p. 73 (which also gives the names of all students)

In addition, there were students who at their own expense received medical education abroad. They either, like their government-sponsored colleagues, went to Europe, or went to nearby Beirut to study at the renowned American University of Beirut, which had a medical school. In 1866, the Syrian Protestant College (later known as the American

256. Rahnama 1333, vol. 1, p. 72-73.

University of Beirut or AUB) established a school of medicine in Lebanon. In 1902, it expanded its scope by building a 200-bed hospital, which had wards for gynecology, obstetrics, and children's diseases. In 1905, the School of Nursing – the first of its kind in the Middle East – was founded. In short, the AUB medical school, which had schools of medicine, dentistry and pharmacy, had excellent practical training facilities as well. It trained physicians, and later also nurses and midwives, from all over the Middle East, including Iran.[257]

DISCUSSION

The Dar ol-Fonun did not produce physicians, but at best practical nurses or *behyars*. Therefore, it cannot be called a medical school before 1928, when a rigorous curriculum and a work program that was more oriented toward practical medicine was established. The Urumiyeh American hospital school was the real first real medical school in Iran, which, as of 1885, produced competent physicians, who not only had thorough theoretical knowledge, but also practical experience in hospital and dispensary care as well as in performing operations. The American missionary hospitals in Hamadan and Tehran also produced well-trained doctors, who, perhaps were less grounded in the theoretical aspects of medicine than their counterparts from the Urumiyeh medical school.

Therefore, the Tholozan and/or French influence on the introduction of Western medical science into Iran is much exaggerated. Most of the teachers at the Dar ol-Fonun were not French. Rather than French physicians, this French orientation was due to the fact that, because of political reasons, Iranian students avoided studying in Great Britain and Russia, and thus mostly went to France. Moreover, French was at that time the common language for foreigners in Tehran and at the Dar ol-Fonun. The result was that French language primacy effectively limited access of the Iranian intelligentsia to other language sources of information, because even translations into Persian were mostly from French. But this did not mean that French physicians played a

---

257. Dodge 1958.

major role in the medical field. In fact, in my view, other teachers at the Dar ol-Fonun such as Dr. Polak and Dr. Schlimmer did more to introduce Western medicine into Iran than Dr. Tholozan, because they wrote more influential and a much larger number of medical texts in Persian than Tholozan, whose scientific output was mainly aimed at the medical community in Europe. Moreover, during Tholozan's lifetime, the number of British and American physicians far outstripped the one or two French physicians in Iran. Also, the British and American physicians worked all over Iran (and in greater numbers), which the French did not.[258] It was only after the establishment of a medical faculty at the University of Tehran that with the help of a few foreign as well as many foreign-trained Iranian physicians that the second real medical school of Iran began. Its example was soon repeated in other cities such as Shiraz that received their own medical school.[259]

Many of the students, certainly those who had been sponsored by the government, worked at the medical faculty of the Tehran University after their return from study abroad.[260] However, it would appear that the medical school of the American University of Beirut was the school of choice for most Iranians wishing to study medicine. In 1933, it was reported that "there are about 300 Persian doctors engaged in Practice in Teheran. Of these about 10 hold European diplomas, 80 are graduates of the University of Beirut (Syria) and the rest are locally trained."[261] Although it would seem that the number of physicians trained in Europe may have been underreported,[262] nevertheless the role of Beirut graduates is rather significant. This seems to be an important subject for another book or article by an interested student of modern medicine in Iran.

---

258. Ebrahimnejad 1998, p. 66; Floor 2012; Idem 2018.
259. Azizi ed. 2014, pp. 231-38.
260. Rahnama 1333, vol. 1, pp. 73-74.
261. Garrison 1933. These data may have been made available to him by Dr. Cyril Elgood, who was physician to the British legation at Tehran from 1925 to 1931 he, as Garrison reports that he was indebted to him for information.
262. See, e. g. *Salnameh-ye Pars* 1308, part 7, pp. 7-9.

However, the new institutional arrangements did not address the immediate needs of the bulk of the Iranian population. Despite the laws to have traditional physicians become licensed, despite the training at the *Madrasheh-ye `Ali-ye Tebb* and later the *Daneshkadeh-e Tebb* as well as the students sent abroad, most Iranians still had no access to modern medical services. For example, to address this issue in Fars, as a result of the agreement between the leaders of the 1945 tribal uprising and the government, a Village Doctors School (*Amuzeshgah-e `Ali-ye Behdari*) was established in Shiraz in October 1945.[263] In Mashad, "There is also a 'medical school' for 'physicians' assistants,' which trains young men as doctor's assistants or village doctors to meet great demand. However, "instruction is given only by busy physicians in private and hospital practice, and it has to depend on the class rooms and laboratories of one of the city high schools, and on odds and ends of rooms in the Shah Reza hospital, for its housing." In 1946, this school acquired its own building so as to house its class rooms.[264] This shows that despite government efforts to increase the number of physicians there were large segments of society that still did not receive appropriate and effective medical care. Also, that there was a great demand for better medical care. This problem remained a headache for subsequent governments, although significant progress was made in the decades thereafter.

---

263. Ghorban 1989, pp. 13-17; Farahmandfar 1384, pp. 118 (with the text of the agreement). On the tribal uprising, see Floor 2016, p. 462.

264. RG 91-20-2, Mashad Medical Report 1944-45; Idem, Mashad Medical Report 1945-1946; Government of Great Britain 1945, p. 411 ("a medical college attached to the Mashhad hospital trains dressers and assistants for work in village dispensaries. All too often hospitals lack men capable of using their equipment.")

Appendix

Sir R. Hoare to Sir John Simon, Tehran, November 13, 1934

Sir,

The following curious story has just come to my notice: it may possibly be a symptom of the dissatisfaction which must exist somewhere in Persia, and may even presage more serious disorders to come. I therefore have the honour to bring it to your notice.

For some time past the students at the school of medicine, which is supervised by the Ministry of Public Instruction and is directed by a Persian doctor named Dr. Bakhtiar, have been inclined to show their dissatisfaction at the teaching and methods of their director. Dr. Bakhtiar, an uncouth but energetic man, has worked himself up by prodigious efforts from a very humble origin, and has been through a full medical education in America ; he holds strong views on the desirability of hard work and thorough training.

3. The usual course of medical training at the Persian School of Medicine has hitherto lasted five years. Dr. Bakhtiar holds the opinion that an extra year is necessary. Without submitting his proposal to either the students of the faculty of medicine, he, by direct but irregular methods, succeeded in obtaining the consent of the "Shora" (the High Council of Public Instruction) to his proposal for the sixth year, this meant that those students who were just completing their fifth year, and were looking forward to earning money through regular practice, suddenly found that they were obliged to support themselves for another year.

4. The dissatisfaction came to a head about ten days ago. Pickets had been placed outside the medical school with a view to stopping the students from attending any classes therein. Dr. Bakhtiar, after consulting with the Inspector-General of the Ministry of Public Instruction, sent for the police and instructed them to put the picketers in prison. The police carried out these instructions.

5. A crowd of students then besieged the Ministry and the Acting Minister. Mirza Ali Asghar Khan Hikmat, came out and delivered a speech on the steps of the building of the Ministry. The inspector-general was dismissed, the five years' course was reinstated, the prisoners were released, and Dr. Bakhtiar's classes were, it is believed, discontinued. The students, having taken the opportunity of smashing the windscreen of Dr. Bakhtiar's car and taking off all four wheels and throwing them in the gutter, dispersed.

6. Hikmat, incidentally, made another change. Dr. Blair, of the American Mission Hospital, had been giving anatomy lectures—another of the innovations of Dr. Bakhtiar. The lectures were not very successful, in the absence of corpses; the size of the class, which numbered 200, was also an obstacle to proper teaching. Hikmat announced that the classes were to be discontinued. The fear that the clergy of Tehran, whose dislike of such irreligious activities as surgery is intense though at present inarticulate, might cause trouble is said to have been one reason for Hikmat's decision in this matter. The result of this shrewd stroke is that Hikmat's position is a little stronger, the students are satisfied with less to do, Dr. Blair is relieved of an irksome duty, and the present batch of young Persian doctors will know nothing about anatomy.

7. The students have now returned to their studies. Some think that the ringleaders will eventually learn that the authorities will have the means of getting their own back by dealing with the recalcitrants singly, when the effect of their victory has evaporated. As I write, I also hear that there is no real intention to rescind the decision to have a six years' course instead of five. What ever the truth of this odd affair is, it is certain that young Persia has, at last, shown a certain tendency to rebel against arbitrary imprisonment.

I have, &c.

R. H. Hoare

Source: IOR/L/PS/12/3481, Foreign medical practitioners in Persia.'

11

THE BEGINNING OF IRAN'S NURSING SCHOOLS

The profession of nurses, let alone female ones, did not exist in Iran. The American missionary hospitals, which needed them, had no choice but to create the profession by starting their own nurses' training schools. Later, these stood as model for the short-lived government attempt to begin nurses' training schools (1936–40) and schools later established by other hospitals. Thereafter, the missionary hospitals continued training nurses, which were often lured away by better pay in other public or private medical institutions. When the missionary hospitals closed in the 1960s, the existence of the nursing profession and standards for training and performance was one of their important achievements and contributions to Iran.

Introduction

Treatment of patients in a modern hospital requires having a trained nursing staff. Although the *Dar al-Shafa* or the hospice of the Imam Reza shrine in Mashhad employed both male and female orderlies or *bimardaran* in the Safavid period, they were not professional nurses as Sureshjani posits.[1] They, like their forerunners in the Roman Empire, in medieval Europe, or medieval Tabriz, were servants or caretakers (*khadem* or *qayyem*), i.e. they had neither training in medical subjects nor were they subject to certain standards of know-how and performance. In fact, the kind of care they provided was probably less than

1. Sureshjani 1395, p. 81. This also holds for the servant (*khadem*), and orderly (*sa`i*) employed in the *Dar al-Shafa-ye Mozaffariyeh* in Astarabad in 1515, see Setudeh 1366, vol. 8, pp. 184-86.

that given by family members at home. The difference was that the caretakers did so within a structured pre-modern medical institutional environment. Modern professional nursing was begun by practitioners such as Florence Nightingale and Clara Barton. They not only insisted that certain rules (such as hygiene) needed to be respected by nurses, but also that they should be trained and educated in the basics of medicine to do a more effective job than a traditional caretaker was able to do. The purpose of this training was to improve the quality of healthcare by ensuring that the nurse was an essential and effective extension of the physician. To that end schools for nurses were established in the UK, USA and elsewhere.

However, nothing of the nature existed in Iran although *bimardaran* were employed in the *dar al-shafa* of Mashhad in the 19th century.[2] This is quite clear from a manuscript written in 1852 that provides a job description of male nurses (*parastaran*) in a proposal for a military hospital in Tehran. The author of the manuscript emphasizes the importance of nurses, because "From the point of view of the public, working at the hospital and nursing patients is quite difficult, because laymen think that all diseases are contagious and believe that whoever works in a hospital falls sick after a short period." However, for patients to have proper treatment there should be one nurse per two or three patients. One group of nurses has to be permanently at the hospital, the other group should be hired from the regiment that sends sick soldiers. Although the author also writes that nurses should be trained, he does not give any further detail about that important subject. He divided the nurses into three categories. The first category consists in the chef and the cook. To the second category belong those who prepare and distribute food and drugs; they also have to take care of ventilation in the room. The third category consists in those who clean the rooms of the hospital, wash clothes and bed sheets. They also need to keep the patients warm by lighting a fire, get them water and help those who cannot move. The task of the chief nurse (*sar parastar*) is to begin the day with prayer, next check whether all nurses are in the kitchen, then finish prayer in the patients' room and

---

2. Sureshjani 1395, pp. 340-41, `Ataradi 1371, vol. 2, pp. 501-02.

with the assistance of the nurses have the patients pray as well. He further had to order the nurses to clean the rooms before the morning and evening visits of the physician and after lunch. He had to be aware which beds are free, when the doctor needs additional beds. He should see to it that all patients have food served, and after lights out in the evening he has to inspect the rooms. Before retiring for the night he should make an inspection and assign night duty to a nurse. Finally, he should be present when the duty nurse is being replaced so that patients are never without a nurse.[3]

Some of the tasks described here also were and are carried out by what I call 'real' nurses, i.e. people trained (to know why what to do and when) and, therefore, an effective extension of the physician in the hospital care of patients. However, the text can also be read that all the listed tasks were not actually happening, which was the reason why the author was so careful to list all tasks to be performed. Also, clearly none of these nurses had received any training and despite the author's stressing the need thereof, he merely mentions that requirement without mentioning anything else on the subject, which is telling. Clearly, it was no wonder, as is clear from what follows, that Western physicians had difficulty finding men or women willing to work in the hospital and being trained to become a nurse. For it was initially only in the American and British missionary hospitals in particular that formal training programs were established to train nurses for use in their own hospital. Because these nurses were lured away by higher offers of pay in other medical institutions or by marriage these same hospitals had to continue training nurses, because there were never enough of them.

The problem of nurses

American missionary physicians pioneered the launching of the training program of female nurses in their hospitals in Iran. The other hospitals, Russian and Persian mostly relied on male orderlies, while

---

3. Ebrahimnezhad 2004, pp. 191-93.

they also had relatives take care of the patients. In short, there was a structural shortage of medical caretakers, let alone nurses, a profession that had not existed in Iran prior to the arrival of the European medical missionaries. American registered nurses also were few in number and the first ones only arrived in the 1910s, and sometimes they were transferred from one hospital to the other. Nevertheless, the untrained medical orderlies needed training and supervision. Therefore, often, the physician's wife worked as matron, such as those of Dr. Funk (Hamadan), Dr. Hoffmann, Dr. Lichtwardt (Mashhad), and Dr. Packard (Kermanshah) who all were registered nurses, or sometimes, even the doctor herself, such as in case of Dr. Mary Smith (Tehran).[4]

From the very beginning of the missionary medical work the availability of trained and competent medical support staff was a problem, one that continued to bedevil the hospitals throughout their existence. When in 1880 the Westminster Hospital of Urumiyeh was built patients were not cared for by trained nurses, but only by their own relatives or hospital servants, all untrained helpers.[5] It was only in 1893 that Dr. Emma Müller started training a nurse in the Urumiyeh hospital.[6] This was as yet neither a formalized nor a continuous activity. How bad the medical caretaker situation was is clear from the situation in 1892, when even school boys had to be used as hospital caretakers to help with the large number of patients during the outbreak of a cholera epidemic in Tehran. During 1897-1905, Dr. Mary Smith was both matron and physician in the Tehran hospital, which was not

4. RG 91-19-27, Medical Work Hamadan 1932; Presbyterian Church 1906, pp. 289-90. In 1901, the CMS hospital employed a Canadian nurse, who transformed its nursing practice. Waterfield 1973, p. 158. In 1910, the CMS hospital in Kerman had two female nurses and continued to employ British female nurses. Administration Report 1910, p. 33-34. The Swedish gendarmerie also had a nurse. On 3 April 1914, Dr. Rönne and his wife, a nurse, arrived from Bushehr in Bandar Abbas on their way to the Gendarmerie in Kerman. Political Diaries vol. 5, p. 470.

5. RG 91-20-7, Last annual report of the Cochran Memorial Hospital, Rezaieh 1934.

6. Presbyterian Church 1894, p. 188.

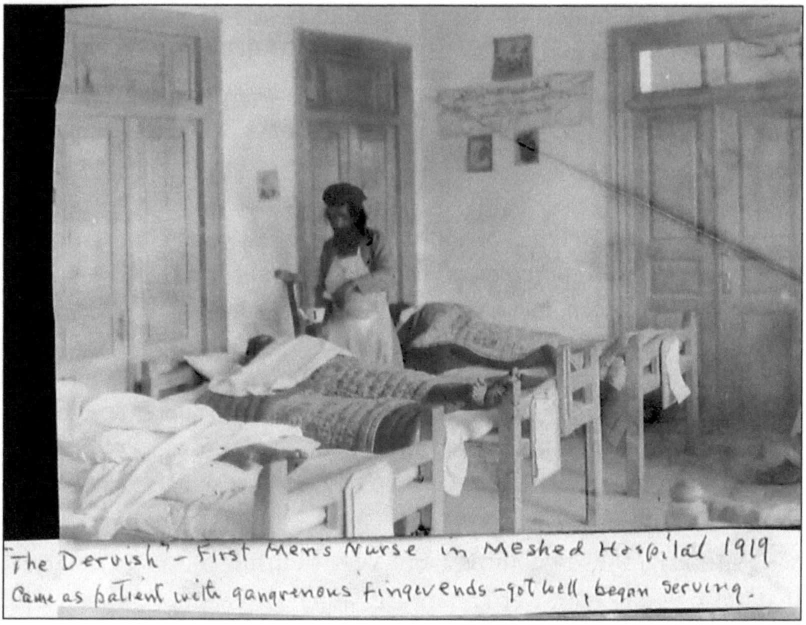

"Darvish," the first male nurse of the Mashhad American Hospital, 1919. He came as a patient, got well and stayed to serve.

an optimal use of her time or qualifications. Therefore, the Tehran mission asked for a matron to free up the physician.[7] In short, the nurses' problem was great, because there were none.

Therefore, certainly in the beginning, medical support staff often consisted in often a few women willing to do this type of work. In 1914, in Hamadan, Dr. Mary Zoeckler hired an older woman who was looking for work, had the right attitude and quickly learned the hospital ways.[8] In 1920, a graduate of the Presbyterian mission school worked as matron nurse, while the assistant matron, a girl of 17, was in charge of house-keeping.[9] Not only was there a lack of caretakers, they often did not stay long. As women, they had less freedom than men, and, if unmarried, they left the profession when they entered matrimony.

---

7. Presbyterian Church 1906, pp. 289-90.
8. Presbyterian Church 1914, pp. 329-30.
9. Presbyterian Church 1921, pp. 332-33.

Each hospital and physician tried to find a local solution. Dr. Cook, who began medical work in Mashhad in 1915, worked with one untrained Iranian assistant.[10] Dr. Hoffman, who took over from him in 1916 received help from some members of the local medical community.

> The 'Chief Doctor,' - Sadr-ol-Atteba, sent a young man who had been his apprentice to be my assistant. Mirza Hajji Agha, about eighteen, had about a ninth grade education, knew some Russian, but no English. [...] Then Dr. Moosa (Moses) Khan sent his nephew, Mirza Morteza, to be my second assistant. Those two worked for a nominal wage, on the apprentice basis. I taught them to take temperatures, give injections, administer chloroform anesthesia, scrub up and assist at operations.[11]

Although these gestures were very helpful, the fact remained that these young men were not professional assistants.[12] In later life, Hoffman summarized the situation during that early period as follows:

> In the early days the mirza or young apprentices gave medicines and did surgical dressings. Then these two were employed as orderlies and several women were found, ex-patients, to work as 'nurses.' One orderly, Yahya had been a 'doctor' in Shahrud. His son served as a mirza, then became a doctor and practiced in Shahrud.[13]

In Rasht, prior to 1918-19, Dr. Frame had no trained nurses for his hospital. During the 1918-19 period, at first, he had to use women as nurses, whose experience had been in the Russian military. These were soon replaced by Armenian girls, who were very efficient, despite a minimum of theoretical training. Some of them continued working in the hospital thereafter.[14] He continued to use local girls for work in

---

10. Presbyterian Church 1917, pp. 301-02.
11. RG 231-1-6, Hoffman, Pioneering in Meshed, p. 36.
12. RG 231-1-6, Hoffman, Pioneering in Meshed, p. 38.
13. RG 231-1-6, Hoffman, Pioneering in Meshed, p. 58.
14. RG 91-19-9, Resht Report Medical Work 1932.

the hospital, but there was no training for nurses. The first informal attempt to do so happened during the fall and winter of 1919-20, when Frame gave his nursing staff three hours/week lessons about various diseases. He also organized monthly social evenings, because he hated to see the staff scatter, because he was leaving on furlough.[15]

In the Tehran hospital, both male and female helpers were employed as of 1890s. During 1917-19, when the hospital was closed for males, the female ward remained open. It was led by Dr. Mary Smith, who intermittently was assisted by an American trained nurse. Both of them taught Iranian helpers through on-the-job training.[16]

The first school of nurses

It is not clear which US hospital pioneered the formal training of nurses, it was either that of Tabriz, Urumiyeh, or Tehran. As in any other hospital in Iran, Urumiyeh, where American physicians had not only built the first hospital built and operated on modern principles of hospital care (1882) in Iran, but also pioneered the first modern medical school (1885) also was in need of trained nurses. Therefore, in 1912 it asked for an American nurse to train the helpers in the hospital.[17] In 1917, there were three young women in training for nurse, both practical and theoretical, but it is not known when they began their training.[18] It is not known either what the early curriculum was, but we may assume that the trainees entered a kind of apprenticeship program that used the student nurses for their labor and trained them to maintain cleanliness, orderliness and close observation of patients. Students received only a limited amount of classroom education in the form of lectures on patient care and related subjects, while being on-the-job,

---

15. RG 91-19-9, Resht Report Medical Work 1919-20.
16. De Warzée 1913, p. 171; Presbyterian Church 1919, p. 259; Idem 1920, p. 310; Griscom 1921, p. 239. Hence there were two dispensaries (male and female) at the same hospital. Presbyterian Church 1921, p. 326.
17. Presbyterian Church 1913, p. 238.
18. Presbyterian Church 1918, p. 291.

as their training advanced, they increasingly carried out most patient care activities offered in the hospital. The result was that in addition to the traditional care taking, increasingly nurses established a clean, orderly work environment that made more complex and invasive surgery possible. With additional training and experience they were also able to carry out more complicated treatments and medication, as is clear from actual hospital practice.

The nursing school was discontinued in 1918, due to the occupation of Urumiyeh by Turkish forces as well as the following massacre of Christians and the expulsion of the American missionaries. Because I have been unable to establish when training began in Urumiyeh it may well be that the honor of starting the nursing school goes indeed to Tabriz, where, in 1915, the formal training of a few nurses started. Subsequently, in 1916 a three-year nursing school was established in Tabriz,[19] whose operation was interrupted by the departure of the American staff for Hamadan in June 1918. In Tehran, the first formal nurse training was begun in 1916, which was continued, with some interruption, until the 1960s. Ms Myra Sutherland was in charge of the nursing and the operating room. She left on 1 April 1916 to get married. Ms Faye Fisher took over some weeks later, being in charge of care for women patients, operating room supplies, sterilizing, etc. for the two last months of the year.[20] Ms Fisher also started a training class for nurses with four graduates (three Armenians, one Moslem). In 1917, Ms Fisher had to leave for health reasons, but she hoped for a new nurse to come to train them.[21] The young nurses, who had begun their training under Ms Fisher, were disappointed that the promised nurse from US did not come. Dr. Smith promised to teach them four days a week and help them in any way she could. They were made responsible for the women patients, the preparation of surgical dressing, sterilizing and getting ready for surgery and the

19. Salsali 1991, p. 190.

20. Presbyterian Church 1917, p. 296.

21. Presbyterian Church 1918, p. 280; RG 91-19-11-1, Historical Sketch of Teheran Medical Work.

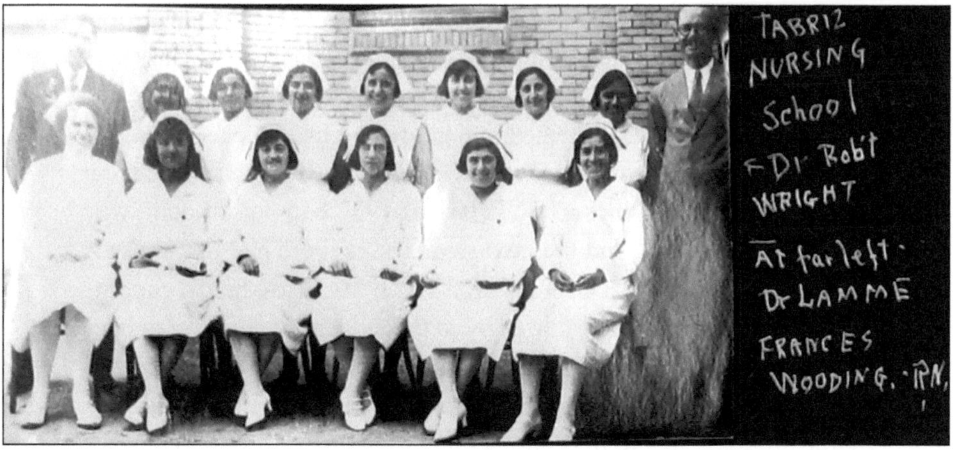

Class of nurses at Tabriz hospital

instruments for operation. Thus, it was not a lost year to them.[22] In 1919, the nurses' training completed its third year and graduated in June, the first in the hospital's history.[23]

Continuation after WW I

Although the medical missionaries were in regular contact with each other the formal training of nurses for the time being remained limited to Urumiyeh, Tabriz and Tehran. In the other US hospitals (Hamadan, Kermanshah, Mashhad, and Rasht) nurses' schools started only in the 1930s.

When the American missionaries returned to Urumiyeh in November 1922 conditions were such that the training of nurses had to be postponed. Ms Pease, an American nurse, who arrived in 1925, would begin a nursing training class as soon as she had mastered Persian.[24] In 1927, the nursing school was re-established and two nurses graduated two years later. The second class began in 1929 and graduated only one nurse. They were taught by Ms Pease, Dr.

22. Presbyterian Church 1919, pp. 259-60.
23. Presbyterian Church 1920, p. 310.
24. RG 91-20-7, Medical Report Urumiyeh 1926.

Ellis, Dr. Cochran and Dr. Müller. The new hospital had a class room that made training of nurses more efficient. In 1930, "Two classes of nurses are in training and a local physician helps in the dispensary and hospital work." In 1931, the hospital graduated its first class of nurses this year and from now on the medical work in Rezaieh should enter a new phase of usefulness." The class of 1932 had one student, who graduated in the fall, and the next two classes there had respectively two and four students. During March 1933, Ms Pease held a capping exercise, i.e. to give an opportunity to the student to synthesize what has been learned in the program. This capping exercise perhaps was the first one in Iran.[25] As in the pre-war situation nursing was done by the students of the first and second years of training. When the number of students was insufficient for the nursing needs of the hospital one or more untrained helpers would be hired.[26] When in 1934, the Cochran Memorial Hospital had to be closed, the nursing school was also closed and a certificate was given to the last class, even though they had not yet finished all work.[27]

In Tabriz, the missionaries already returned in 1919. As of that year, the nurses' training class was under Ms Wells and included three women from the Urumiyeh hospital, who had been in training there prior to the evacuation.[28] In 1920, the first class of nurses graduated; the first in W. Persia.[29] In 1921, Ms Wells continued training nurses, to wit: four Iranian young women (two Armenians, one Assyrian, one Russian-Georgian), while also three Armenian young men were employed to care for male patients.[30] In 1925, another class of nurses graduated from the three years' training course in the Tabriz hospital,

---

25. RG 91-20-7, Cochran Memorial Hospital Report 1933; Presbyterian Church 1932, p. 175; Idem 1933, p. 178.
26. RG 91-20-7, Cochran Memorial Hospital Rezaieh 1932.
27. RG 91-20-7, Last annual report of the Cochran Memorial Hospital, Rezaieh 1934.
28. Presbyterian Church 1920, pp. 331-32; Idem 1921, p. 344.
29. Presbyterian Church 1921, p. 347.
30. Presbyterian Church 1922, pp. 377-78.

and among the new class there were two Moslem girls.[31] In June 1928, three nurses graduated,[32] and the 3-years course in nurses' training that had full grades for each class was continued in the decades thereafter.[33] There was a good reason for that, because graduate nurses from the training school were in increasing demand for private work in the city as well as in the other missions, companies, and private and government hospitals in Iran.[34]

After a brief interruption in the training of nurses in Tehran, nurses training started again. In 1933, in the absence of a US nurse, Ms Haikows Minassian, a graduate from the Tabriz Christian hospital took over. She supervised nurses, did the hospital records and also did nursing.[35] Because in 1934, there still was no US nurse, Ms Hikowe Boghasian, continued as head nurse. There were also two new hires, Ms Hosmik Karapetian, a last year's graduate from Tabriz, and Ms Vartanush Minassian, who, after graduating from Tabriz, worked some time in Mashhad and Kermanshah. She only worked in the Operating Room (OR) and the dispensary. Ms Astqiq Hosepian, the other OR nurse was crippled most of the year by an eye infection. In December 1934 another class of two nurses graduated.[36] In 1935, it was proposed to begin a new training school for nurses, together with the mission's Sage College (a high school), which was important for the Christian Hospital, because in this way it might keep its comparative advantage to the national hospitals. There was a great demand for well-trained head-nurses in many of the new government hospitals that were being opened in the country. Also, there was a growing demand for private nurses. At the same time, there were neither standards for nurses nor what these should be. The government veered toward inadequately

31. Presbyterian Church 1926, p. 222-23.
32. Presbyterian Church 1929, p. 103.
33. Presbyterian Church 1930, p. 194.
34. Presbyterian Church 1932, p. 175.
35. RG 91-19-11-1, Report Teheran Hospital 1933.
36. RG 91-19-11-1. Report Medical Work Teheran 1934. Two nurses married and were replaced by graduates from the Tabriz school. RG 91-19-11-1, Report Tehran Medical Work 1934-1935.

training immature girls, which would result in poor service and low appreciation of nursing, which was an important part of modern medicine. With the establishing of a nursing school the Christian Hospital might have a chance to show the need and value of better training.[37] Although the records provide no information on the Tabriz school's training program, we may assume, given the development of the nursing profession in the USA that it followed the standards laid down by the American Nurses Association or those of the nurses licensing board. This meant more theoretical class room training and less hospital work for the trainees, as is clear from the situation in e.g., Kermanshah (see below).

Ms Fulton arrived in September 1935 to be supervisor of nursing and director of the school of nursing. Mrs. Blair also taught some classes in the nursing school, kept records, and worked in the men's OR and wards. Mrs. McDowell worked in the pediatric clinic and took care of feeding several patients who needed a special diet. The training of nurses was necessary, because, apart from their small number, attrition was high. In 1935-36, three nurses left to marry, a fourth went into private practice, a fifth was incapacitated by eye trouble, and the sixth left for other reasons. Fortunately, the hospital was able to hired six new nurses (two from Tabriz, three from Rasht and one Swiss girl).[38] The start of a class in nursing in 1935 was one of the high spots in that year. It was temporarily discontinued in the absence of a US nurse, but resumed in October 1935, in collaboration with Sage College with two students. However, one left and became a bookkeeper with the Anglo-Iranian Oil Company (AIOC). The capping exercise for the remaining girls was held in June 1936.[39] In 1937, "A new school for nursing with higher professional standards than have been possible before in Iran has had its inception at the mission hospital in Tehran during the year, the students are taking

37. RG 91-19-11-1, Report Tehran Medical Work 1934-1935.

38. RG 91-19-11-1, Medical Report Teheran 1936.

39. RG 91-19-11-1, Medical Report Teheran 1936.

part of their work at the hospital, and some of their scientific courses at [the] Nurbakhsh [high-school]."[40]

Hamadan

The missionaries could not change local social conditions, but they tried to increase the supply of nurses. Therefore, Hamadan, like the other American Missionary hospitals, began training its own nurses to cover the shortfall in that regard. Hamadan began later than the other American hospitals; in fact it was only in 1931 that the first class of nurses graduated. The student-nurses received both regular class room schooling as well as on-the-job training, because they were used in the daily work of the hospital. The training program evolved over time.[41] In 1932, the new class had only two new students and in that year there was no graduation of nurses.[42] In 1933, the hospital had only one graduate Iranian nurse of its own school, three students, but as yet no new recruits.[43] In 1934, Hamadan had only a temp nurse, whose strength and eye difficulties prevented her from full instruction, so Dr. Funk had to give classes as well. There were two graduates in June; the third had been dropped for insubordination. However, no new class was started. In that year, the nursing staff was composed of: one former graduate, one of Hamadan's training school, one from Urumiyeh and one slightly trained nurse from the Adventist hospital in Soltanabad. Because of staff constraints the hospital was unable to give her additional training. Therefore, Dr. Funk hoped for a permanent US nurse.[44] In 1935, the nursing problems were partially resolved with the arrival of Ms Pease (from Urumiyeh), who took over hospital supervision and nursing. Two nurses who graduated from the Hamadan nursing school left, but two graduates from Rasht joined the hospital staff. However, there were no pupils in the fall to start training. Thus,

---

40. Presbyterian Church 1938, p. 48.
41. RG 91-19-27, Hamadan Medical Report 1933.
42. RG 91-19-27, Hamadan Medical Work 1932.
43. RG 91-19-27, Hamadan Medical Report 1933.
44. RG 91-19-27, Hamadan Medical Report 1934.

there was only one graduate nurse since September, when the last of the old students finished their training. Sometimes there were three or four, in May only two; and fortunately Mrs. Lichtwardt was in particularly helpful in supervising the OR.[45] In 1935-36, the nursing staff consisted of Ms Pease as supervisor with four Iranian graduate nurses and Mrs. Lichtwardt assisting in the OR. However, Ms Pease was transferred to Tehran to teach at the Nursing School and Mrs. Lichtwardt substituted for her. One additional male orderly was hired and patients probably had a better type of nursing than ever before. The problem of getting nurses remained a big one as there were only four training schools and they were all in demand not only by mission hospitals but also by government institutions.[46]

KERMANSHAH

In 1932, Ms Fulton R.N.[47] opened a Nurses Training School in Kermanshah. The doctors and their wives, who were R.N.s, helped with the teaching and Ms Gertrude Benz taught English.[48] In that year, the hospital had three trained nurses from Tabriz, and six new trainees. Over a three-year period, the student-nurses received lessons in ethics, practical nursing, personal hygiene, dietetics, bacteriology, materia medica, anatomy, physiology and English; all subjects were taught by the American medical staff. After a six-month probation period, the student-nurses learned nursing skills, both on the job and in theory,

45. RG 91-19-27, Medical Report Hamadan 1935.

46. RG 91-19-27, Healing in the Home of Avicenna 1936.

47. R.N. or registered nurse indicates that the person in question has graduated from a government accredited training program and is licensed to work as a nurse.

48. RG 91-19-28, Kermanshah Westminster Hospital News vol. 1/3 -15/09/1932. ("We have 3 graduate nurses, 2 Armenian one Moslem, all from the Tabriz training school. One is in charge of the second floor, the other two alternating in the operating room and night duty. Also trainees: 4 Christian (3 Assyrian, 1 Armenian) and 2 Moslems. The traines are on the floor above the US nurse; we will have to add later two more rooms. The plan is to have a school of 12 student nurses with classes of four.").

and after three years received their diploma, nurse's cap and a pin.[49] Of the six students who began, four finished training school, one dropped out due to illness, one was let go due to lack of aptitude.[50] Although nursing care improved after the arrival of Ms Margaret Yohannan from Urumiyeh, it still was not feasible to have nurses provide nursing care to male patients without the presence of a supervising nurse. During four months, twice per week nurses were trained in the lab to learn about bacteriology and chemistry.[51] In 1934, the nursing class consisted of four trainees (two Christians, one Jewess, one Kurd). Dr. Jenny Stead came from Faraman to give 3-weeks training in gynecology and held a women's clinic. The entire year there were three nurse graduates, all from Urumiyeh.[52] In 1934-35, the nursing staff suffered from malaria and to avoid further problems all nurses received the typhoid vaccine.[53] The hospital hired two graduate nurses; one of whom was the product of their own training. In the second half of 1934, Ms Fulton was transferred to Tehran to begin nurses training there. This created a problem, because there were five nurses in three classes. Moreover, new students came, so there were then 10 nurse students. To solve the problem created by Ms Fulton's departure, her responsibilities were taken over by Mrs. Packard and Mrs. Bussdicker, both R.N.s. Mrs Packard for 10 years had been the head of the Tabriz nursing training school; to relieve her, Mrs. Bussdicker taught the Packard children, who were home schooled.[54] In June 1938, the nurse

---

49. RG 91-19-28, Kermanshah Westminster Hospital Report 07/03/1933; Arasteh 1970, p. 124. Of course, all these subjects were simplified for the trainees, since they only had elementary education. As the educational level of trainees increased so did the level of training.
50. RG 91-19-28, Kermanshah Westminster Hospital 1933.
51. RG 91-19-28, Kermanshah, Report of Westminster Hospital 1933-1934.
52. RG 91-19-28, Kermanshah, Report of Westminster Hospital 1933-1934.
53. RG 91-19-28, Kermanshah,The Westminster Hospital Annual Report 1934-35.
54. RG 91-19-28, Kermanshah, The Westminster Hospital Annual Report 1934-35 (with photo of the hospital); Idem, Kermanshah Medical

in charge of surgery and the hospital's druggist left, while a graduate nurse left to join Dr. Sarfeh for better wages, while another graduate nurse left to Khorasan. Fortunately, on 17 October 1936, Ms Estelle Chambers RN arrived and on 29 October, Dr. Zoeckler. The work load was heavy often running into the afternoons, and sometimes there were 14 operations in one day, but the work got done.[55]

MASHHAD

In October 1918, Dr. Hoffman had "three assistants, as in former years."[56] In 1919, he carried out operations with only locally trained helpers. Unfortunately, one of these two assistants left to Tehran to study in the "Medical School' there and the other was not in good health. He tried two replacements, but that did not work out, so that they were let go after two weeks.[57] As of 1920, Mrs. Hoffman and Mrs. Lichtwardt, who were both RNs, and Khanom Sharifeh, assisted in the hospital, OR, and dispensary.[58] However, these were married women and, therefore, it was no surprise that in 1921, the nursing problem awaited a solution.[59] Although in 1928-29, the hospital had two Armenian nurses, three US persons of a staff of 30 persons, the physicians felt that their nursing service was still inadequate. A second Armenian graduate nurse from the Tabriz training school was hired, and later, in 1929 when Ms Nelson returned from furlough, plans were made to start the systematic training of the Iranian nurses already employed, both men and women. Daily classes were given by Ms Nelson about patient care. Most teaching was elementary, because the Iranian nurses had little education and some were illiterate. As a result, the standard of nursing improved.[60] In 1929-30, Ms Nelson was helped by two Armenian nurses from the Tabriz hospital; she also

---

Report 1936.

55. RG 91-19-28, Kermanshah Medical Report 1937.
56. RG 231-1-2, Hoffman to Parents, Meshed 02/10/1918.
57. RG 231-1-6, Hoffman, Pioneering in Meshed, pp. 46-49.
58. Presbyterian Church 1921, p. 338.
59. Presbyterian Church 1922, p. 371.
60. RG 91-20-2, Mashad Medical Report 1929.

trained non-graduate Iranian nurses, which was slow-going because most were illiterate. At that time the nursing staff consisted in: two Armenian nurses from the Tabriz hospital; five Iranian married women, some with home responsibilities; four men, two Mirzas, who did not do nursing, but gave out medicines and did dressings on male patients and the US nurse, or 14 persons in total. The Armenians nurses did dressings and gave medicines to the women, so there was no need for the Mirzas to go into the women's wards as was done before. They also assisted in the OR and dispensary and helped oversee ward nursing.

Three months in the fall of 1929, the US nurse had classes in practical nursing for both men and women nurses, but only three out of nine had ever gone to school and were literate. Consequently, instruction was mostly oral and repetition.

> Introducing them to this remarkable machine of the human body of which they knew very little, to its care in health and sickness, the danger of germs, necessary foods, air, water, and hygiene, general cleanliness, and practical nursing of each kind of disease, the idea was to try to get the nurses to put themselves in the place of the patients, to develop quick eyes, and sympathy for each individual patient. Such answers as "we have two livers, a black liver and a white liver," "but we can't give that patient water, he has been operated on and the water will go to the site of the operation," or "she has a hot disease and can't eat that food, or that diet is hot and he has a cold disease", and when a 'rag" (Persian word) meaning a vein, artery, nerve, lymph vessel, to the most of them, and an "azoleh" may mean muscle, sinew, tendon to the uneducated, and how there is much for them to unlearn , and more patience is necessary.[61]

---

61. RG 91-20-2, Mashad Medical Report 1931. This description shows how difficult it was to train candidates, who had little or no education, but at the same time it also show that the US staff did their utmost to make medical subjects comprehensible, so that the trainees had sufficient understanding to be effective nurses and helpers of the physicians.

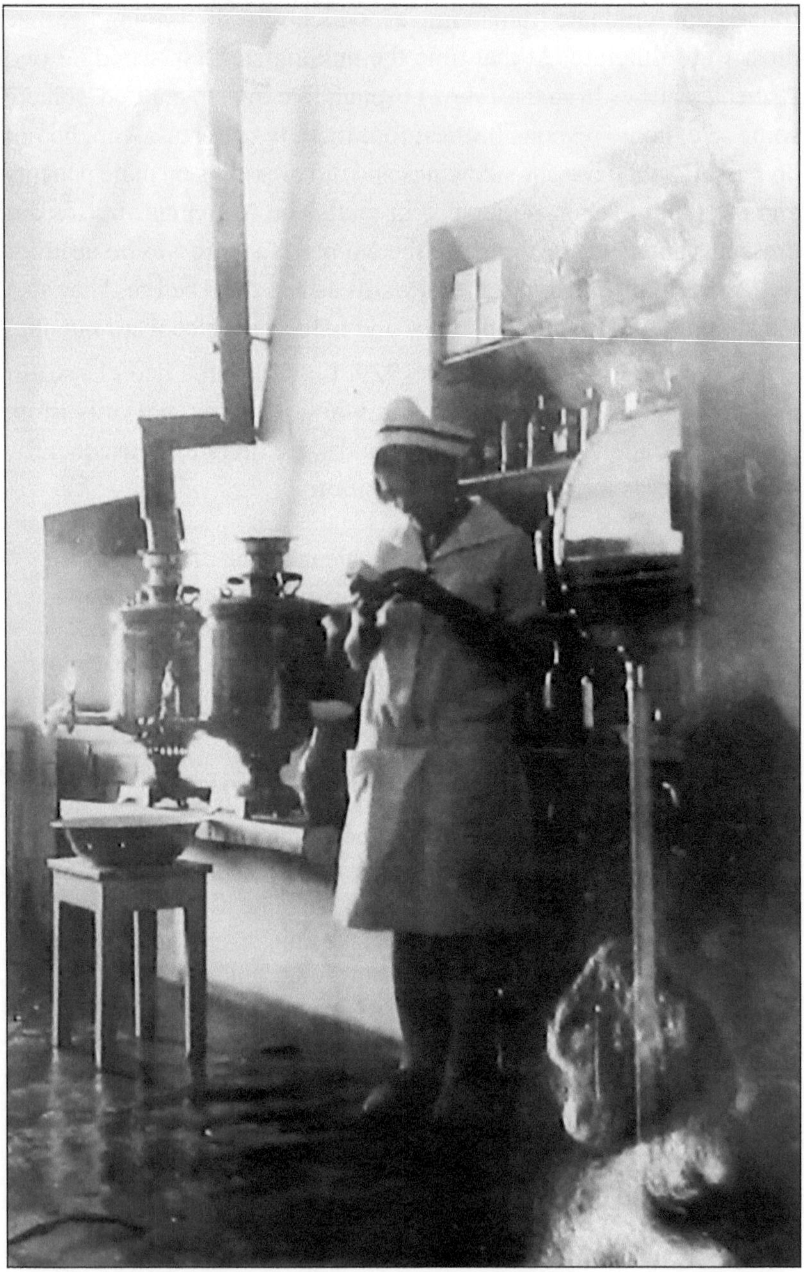

Ms Vartanush, graduate nurse of the Tabriz school of nursing in the sterilizing room of the Mashhad American Hospital, 1930.

In 1929-31, there were three graduate nurses (Ms Mabel F. Nelson; Ms Virginia Sahakian; Ms Vartanush Minassian), besides 25 male and female employees (nurses, orderlies, cooks, doormen, laundresses, a gardener and an engineer).[62] In 1931-32, there was only one nurse.[63] In 1933, nursing improved when Ms Mary Muradian and Mokhtara Khanom were employed, who came from Tehran and refused to wear the veil. For several months instruction was given to three female nurses in the dispensary and OR, but the most dependable died, while another left due to her husband.[64]

Rasht

After his return in September 1921, Dr. Frame's hospital was in great demand. Therefore, Frame stressed the need for a trained nurse to take over the management of the hospital and the nursing staff.[65] When Ms Ellen Dorothy Nicholson RN arrived in 1924 in Rasht, she started organizing the nurses' service efficiently and began training classes for nurses. The objective of training the hospital's own nurses was "not with the idea of developing professional nurses but of meeting our needs and helping as many young women as possible to get a wider knowledge of care of the sick, etc." At first, only Armenian girls would accept to work as a nurse, but in the summer of 1929, when three experienced nurses left because of marriage, for the first time Moslem girls applied to become nurses. Frame hired five nurses, four Moslems and one Armenian, for intensive training before Ms Nicholson left on furlough. He commented that, "The mere fact that these girls can work with unveiled faces for men as well as women patients indicates a great social revolution." As head nurse, in her

62. RG 91-20-2, Mashad Medical Report 1931.

63. RG 91-20-2, Mashad Medical Report 1940-41.

64. RG 91-20-2, Mashad Medical Report 1932-1933. Classes were given in the nurses' home situated in the grounds of the hospital. It was a two-storey building and the class rooms were on the second floor. Khakestar 1395, p. 182.

65. RG91-19-9, Resht Medical Report 1921-22; Idem, Resht Medical Report 1919-20.

absence, he got a graduate nurse from Tabriz, who did not know Persian; as matron an Armenian woman, who, before Ms Nicholson arrived had been matron. As night supervisor, because Moslem girls were not allowed to remain alone, a Russian Protestant woman, who had joined the local church a few years earlier. Frame was unable to give any formal nursing instruction, but he held a staff meeting once week, where he discussed hospital problems and special needs of certain patients and incidentally smoothed some personal matters. The new staff cost more than expected, resulting in an operational loss, while they also were less efficient.[66]

The change in the composition of the nursing group went very fast. In 1931, instead of Armenian nurses there were 6-7 Moslem ones of all classes of society. Given their social background they had little training in personal responsibility or administrative work; no standard education or adequate training in English, while there were no textbooks on nursing in Persian. Therefore, Ms Nicholson not only had to train them in nursing, but also had to supervise their work closely and give them the essentials of a little English. What was of particular interest was that these nurses brought in new patients.[67] In 1932, there was the first formal graduation of nurses with two Moslem girls. In the past decade many nurses had been trained in the hospital, some of whom found work elsewhere after leaving. However, these nurses had not received any routine lessons for any long period of time and were not given 'diplomas'. Also, these nurses had all been Armenians. In 1929, a Moslem girl of high society standing wanted to learn nursing; another Moslem and Armenian girls also came, but the Armenian girl failed to finish the course. Not only was the graduation noteworthy because the two graduates were Moslem girls, but "they appeared

66. RG 91-19-9, Resht Medical Report 1929; Idem, Resht Medical Report 1930. In 1928-29, the hospital had two Iranian Moslem orderlies, one for day and one for night work, three Armenian nurses, and a Turkish boy, who worked half time in surgery and did the sterilization of equipment. RG 91-19-9, Resht Medical Report 1927-1928.On the reluctance of Moslem families to allow their daughters to train as a nurse, see Ta`eb 1384, p. 53.

67. RG 91-19-9, Resht Medical Report 1931.

before a mixed audience with unveiled faces while the health officer of the province made the chief speech and the governor presented the diplomas." One was employed in national hospital, the other as a doctor's assistant in the city.[68]

Although the supply of suitable candidates for nurses was limited selection was strict. One of the nurses who had received her training in Rasht in the mid-1930s, Ms Fatemeh Tavana'i, told that she first had an interview with Ms Nicholson, who told her how difficult the life of a nurse was with nights without sleep, difficult patients, and the supervision of patients, which all required sacrifice on the part of the nurse. She told Ms Tavana'i if she wanted to become a nurse she had to forget about amusements and social life, and that when on the job she had to forget about family and friends and only have thoughts and attention for the patients. Also, nurses always had to be kind, patient and tolerant and realize that they did not belong to themselves, but to the hospital. Ms Nicholson then gave Ms Tavana'i two weeks to think about it, and then decide whether she still wanted to be a nurse.[69]

In July 1932, there was a class of eight nurses, but in October one Armenian nurse left. She was replaced by a Moslem girl. In April 1933, two nurses graduated and four new ones were accepted for the new class. The student-nurses were all young, just having left school and were all serious. Therefore, Frame was pleased that teaching facilities had been improved. At that time, the hospital had 10 nurses: seven Moslem, two Jewish and one Armenian. In that year Frame also arranged for the availability of a sleeping room for the night nurse, which, although far from quiet, was well worth the investment.[70] In the spring of 1934, three nurses graduated. In the summer two of them were employed, until a new class began in the fall. Frame commented that it would be better if the hospital was able to retain these graduates indefinitely, but in a small hospital there was

---

68. RG 91-19-9, Resht Medical Report 1932. The Christian hospital invited representatives of the Ministry of Health and Education to participate in the examination of the nurses. Ta`eb 1384, p. 53.

69. Ta'eb 1384, p. 66.

70. RG 91-19-9, Resht Medical Report 1933.

neither the work nor the money to warrant maintaining a graduate staff, in addition to nurses in training.[71]

In the late fall of 1934, there was a class of four new students. Because of illness and other reasons the number of student-nurses was smaller than usual. The senior class had been depleted by illness, so that only one graduated next fall. Besides the senior nurse, there were four juniors and four freshmen. Only one senior nurse was kept as well as two of graduates of 1933 on a one-year's contract. However, the Hamadan Christian hospital needed nurses so they were released. Ms Nicholson did the major part of the training, but the doctors also gave classes. Also, one of the teachers from the government school taught chemistry.[72] On 6 April 1936, five nurses graduated. The governor of Gilan and director of Health Department held brief speeches in the auditorium of the Girls School. Next year, Frame wanted them to complete their work in the fall, when the new class of students was admitted. For with the current system, he lost his supply of nurses until he had accepted a new class. During this time he contracted for one year two former graduates, but one them left after one month by marrying. Three graduates signed with the Tehran Christian hospital. Two former graduates worked for the Military Hospital in Rasht, the first time that female nurses were accepted there. Its head surgeon would have liked to hire more but none were available.[73]

---

71. RG 91-19-9, Resht Medical Report 1934.

72. RG 91-19-9, Resht Medical Report 1934-35.

73. RG 91-19-9, Resht Medical Report 1935-36. Probably one of the graduating nurses was Fatemeh Tavana'i, who mentions this graduation in the presence of the governor and her training and experience as a nurse in an interview to a woman's magazine. Ta`eb 1384, pp. 65-69. For the names of other nurses, see Idem, p. 54.

Government of Iran begins nursing schools

What hospitals really needed most were trained nurses. Apparently, the government of Iran had similar ideas, for, in early 1936, Dr. McDowell served on a government committee preparing the curriculum for the School of Nursing, of which the government intended to initially establish three.[74] A two-year program of study was developed and the entry-level requirement for these schools was a minimum of nine years of general education. `Ali Asghar Hekmat, the Minister of Education wanted to establish five schools for nursing, viz. in Tehran, Tabriz, Isfahan, Mashhad and Shiraz. Because there was a lack of qualified nurse educators in Iran, the US missionaries were asked to participate. "We do not ask for anyone's services gratis" said the Minister, "but shall pay everyone that helps."[75] The Tehran missionaries were surprised by the end result in August 1936; it called for three nurses from the Presbyterian mission to act as principal of each school. The schools were to be located in Tabriz, Mashhad and Tehran. Hekmat formally asked for US help in establishing the government nurses' schools and when told that it had been decided that this was not possible he expressed his bitter disappointment. He also said that the Shah had approved of the project and the hiring of American nurses. "Now then, especially in view of the relations between the American Government and the Iranian Government at the present time, if you do not as requested, I fear it may be very bad." As a result, the missionaries in Tehran discussed the result of this meeting with Hekmat, who wanted a follow-up meeting with Dr. Blair and Ms Fulton. During that next meeting the American side made it clear that they could not made a firm commitment, even for three nurses half time, without approval from the Presbyterian Board. However, for the next fiscal year an allocation would be made to possibly make two nurses available half-time. Given the likely negative repercussions for the work of the American missionaries if they did not respond positively the Iran Presbyterian Mission decided to give a favorable

---

74. RG 91-19-11-1, Report Teheran American Hospital 1937 (Ms Margaret Oman helped out over the summer).

75. RG 91-20-2. Mashad Medical Report 1935-1936.

reaction. Also, because Hekmat had arranged that medical and school supplies for the US missionaries were exempt from customs duties, which represented a value of 80,000 rials.[76]

The schools were scheduled to begin in the third week of September, but were actually opened on 1 October 1936. The Ministry of Education paid the Iran Mission for the half time of three US nurses and provided an Iranian assistant per school. However, between practical instruction and supervision, administrative duties, preparation of lessons for both immediate use and printing, they had very little time and strength left for hospital responsibilities.[77] Ms Wilma Pease arrived in Tehran in August 1936, but then went to Mashhad to start the government nursing school there, which demanded her full time. This was a heavy burden for the hospital, the more so, because Ms Nicholson went on furlough. The arrival of Ms Hoeldeck, a German nurse, whose father was employed by the Iranian government, gave some relief. Ms Pease returned in May 1937, just before Ms Fulton left on furlough.[78]

The government made further arrangements to employ three US special term nurses, one to take over the Tabriz school, the others to open schools in Isfahan and Shiraz. The number of students was small, in Tehran only eight. Classes started in the government hospital for women (*bimarestan-e nesvan*), which also housed the School for Midwives. After one month the school was transferred to the Vaziri Hospital and in winter to the American Hospital. Until spring the didactic classes were mostly taught by Dr. Saleh, a graduate of the Syracuse medical school, which were given in the Vaziri Hospital. Thereafter they were given in a government high school about 10 minutes walk from the American Hospital. Training was on a day school basis, but two students whose homes were far away stayed in the crowded Nurses Quarters part of the year as did the nurses assigned in rotation to evening duty.

---

76. RG 231-1-5, Gifford [?] to Allen and Wysham, Tehran 17/08/1936, Government Nurses' School Project.
77. RG 91-19-11-1, Report Teheran American Hospital 1937.
78. RG 91-19-11-1, Report Teheran American Hospital 1937; RG 91-20-2, Mashad Medical Report 1936-1937.

Table 7: Curriculum of the Two-Year Nursing Schools approved in 1316/1937

Subject	No. of class hours
Anatomy and physiology	96
Microbiology	16
Pharmacology	35
Preparation of solutions	8
Internal diseases	32
Contagious diseases	16
Tuberculosis	2
Nervous diseases	3
Pediatrics	12
Child-nursing	4
Diseases of eyes, ears, throat and nose	4
Nursing procedures	2
Ethics in nursing	12
Personal hygiene	16
History of nursing	12
Scientific teaching for patient's nutrition	24
Cooking	8
Nursing procedures	18
Practical nursing	84
Conduct in operating room	12

Subject	No. of class hours
Surgery	32
Foreign language	114
Women's diseases	4
Midwifery	24
Nursing of mothers and infants	16

Source: Seven-Year Development Plan, vol. 2, Exhibit A-5.

The school had all kinds of problems - misunderstanding of official relations by people who had never been in government employ; misunderstanding of the concept of modern nursing by students and officials, lack of text books in Persian, insufficient equipment for teaching, etc. etc. However, the Minister of Education took a personal interest and backed the teaching nurses all the way. Students raised on the idea that manual work was only for servants were learning with their hands what nurses had to do for patients, and began to take pride in it. In 1937, they started to take turns in clinics and the OR. The capping exercise was on 11 May 1937, just when Ms Fulton left on furlough, in the auditorium of the Women's Club of Tehran.[79]

The nurses' school in Mashhad started in October 1936 in the Shah Reza hospital (14 students), but in the beginning of the second year it was moved to the Irandokht high school (8 students), and then to the American hospital. The Shrine authorities did not like this fearing that the students might be converted to Christianity. Admission requirements for the school were having: a ninth grade diploma, minimum 16 and maximum 25 years of age, while girls had to be unmarried and of good morals. During year one students received lessons on subjects detailed in Table 7, while during the second year the emphasis was on the practical side of nursing. The entire study lasted three years

79. RG 91-19-11-1, Report Teheran American Hospital 1937.

and in 1938 the first eight students graduated. On 6 April 1938 the capping exercise took place. In 1939, seven students graduated and in 1940, the contract of Ms Degner expired. Thereafter, the school was continued by Iranian nurses.[80]

The government nursing school apparently did well. The Ministry of Education was very pleased with Ms Pease and gave her a medal. Dr. Blair commented, with some pride:

> Considering the age and background to the girls it was amazing how well some of them have done. They have developed poise and dignity and hardly resemble the girls who entered two years ago. One of the first year class is so particular to be accurate in her observations that she reads and records temperatures to one hundredth of a degree! I overheard one of the examiners remarks that the pharmacology examination papers of the nurses would do credit to the medical school.

The women's part of the hospital of necessity revolved to a certain extent around the Nursing School. Given the size of the class and the number of beds the hospital had difficulty giving enough work and enough kinds of work. Financially the school was quite a burden, because equipment was broken and wasted, also, board and room had to be provided to a great extent. Dr. Blair wrote that it was difficult to calculate how much it actually cost, but he thought that it cost the hospital more than it got in return. At the end of the 3-year contract this had to be taken into account if the arrangement were renewed.[81]

In 1938, the organization of nursing schools under the Ministry of Education, in which mission nurses and hospitals participated, was most important and of significance. This was a project with varying success due to inadequate ideas of the work, insufficient education, and many students had to live at home. Despite these problems, there

---

80. Khakestar 1395, pp. 215-18. Although the government program was two years, Khakestar states that in Mashhad it was three years. Perhaps he and/or his sources were misled by the 3-year American program that had been in place before 1936.

81. RG 91-19-11-1, Report Medical Work Teheran 1937-1938.

also was that of the drafting of the course layout and translation into Persian."[82] The first capping exercise in 1939 drew many interested people. Practical work had to be shown, taking temperatures, preparing for operations, making beds with 'hospital corners', helping patients to overcome their fears, and other daily problems. What took the house was the bathing of a life-size demonstration baby doll." A major problem was keeping graduate nurses, because the AIOC and other modern industry were developing their own health clinics and hospitals for their staff. This was good for the country, but undercut the service that the Mission hospitals could render. Hamadan "tried a several months' experiment in training practical nurses, which had a fair degree of success."[83] Because of the dissolution of the Government School of Nursing in 1940, it was not clear whether the teaching contract would be renewed. Nevertheless, Ms Fulton gave post-graduate work for nurses with Tehran Hospital. Despite this change, in Tehran eight and in Tabriz five girls graduated from the government training course in that year. Furthermore, seven girls graduated from the Mission Nurses' Training School in Rasht, which was recognized by the government.[84]

In addition to the three schools managed by American missionary nurses, there was the school of nursing established in Shiraz. In 1937, `Ali Asghar Hekmat, the Minister of Education, organized the assistance of an American nurse, Ms A. Setzlar, to start a nursing school in Shiraz. A small building near the CMS hospital, where its students attended demonstrations, was rented as the teaching locale. To overcome the problem to find girls willing to become a nurse Dr. Ghorban called on parents of girls, who had graduated from the ninth grade and persuaded some of them to allow their daughters to attend the training at the *Amuzeshgah-e Pezeshkyari*, or the School of Nursing Assistants. Finally, six girls attended the two-year course, who were trained by Ms Metzlar, assisted by Ms Molly Williams, the CMS nurse, while Ms Soghra Namazi acted as interpreter. Dr. Ghorban

82. Presbyterian Church 1939, p. 61.

83. Presbyterian Church 1940, p. 64.

84. Presbyterian Church 1941, p. 72.

taught some anatomy, physiology and medical terminology. When Ms Metzlar had to return to the USA because of WW II, the school was closed. Until then 20 nurse assistants (*pezeshkyar*s) had been trained, who worked in the Sa`di Hospital and the Health Department.[85]

It would seem that in 1940 the government discontinued its five schools of nursing. Perhaps it was because too few prospective nursing students showed an interest to pursue this profession. All nursing schools had problems attracting candidates, because there were few 9th degree school graduates, and of that small group very few who wanted, or were allowed, to become a nurse. This had to do with the fact that in Iran women were prohibited to engage in any social activities that required close contact with men outside their family (not belonging to the *maharem*). However, in nursing this was almost impossible, thus constraining the availability of prospective nursing students.[86] In any events, the government continued with a school for nurses (*pezeshk-yar*s) that was operated by the University of Tehran, while the Army also had it own school.[87]

Tehran

After the dissolution of the Government School of Nursing in 1940, Ms Fulton had to restart the Mission Nursing School from scratch. She took in a new class of five students (with an 11th degree school education), two of whom dropped out, the remaining three completed their first year. Two other students with only a 6th class education were accepted in 1941; they were studying 7th–9th class subjects under an Iranian teacher, but were also part-time working in the wards and studied practical nursing. This was an experiment. For the first time the Mission Nursing School was able to teach chemistry with a lab course thanks to the lab equipment inherited from the Nurbakhsh School for girls in Rasht that closed in 1939. A Sage College (Tabriz) graduate, Ms Soghra Azarzi taught the course. Dr. Varjavand and Dr.

85. Ghorban 1989, pp. 11-12; Administraton Report 1938, p. 18.

86. Hajbagheri and Salsali 2005.

87. Karamati 1999.

Hoffman gave some didactic courses, but Ms Janet Fulton bore the greatest teaching burden. The housing of the nurses was unsatisfactory, as it was located in buildings not intended for such use, and there was a real need for a Nurses Home. Nursing under Ms Fulton was carried by 10-15 graduates, three student nurses, two sub-nurses and half a dozen 'practical' nurses or maids.[88] In 1940-41, there was one class of two nurses. The Tabriz hospital had more experience, because it had a regular training school and the Tehran hospital used five of their graduates; these graduates were in demand by everybody. Non-trained orderlies had to obey the nurses. A requirement for entrance was 8th grade with knowledge of English; the Tabriz school required 12th grade.[89] In 1941-42, the hospital nursing staff consisted of 24 nurses - 11 graduates, 10 students, and three practical nurses. Ms Janet Fulton continued to run the school of nursing in Teheran, where the three senior nurses had already better command of English, so that they were able to use US text books for many of their courses and thus got broader view of the nursing principles than was possible before. The school staff was also bigger in that year. Drs. Varjavand and Hoffman gave medical lectures. A German lab technician gave a course in bacteriology; a Sage graduate, who was attending medical school, taught a course in chemistry. Ms Jane Doolittle did much to prepare Persian outlines of the course materials and helped for the anatomy course and taught it. An Iranian medical school student spent many hours of special teaching filling the gaps for a couple of students admitted without a ninth class diploma. That year two male students were admitted to the nursing school for service in the men's ward.[90] In 1949, in Tabriz, the Sage school of nursing started and there was an increasing interest among Iranians in nursing. One US and one British nurse were invited by the government to survey the nurse training situation and make recommendations.[91]

88. RG 91-19-11-1, Report American Hospital Teheran 1940-1941.
89. RG 231-1-2, Hoffman, no date.
90. RG 91-19-11-1, Teheran Medical Report 1941-1942.
91. Presbyterian Church 1950, p. 46.

The Impact of the Government Nurses' Training School Elsewhere

Hamadan

In 1937, Ms Pease moved to Tehran as supervisor of nurses there and later to Mashhad (see above). Mrs. Lichtwardt subbed for her. One assistant was dropped, because of unsatisfactory work; two nurses were obtained from the Tabriz nursing school to replace two Rasht nurses, who resigned at the end of their contract. Again, the need for a US nurse was stressed.[92] In 1938, there were many nursing changes; the only holdover was Nevart Khanom, who already had worked in Hamadan for two years. Two nurses followed Ms Pease to Tehran and one went to the AIOC at Abadan. The hospital was shorthanded as graduate nurses were almost impossible to find. Therefore, two inexperienced young women we hired as practical nurses and in spring another two. Although they worked out fine, the hospital staff was unable to give them nurses' training. In September 1938, Ms Gudhart, formerly of the Lutheran mission in Sowjbulagh, joined the nursing staff. She was night superintendent for most of the year. With her was a practical nurse formerly of Mashhad. In the late fall a graduate nurse from Tabriz came, but after three months she returned to Tabriz. Ms Enderson lived in the US nurses' quarters and helped looking after the home life of the nurses.[93] In 1939, the hospital did no longer have a US nurse, because Ms Harvey had gone to Mashhad, so that Mrs. Lichtward supervised nursing. The hospital had only one graduate Iranian nurse, from the Tabriz hospital.[94]

In the women's hospital, there was fortunately an Armenian graduate midwife, trained in the American University of Beirut. In the men's hospital a graduate of the missionary Tabriz school was in charge of nursing and surgery, but what was still was needed was

---

92. RG 91-19-27, Hamadan Medical Report 1937.
93. RG 91-19-27, Report Medical Work Hamadan 1937-1938.
94. RG 91-19-27, Christian Healing in Hamadan 1939.

a US nurse for general supervision.[95] In October 1942, Ms Gertrude Winkelman, the long awaited US nurse came, who had spent one year in the Miraj hospital in India awaiting the opportunity to go to Iran. At the end of the year, another graduate nurse came, who was trained in the Kermanshah hospital. Thus, with 1 US nurse, 2 graduate nurses, and five practical nurses, the nursing staff situation was much better than before.[96] In 1943, however, Hamadan did not have a nursing school. To continue the Nursing School Ms Winkelman was transferred to Mashhad in 1945.[97] Mrs. Arthur Muller supervised the nurses and Ms Enderson was general superintendent.[98] Despite all these efforts, the lack of nursing staff remained a problem. For most of the year there was only one graduate nurse, and only in May 1947 the hospital was able to hire another one. This put a heavy burden on Ms Pease and the one lone Iranian graduate nurse, who both often worked 12-16 hours. Moreover, as expected, one of the best practical nurses married. Meanwhile, Ms Pease tried to work in the new girls with varying degrees of success. One left to Kermanshah to study nursing, when she just became useful. Another one was very clever, but only spoke Russian. Given this situation, Ms Pease felt she was unable to start a regular nursing school. Therefore, a plan was drawn up for a 2-year practical nurses training, however, the Hamadan Mission Committee did not agree, so the plan was shelved.[99]

KERMANSHAH

When in 1936, the Ministry of Education decided to start nurse training schools in Tehran, Tabriz and Mashhad it allowed the Westminster Hospital in Kermanshah to continue to operate its nurses training school, adhering to the government program. The only inconvenience was that the government required a two-year training, whereas the Westminster Hospital of Kermanshah had a 3-year program, which it

95. RG 91-19-27, Healing in Hamadan 1940.
96. RG 91-19-27, Report Medical Work Hamadan 1943.
97. RG 91-19-27, Report Medical Work Hamadan 1944-1945.
98. RG 91-19-27, Report Medical Work Hamadan 1944-1945.
99. RG 91-19-27, Hamadan Medical Work 1947-1948.

preferred. However, by adhering to the government rules, it ensured government recognition of the diploma of their graduates. Unfortunately, Ms Chambers was not available for five months, because she had left to help out in Rasht. She returned on 1 September 1936 and took charge of the nurses training school. In the afternoon nurses took classes from 2-6 p.m. In 1937, four nurses graduated, two of whom stayed in Kermanshah, one went to Mashhad and one to the AIOC in Abadan. This left six nurses in two classes.[100]

Of the fourth class of nurses two graduated. One left to the AIOC, the others continued working in the hospital. Thus, by 1939, the school had graduated a total of seven graduates since 1932. The recognition of the Westminster Hospital nurse training school by the government meant that it only could admit girls who had graduated from the 9th grade. This posed a problem, because in 1939, there were only about 20 graduates in Kermanshah, of which the hospital was only able to induce one to come. Some graduates continued to 10th grade, some married; also, nursing was looked down upon; parents didn't want their girls to sleep outside the home or do night work. But the hospital badly need nurses. Therefore, it allowed three sixth class graduates to join the nurse traning school on condition that they would continue to study and get their 9th grade diploma and only then they would get their US diploma. Unfortunately, there was a high attrition rate of both students and graduate nurses. The head of the training school opined that the nurses didn't come because they had the idea of service, but rather came to get away from home and when trained, knowing English and the typewriter they received attractive offers with easier work and better pay. Marriage was another reason why nurses left their service. On 1 April 1939, three nurses graduated and received their caps and pin. To make living conditions in the nurses quarters more attractive, a basement store room was transformed into a dining room and the former dining room became a reception and sitting room for nurses. A library and study room were next to the hospital office. There also

---

100. RG 91-19-28, Kermanshah Medical Report 1937; RG 91-19-28, Report Westminster Hospital Kermanshah 1938.

were badminton rackets, but not a court.[101] On 29 May 1939, three nurses graduated, while on 15 September four students began nursing school. A skeleton had been received for teaching purposes.[102] In the summer of 1940 four nurses graduated after three years of school. All continued working in the hospital, but it meant more claim on its budget. However, they were needed, the more so, because the next class of nurses was disintegrating. In 1940, the hospital employed four graduate nurses, three practical nurses, four student nurses, and five orderlies.[103] In 1940-41, the new class had four students (two Jewish, two Assyrian), but that gain was negated by the departure of three graduate nurses to Abadan, where they earned 800 rials per month plus 250 rials for food and room with clothes. One would-be student left to become a nurse-maid with a family at the AIOC refinery for 350 rials per month with full maintenance.[104] The two graduate nurses were the highest paid with $30/month plus maintenance. The two male assistants received $30/month, but no maintenance; the cook received $20 plus food; the rest of the Iranian staff $18.75/month plus one meal. In total, the Iranian staff numbered 27. Student nurses only receive maintenance.[105] In June 1943, there were 10 student nurses, of whom seven were expected to finish next summer; the other three still had another year to go.[106]

Mashhad

The government school for nursing in Mashhad started in 1936, which was led by Ms Pease RN, which demanded the nurses' full time, so that the doctors also had to help them. Moreover, Ms Nicholson went on

---

101. RG 91-19-28, Report Westminster Hospital Kermanshah 1938-39.
102. RG 91-19-28, The Westminster Hospital Bulletin. vol. 2/1. October 1939.
103. RG 91-19-28, Report Westminster Hospital Kermanshah 1940.
104. RG 91-19-28, Report Westminster Hospital Kermanshah 1940-41.
105. RG 91-19-28, Social and Education Project 1944-45 (100 rials = $3.2).
106. RG 91-19-28, Report Westminster Hospital Kermanshah 1943.

furlough.[107] Despite the school of nursing, the hospital's greatest need remained educated nurses. In 1936, the Mashhad hospital had only one, a German nurse. The school that had begun under Ms Pease in October of that year had great difficulty, due to the absence of facilities for nursing. It began with 16 students, but as they had no idea what nursing was five dropped out after the first few months. Then two of the best moved elsewhere, when they were made to work five hours' of steady work, they complained that it was too hard work and one girl quit. This left half of the group, of uncertain enthusiasm, and only having 7th and 8th grade education. But the public capping of 10 of them in 1937 with a public event with the Minister of Education and the governor-general was impressive and was aimed to stimulate them.[108] Ms Pease had to work under almost impossible conditions at the Shah Reza Hospital, which was continued by Ms Nicholson until October 1937, when Ms Emma Degner, a 3-year US contract nurse employed by the Iranian government came and took over. She prepared eight girls to graduate in this fall of 1938 after a 2-year course. The missionary doctors helped her out as much as possible. However, as of 1938, the US hospital was free from having to teach at the government school of nursing. Ms Nicholson was in charge of the government school of nurses until October 1938. Then she assisted the US hospital till December, while she remained for another three months to find half a dozen girls and teach them and the hospital's other 'practical' nurses enough to continue and then left to the US to marry. The Christian hospital had no graduate nurses at all, because the AIOC hired all the available ones, mainly graduates from mission schools at salaries that were twice or three times higher.[109]

To have a regular training school for nurses in Mashhad like in Tehran was not possible. Nevertheless, the nurses employed there had acquired a good level of practical experience. An Armenian graduate from Tabriz was in charge of women's wards and assisted in the OR. Drs. Hoffman and Cochran worked all year and Mrs. Hoffman worked

107. RG 91-20-2, Mashad Medical Report 1936-1937.

108. RG 91-20-2, Mashad Medical Report 1936-1937.

109. RG 91-20-2, Mashad Medical Report 1937-1938.

as matron and supervised repairs and alterations. Ms Nicholson left in February 1939, so that the nurses had no US supervisor and thus, the doctors were glad with the arrival of Ms Harvey in January 1939.[110] The hospital lost several graduate nurses to marriage, so it had to hire several untrained girls. After Ms Harvey's arrival in November 1939, Ms Ophilia was hired, a graduate nurse, who translated for her in the clinic and taught the girls the elements of nursing care.[111] Ms Harvey had her disappointments in trying to institute more formal training for the nurses. To get better educated girls the doctors encouraged their nurses to study for and obtain the government 6th cycle certificate. They got time off to study and the hospital paid for a teacher in the evenings; as a result, four of them passed the exam. In the fall of 1940, the 'nursing school' started on a new basis; the girls were considered students and were not being paid. They also needed to have 6th cycle certificate.[112] Ms Esther Edgar, a graduate nurse from Beirut, made many improvements in the surgery department and in the men's ward that were under her supervision.[113] When in the fall of 1942, the Hoffmans returned to Mashhad they came with three nurses from the closed Tehran hospital, one graduate (Shamshi Khanom, a graduate of Kermanshah) and two students. The former took over as supervisor in the OR from Esther Edgar. In the men's ward Tuba Khanom was the supervisor.[114] Late in 1942, Ms Harvey started the nursing school. Throughout the remainder of the year the two doctors, Ms Harvey, Father Edwards (later Shamsi Khanom) and Mrs. Cochran taught the two classes in training. The older group of five girls was taking more and more responsibility. The junior class of two received their cap after seven months in May 1943. The same group of teachers also had been giving weekly classes in dietetics, nursing supervision. English was taught by Mrs. Cochran and Ms Harvey to the nurses of the Shah

110. RG 91-20-2, Mashad Medical Report 1938-1939.
111. RG 91-20-2, Mashad Medical Report 1940.
112. RG 91-20-2, Mashad Medical Report 1940-1941.
113. RG 91-20-2, Mashad Medical Report 1940-1941.
114. RG 91-20-2, Mashad Medical Report 1942-1943.

Reza hospital, who were without a supervisor or teacher.[115] A second class of four was started in 1943, and a third of five in 1944. Finding doctor assistants was difficult.[116]

In 1945, the brightest point was the continued progress of the nursing school, and the graduation of students in December, who all remained working in the hospital. There were four in the next class and five in the beginners' class. Ms Harvey left in June 1945 on furlough. In the first six months of 1945, the Christian hospital had seven graduate Iranian nurses.[117] In February 1946, the second class of three graduated; the girls performed a play. Meanwhile, instruction of the remaining class continued, but a new class had to wait the return of Ms Harvey, as Ms Winkelman was still studying Persian. There were eight graduate nurses in the hospital.[118] Ms Mabel Wilson R.N. improved hospital nursing; at that time there were four nurses. Nursing was improved when two Armenian graduate nurses Ms Vartanush and Ms Virginia from the Tabriz nursing school came for 3-year terms. Later another pair of nurses was found, and thereafter again from Tehran.[119]

Rasht

In April 1937, Ms Nicholson was temporarily transferred to Mashhad to take charge of the government school of nursing. Ms Estelle Chambers came from Kermanshah to help the Rasht own school of nursing. At that time, there were three graduates and only four student nurses. The government recognized the Rasht nursing school as an accredited private school of nursing, so far the only such school recognized. Since 1924, the Christian hospital in Rasht had been training nurses, most of whom found employment with Iranian hospitals. The government

115. RG 91-20-2, Mashad Medical Report 1942-1943; RG 231-1-6, Hoffman, Pioneering in Meshed, p. 140.

116. RG 231-1-6, Hoffman, Pioneering in Meshed, p. 140.

117. RG 91-20-2 Mashad Medical Report 1944-45.

118. RG 91-20-2 Mashad Medical Report 1945-1946.

119. RG 231-1-6, Hoffman, Pioneering in Meshed, p. 63.

not having courses or standards of their own winked at the Rashti 'certificates', but now that they had established their own schools required the Christian hospital of Rasht to come up to their standards and submit to supervision. This implied following government courses, "submitting to government inspection and meeting government requirements as a 'school.' This last involves one class room for each of the two classes. One room for the night nurse to sleep. To make room for the school we have built a room in a remote corner of the yard and enclosed a large veranda as a class room." The government required only two instead of three years training that the missionary hospital gave. "It also makes the didactic theoretical part of the training more prominent." This posed some problems to get student nurses for the hospital's own hospital work. Five of the Rasht school's former students entered the government new school, those who had not finished the Rasht hospital course extending their time of training to government standing.[120]

The training program was taught by Dr. Frame (public health, internal and infectious diseases, obstetrics), Dr. Brinkman (anatomy, physiology, bacteriology, diseases requiring surgery), Ms. Nicholson (rules for nurses, writing patients' records and their condition, in English), Ms Benz (diet, cooking easy meals for patients, English), Mr. Ehteshamzadeh (physics, chemistry). Most of the teaching material was in English, brought over from the USA, although summaries were available in Persian. Those students who knew English helped their colleagues who were still studying that language also translated parts of the teaching material and made copies available to them.[121]

Ms Nicholson had received permission to conduct a private school of nursing under government supervision and to send her students to government examinations. To help them, the US hospital staff organized some repertory courses for them. Because at the hospital a foreign language had never been taught, a government requirement, Mrs. Frame took charge of this deficiency. Dr. Frame decided not

---

120. RG 91-19-9. Resht Medical Report 1936-37.

121. Ta'eb 1384, p. 84 (Mr. Ehteshamzadeh was a school teacher in Rasht).

to take any new students during Ms Nicholson's absence.[122] On 1 October 1938, the government held its first exam of the hospital's four nurses, who all passed. The second exam was held in June 1939, and the hospital's three candidates passed.[123] In the fall of 1939, seven nurses received the government diploma, "these being among the first awarded in five schools of Nursing throughout the country." A new class of four started in October. For the first time, blue dresses and white aprons were made as uniforms for our students through Ms Benz's effort. Until then the student nurses had not worn any distinct dress. The nursing staff in 1930-40 consisted of: five graduate nurses, four students, three nurse helpers, and three orderlies. Dr. Frame tried to stick to a normal working week, but on average they worked 54 hours. The nursing staff did surgery supervision, actual ward work, responsibility for night work, including obstetrics, helping each day in the dispensary and dressing room, regular care of patients, and all this, during the 9,314 patient--days. The nurses were all Rashti girls and lived at home. For day sleeping of the night nurse there was a room. The hospital nursing school with government recognition tried to get as many girls from the best families of the province.[124]

In 1940-41, it was expected that a number of nurses would leave in the fall. Two of the older ones wanted to go to the Midwifery School; four students were under the government program and would take exams in September and finish their course in October. These nurses and the junior ones were all taught by Dr. Frame and Dr. Kibbe, Ms Nicholson and Ms Benz. In 1941, one of the hospital's best graduate nurses left, but three additional student nurses joined the four of the previous year.[125] Ms Benz was in charge of the classes for nurses and in April 1942, when she went on leave, Mrs. Browning took over. In October 1942, four nurses graduated; one of them stayed working in

122. RG 91-19-9, Resht Hospital Report 1937-38.

123. RG 91-19-9, Resht Hospital Report 1938-39. Om graduation the nurses received a medal with a cross and the text "Sympathy binds us." In the margin of the medal was written: American Mission Hospital Iran. KA [year] Rasht. Ta'eb 1384, p. 84.

124. RG 91-19-9, Resht Hospital Report 1939-40.

125. RG 91-19-9, Resht Hospital Report 1940-1941.

the hospital. Three students were accepted, while there were three in the senior class. Ms Nicholson still had government permission to conduct the School and the Department of Education continued to receive the hospital school's reports and plan for exams.[126]

In 1942-43, the government recognized nursing school was continued, although its teaching staff was somewhat depleted. Dr. Adelaide Kibbe-Frame taught a few afternoons, Ms Wilder taught English, personal hygiene and dietetics. Ms Benz helped in many ways. The Iranian nurse, who for years taught anatomy, married and left to Tehran. Mrs. Kar was able to teach in four languages, but not in Persian. The government was still interested and examined three girls who completed the 3-year class in September 1942. To have fair standards of nursing the Rasht school accepted classes every year and therefore, this government contact was useful.[127] In the fall of 1943, nurses did the exam and were graduated by the department of health and education. The examining Iranian doctors were surprised that the girls were able to reply so comprehensively. They also seemed to enjoy visiting the hospital and observing the girls at practice in patient care. They received their awards at the annual presentation of high-school diplomas. The Christian hospital had six students that year, four of whom passed their exam in September. One of the graduates was in charge of the in-patient department, one of surgery, one in the dispensary and another on night duty. Orderlies did most of the work for the men, but unschooled men for this department were often unsatisfactory and the doctors looked forward to the day when the girls would do practically all of the work in the men's department. The girls slept at home and left before dawn to be at the hospital at 7 a.m. for handover. Two classes were taught by the very busy and lone US doctor, Dr. Kibbe-Frame (her husband Dr. John Frame had died on 11 June 1942). Ms Wilder taught English for six months and all other classes were taught by Ms Nicholson. Over the years, the Christian hospital in Rasht had sent many well trained girls out in the community; they were working in the City and Maternity hospitals, in private practice and as assistants to doctors in the city.

126. RG 91-19-9, Resht Medical Report 1941- 1942.

127. RG 91-19-9, Resht Hospital Report 1943.

Some went to Tehran. However, to have sufficient and competent nursing the hospital needed a nursing school.[128] In 1948, besides four graduate Iranian nurses there were 11 students, all of them having 9th grade or better.[129] Dr. Hoffman wrote: "The very best feature of the hospital work is the availability of well educated girls from good families as nursing material, in spite of the hospital's total lack of facilities housing them." In 1949, the Rasht school had a class of six graduates. The nurses lived at their parents, but it was not possible to properly train and control them, unless they lived at the hospital, thus a nurses' home was needed.[130] Although the school was not officially recognized the nurses that the school graduated were immediately hired by government hospitals. For example, in 1947, the nursing had graduated 13 nurses, three of whom worked in the National hospital, three in the military hospital (1 married) one in a Tehran hospital; five in the missionary hospital (three of these were taking the government exam), one got married, and only one was out of work.[131] After Ms Nicholson's departure in 1947 from Rasht, the nursing school was led consecutively by Ms Eunice Barber, Ms Emma Degner, and Ms Guan Belgum, until the closure of the Christian hospital in 1962. During that period the school graduated at least 10 nurses each year.[132]

The AIOC

In 1941, the AIOC, which had hired quite a number of the nurses from the American nurses' schools, decided to open its own school (*amuzeshgah-e parastari*) for both men and women after the government closed down its nurses school program. The training course lasted three years and candidates needed to have a 9th degree school education.[133]

---

128. RG 91-19-9, Resht Hospital Report 1944.
129. RG 231-1-5, Hoffman/Rasht to Friends, 12/09/1948.
130. RG 231-1-5, Personal Report 1949 and Hospital Report Resht.
131. RG 231-1-5, Memo Medical Needs Rasht Hospital undated, probably 1948.
132. Ta`eb 1384, p. 55.
133. For details on its study program, see Appendix 2.

THE SITUATION AFTER WORLD WAR II

At the end of the 1940s the nursing situation was still problematic. This is, for example, clear from the situation in Shiraz, where a program for the training of village nurses (probably a first for Iran) had started for girls who had a 6th-grade education. Its annual graduation rate aimed for 20 per year.[134]

Table 8: Curriculum of the nurse-aide (*behyar*) training program in Shiraz:

Two months	Morning	Afternoon
Three months	Working the rooms of patients, household work, cleanliness, preliminary care	General information on anatomy and physiology, contagion and disinfection
Three months	Clinic training; medical training	Internal diseases, nutrition of healthy people and patients, housing hygiene, hospital hygiene, drug-making and medical elements
Three months	Surgery	Some elementary information on surgical and medical science, combat against disease
Two months	Infectious diseases	Prophylactic medicine; control of infectious diseases
Two months	Child dispensary	Pediatrics and principles of child growth

Source: Seven-Year Development Plan vol. II, Exhibit A-6.

134. Overseas Consultants 1949, vol. 2, p. 17

However, such graduation numbers fell far short of the needs. In 1948, the Ministry of Health employed only 477 male and 85 female nurses. However, many of the older ones were without formal training. Many of them were so-called practical nurses, i.e. those who had received an on-the-job training in hospital. The Army employed some 500 male medical aides, of whom 100 were civilians. There are no data available on nurses employed by the private hospitals, but that number was probably less than 100. Therefore, it is no surprise that the Seven-Year Plan concluded that "there is a need to increase the number of properly trained bedside nurses to replace the untrained ones."[135]

To increase those numbers the Seven-Year Development Plan noted that training schools for nurses (*pezeshk-yar*s) were operated by the University of Tehran and the Army. It further noted that until 1940, the entrance level requirement was six-grades of elementary school, but by 1948 the ninth-grade level was required. Also, the length of study was increased to three years. In 1948, only 25 such civilian nurses graduated and it was intended to double that number in the future. In 1950 the school's diploma was evaluated as a bachelor degree in nursing (*lisans-e parastari*).

To increase the number of nurses a graduate school for nurses, under the auspices of the University and the Imperial Social Services Organization, was about to be opened, for which 11th-grade was required. This school's 3-year study followed the British nursing training program and therefore, British nurses were in charge of the school. Starting in 1952 the school intended to graduate 50 nurses per year. An additional year of public health training would be required for those nurses who would begin working in the public health sector and needed this extra training. Public health nurses and home visitors were needed for home management and child care. Therefore, it was also intended to start a 3-year training program for public health nurses to be jointly operated by the Imperial Social Services Organization, the University and the Rockefeller Foundation. The entrance level

---

135. Overseas Consultants 1949, vol. 2, pp. 16-18.

required would be 11th-grade and the program would provide bedside and public health nursing to prepare them for work in health department and health centers. The aim was to graduate 25 girls per year.[136]

In 1948, the first government-sponsored nursing school was opened in Tehran, the Princess Ashraf School of Nursing (*Amuzeshgah-e `ali-ye parastari-ye Ashraf-e Pahlavi*), which replaced the Tehran School of Nursing (*Amuzeshgah-e parastari-ye Tehran*) which had been established in 1936 (see above). Also, in 1952, a nursing section was established within the Department of Public health. This was the first time that nursing as a profession was officially recognized by the government and became part of its structure. [137] The first university program for obtaining a BSN began in October 1967 at Shiraz University.[138]

In 1957, the government established a two-year college of nurse-aides (*Amuzeshgah-e Behyari*) in Tehran admitting a total of eighty students.[139] Similar steps were taken elsewhere in Iran, such as had already been done in Shiraz. The establishment of a new university that had a medical school as well as two modern Iranian hospitals and a nursing school Shiraz was well positioned to address the medical problems and challenges of Fars province. CARE provided the Namazi Foundation with a Director of the Nursing Services at the Namazi School of Nursing.[140] The first university program for obtaining a BSN began in October 1967 at Shiraz University.

In 1958, the government established requirements for a 3-years female nursing school, which required a 12th grade entrance level diploma and a 2-years *behyar* school for both men and women, with 9th grade requirements. In 1963, there were seven professional nursing schools with more than 5,300 students and nine *behyar* (nurse aide) schools with 300 students. Both schools had more applicants than

---

136. Overseas Consultants 1949, vol. 2, pp. 16-18; Karamati 1999.
137. US Army 1963 p. 154; Karamati 1999.
138. Hajbegheri and Salsali 2005.
139. Encyclopedia Iranica 1989.
140. CARE 1961, p. 6.

they could train, so that with USOM grants a small number (by 1961 more than 20) also were trained in the USA or in Beirut.[141]

The NIOC still operated its own nursing school, which as of 1954 changed its entrance requirement from 9th to 11th grade diploma for the 3-year training course. In 1958 this requirement was increased to a 12th grade diploma, which was in accordance with government requirements. Later these entrance requirements became more demanding and stricter, while the secondary training and labor conditions became more attractive.[142]

The Seven-Year Plan totally ignored the nursing training programs established by the missionary schools, which were the originators and the basis of all further nurses training activities in Iran. In 1948, nursing education was done in four US missionary hospitals. "Its school of nursing continues with a new class of a dozen girls with a 2-years course."[143] Nursing education began a new chapter with the opening of the Sage School of Nursing in Tabriz in 1948. "This school is designed to take in students of higher education than the others and to give more advanced work, at the same time developing the spiritual life of the pupils."[144] This school was so successful that in 1954 the Tabriz missionary hospital continued to carry on the largest nurses' training school in the country.[145]

In 1958, the Tabriz missionary hospital had electricity, 60 beds and 10 bassinettes, also running and hot water and an Iranian flush

---

141. US Army 1963 p. 154. In 1954-55, continued American aid was given to Iran to establish and operate public health services, including public health nursing-midwifery services as well as to finance the employment of American physicians at the Namazi hospital and of nurses assigned to the school of nursing of this hospital. US Government 1956, pp. 435, 1140.

142. For details, see Appendix 2.

143. RG 91-20-2, Mashad Medical Report 1945-46.

144. Presbyterian Church 1949, p. 67. Private organizations such as Jewish Ladies Committee in 1953 opened a Nursing school. The school had a two-year curriculum and was attended by some ten girls. [American Jewish Joint Distribution Committee].

145. Presbyterian Church 1955, p. 54.

toilet. However, the hospital needed repairs; most needed were a new operating room, a delivery room suite, and a nurses' dormitory and class room block. The most urgent financial need was the increased regular appropriation for both the hospital and the school of nursing. The hospital's full time staff consisted in 2 foreign doctors, 2 national (one on study leave); 2 foreign nurses; 12 national (one on study leave); 1 bookkeeper; 2 technicians; 6 finished nurses and 5 orderlies. The most urgent staff need was a business manager, 2 short-term nurses and a dietician. In 1958, the nurses' training school had 13 students. The entrance requirement was 12th grade, which was much higher than at the other nurses' training schools. In that year there were 3-6 first year students; three second year students; and four third year students. After graduation the nurses had to qualify for an official licensing requirement. The Sage school was not an exclusive American affair. Eight Iranian government physicians taught in the school. Also, the nurses observed patients and treatment in the City Neurological Hospital and the Hospital for Mental Diseases. As to preventive medicine and public health both the government and Point IV were active participants.[146] In that same year the hospital decided to further upgrade the nursing school to a standard that might get it official recognition by the government. This meant that the school would be approved by the licensing committee of the Iranian Nurses' Association.[147] The government requirements were: (i) at least three qualified graduate nurses with degrees, if possible, as faculty; (ii) associated with a 100 bed-hospital with a nurses' home; (iii) presence of a chemistry lab, microbiology lab, dietetics lab and a library; (iv) students had to be 18 years or older and have a 12th degree diploma The school had as yet not applied for official recognition, because it did not meet all requirements. However, the school had a 3-year course using the curriculum of the American nursing schools, except for chemistry and psychology. The graduates were in great demand

146. RG 161.3.51, Questionnaire for the Medical Office, 1958, Tabriz, 17/01/1959.

147. RG 161.3.51, Arnold Schneider (Tabriz) to Stevenson and Sundberg (N.Y.), 04/08/1958.

throughout the country, because of their excellent training. However, the government did not want to give the missionary school official recognition, because of its small size. Thus, graduates received a diploma from the missionary school of nursing, but no diploma from the government. Nevertheless, the graduates were eagerly hired by private and government hospitals throughout Iran, they only did not receive government wage increments.[148]

In 1960, the Sage school in Tabriz, established and operated by American missionaries, adjusted its program to government requirements. The length of the nurses' training course remained 36 months, while 17-18 also remained the minimum age. However, now a 12th degree diploma was required. Courses were given in Persian and English. The nursing school had three class rooms with equipment to teach the nursing arts. Although there was no nutrition lab, the missionary's kitchen was used to that end. Although there was no science lab the school had a chemistry lab. The library had 200 books, which were mostly in English. Teaching aids included charts, only one filmstrip, but many slides. Moreover, there were models for eye, ear, heart, torso and skeleton. Also, there were many specimens from operations, films from the USIS and the mission library. The film projector used belonged to the station.

Students had a period of full-time class work before they went to the wards, where they worked 15 hours/week. Class time came out of duty time. Each student during her entire course had to four periods of night duty of three weeks, i.e. 8 hours/night. In 1960, there were 13 nurses in the Sage school. These were 6 first-year students, three second-year and four third-year students.

---

148. RG 161.3.51, Questionnaire for the Medical Office 1958, Resht, 26/12/1958.

Table 9: Curriculum of the Tabriz Sage School of Nursing (1960)

First year	Hrs	Second year	Hours	Third year	Hours
Anatomy, physics	175	English	100	Public health	w/6 wk field experience
Chemistry	50	History of nursing	32	Pediatrics	36
Microbiology	48	Sociology	15	English	100
Nursing arts	175	Medical and surgical nursing	140	Nervous & mental diseases	30
Dietetics	30	Communicable diseases	45	Professional Adj. II	15
Personal & community-hygiene	35	Skin disease	12	Ward management	20
Professional Adj. I	15	E.E.N.T.	20	-	-
Physical education	15	Gynecology	12	-	-
Pharmacology	48	O.R. Technique	24	-	-
Metrology	24	Obstetrical nursing	60	-	-
English	120	-	-	-	-
Psychology	25	-	-	-	-

The teaching staff consisted of Ms Estella Chamber Director SON, supervises, teacher; Ms Wilma Pease director nursing service; ass. dir. SON; and Ms Vivena Gisete ass. dir, nursing service and OR supervisor. The hospital employed 7.5 national RNs and 1 post-graduate in nursing education at Syracuse University. Further, a 4-5 orderlies were employed.

The daily workload of nurses was: 1 hour teaching; 1 hour administration; 4 hours supervision; four hours bedside nursing, but no time was spent on public health. The weekly schedule for duty time nurses was: RNs 5.5 hours/day, 1 evening and 1 night. For assistant nurses the weekly schedule was: 3 days; 1 evening; 1 night; and for student nurses: 11 day; 1 evening and 1 night. The latter two groups were trained on the job. The American Kirkwood Hospital at Tabriz had 61 beds, 40 for men's section (surgical and medical beds for men: 24; for children: 12; and 4 unallocated private rooms). For the women's section there was a total of 21 beds (medical and surgical 16 beds; maternity 5 beds). Even with the school and the regular nurses there were occasional shortages of nurses leading to crisis situations, such as in 1962.

None of the teaching staff lived on the school grounds, but the students did. There were three rooms with three students and one room with four students. There were three flush toilets in the hospital and 3 showers, for students only. In the nurses' hostel three servants were employed. To relax, there was a volley ball court, a tennis court, swings, a ping pong table, a radio, a garden (vegetables, flowers), indoor games and a phonograph. The monthly expense for food per nurse was $16, which was fair in balance and adequacy. The nurses further received one pint of milk/day; fruit once daily and one egg every other day. From 1920 to 1959 a total of 128 students graduated (39 years). In 1958 five graduated. The school kept in touch with graduates via letters, visits and an Alumni Association. Despite this, the school director did not know how many nurses were still working as nurse, but she believed that it was quite a few. She also noted that there was a special need for post-graduate courses, a reorganization of the Alumni Association and guided activities for them.[149]

---

149. RG 161.3.51, Gloria Simpson, Nurses education; Idem, Hospital Tabriz Report 1962-1963.

In July 1964 four nurses graduated from the Sage nursing school and passed the government exam. The staff made it into a major occasion. A group of 55 nurses, all in uniform, marched from behind the hospital to the site of the ceremony and there were seven speakers, including from the government.[150] In December 1964, the Tabriz school of nursing received official recognition by the government and permission to continue to operate.[151] In 1966, the American Kirkwood Missionary Hospital also founded a Midwifery program in 1966 and began to train students in midwifery major. The Sage school existed for another eight years. This institute trained nursing students until 1971 when it merged with Tabriz University.[152]

As a result of the activities of the various nursing schools, both government and private, by 1960, there were some 1,640 trained nurses and 1,000 nurses-aides in Iran, which was the group of health workers that, relatively speaking, were the most in short supply, in fact, they were in critical shortage.[153]

---

150. RG 161.3.51, N.N. to Stevens (N.Y.), 07/14/1964.

151. RG 161.3.51, Memo Sundberg to Stevenson and McGilvray, 06/12/1964.

152. Arasteh 1970, p. 125.

153. US Army 1963, p. 153.

Discussion

Despite the social and cultural obstacles (women's inferior position resulting in limited supply of willing workers, low level of education, no 24-hour availability, marriage, no contact with men outside of the family), economic issues (higher pay in the private sector), and religious constraints (working for infidels, impurity or *nejasat*) the US missionary hospitals were able to train nurse-candidates. Initially, these were mostly non-Moslem girls, but over time that changed and both the number of candidate girls and those of the Moslem persuasion increased and in the 1930s were the majority. Founded in 1916 by the American Mission Hospital, the Tabriz school of nursing was the first nursing training institute in Iran. Therefore, the US hospitals had a model function, one that they purposefully pursued, and not only in the field of nursing. As a result, the government of Iran adopted the US training program (be it shorter and less demanding) in 1936, a program initially led by US nurses. In 1940 the government discontinued this program and the US hospitals had to re-establish their own training programs, where these had been discontinued. They were followed by the AIOC and later by government hospitals and other private organizations.

The training program of the nurses developed and improved over time, of course. In the beginning, the nurses received training on-the-job, with little theoretical education. They mainly learnt to maintain cleanliness, orderliness and to closely observe patients. The result was that increasingly nurses established a clean, orderly work environment that made more complex and invasive surgery possible. With additional training and experience they were also able to carry out more complicated treatments and medication. Although initially standards were not uniform, as of the 1930s these standards reflected those prevailing in the USA. This meant that nurse trainees received more class room education and thus less work in the hospital during training. This development coincided with the availability of girls with better education than during the earlier period, the result of the increase of the number of schools in Iran.

For the mission hospital the schools of nursing were essential, because the student nurses (if there were enough of them) solved the problem of the lack of nurses, because after a few months they were used in the hospital to learn the reality of hands-on nursing. Therefore, the departure of graduate nurses, if possible, was always time with the arrival of a new batch of student nurses. This was because the mission hospitals, due to financial constraints, were unable to keep most of their graduate nurses, although they needed them very much. However, those graduate nurses that they kept often left their service either to marry, to return to their home city, or were lured away by much higher pay by other hospitals or by local physicians.

After the implementation of the Seven-Year Development Plan in 1949 the government tried to increase the supply of nurses by establishing more training schools and institutions. This attention resulted in 1953 in the creation of the Association of Iranian Nurses (AIN) by a group of Iranian nurses, who were educated abroad and returned to the country, with the aim to raise the standard of nursing and to promote the cooperation among nurses.[154] The AIN in consultation with the Ministry of Public Health set and established training standards for nursing schools. The founders of the AIN probably also wanted to get more appreciation for their work, which still was a line of work that many families did not want their daughters to get involved in. Also, the work of nurses, as women, was not given the same kind of societal value and economic remuneration that men enjoyed. Therefore, in 1962 nurses joined strike to prove the value of women in society, but they did not lay down the work in the hospitals.[155] By the early 1960s, despite the progress made in training nurses, it was felt that there was "a need to establish the registered nurse in the eyes of the doctors, since the doctor traditionally has employed only servant-class assistance."[156]

154. Paidar 1995, p. 128.

155. Iran Almanac 1963, p. 411.

156. US Army 1963 p. 154.

Meanwhile, the American missionary hospitals, which had paved the way for the training of nurses, continued to play an important role in training highly qualified nurses. This held in particular for the oldest nursing school in Tabriz, founded in 1915, which in 1948 was modernized and renamed the Sage School of Nursing. Therefore, when in 1971 the US missionaries ceased their hospital in Tabriz the Sage school of nursing was merged with the University of Tabriz as one of its flagships faculties.

APPENDIX I

FACSIMILE OF: RG 91-19-28, Social and Education Project 1944-45; musings about nursing education.

JAN 28 1946
2227
SECRETARIES

Social and Educational Project -- Kermanshah
Hospital

1944-45

Nursing education in Iran has long been known as a part of the medical
work of the Mission -- and justly so, for without our hospitals taking
the initiative in training their own nursing staffs, it would have been
impossible to carry on the work with as high a standard of nursing as is
now carried on in many of our hospitals. However, in line with the new
emphasis on education for nurses in America, more and more, we in Iran
are wanting to make our Schools of Nursing truly educational institutions.

During the years just prior to the closing of our secondary schools for
girls in Iran, two of our hospitals, notably Tabriz and Resht, were able
to draw their student applicants in great measure from those Mission
Schools which was a very happy arrangement, for the girls came with four
valuable assets which are now in large part lacking in students from
the government schools. In the first place, the girl had had a number of
years of close contact with American teachers and methods of teaching.
They had, in a measure, learned how to study and how to think, rather
than to memorize and learn by rote. In the second place, the girl was
usually keen to carry on her secondary education to the tenth class to
get the American School diploma before going on with her nursing course.
This produced a girl with adequate educational background to go on to her
course in the hospital. In the third place, because she had carried
her preliminary education to the tenth class,
she was also older and more mature and able more easily to take the
responsibility thrust upon her so quickly in the professional course.
And fourthly, during her years in the American School he had acquired
fairly good use of the English language and was therefore able to more
quickly learn to use the medical, scientific and pharmaceutical terms
which were essential for her work and could in some degree avail herself
of the help of American text books.

Now look at the typical present-day applicant to the School of Nursing
in Kermanshah. In the majority of cases she has gone no farther than the
sixth grade in her preliminary education. There are several reasons for
this. She is tired of studying. That in itself should disqualify the
girl, for certainly she must be an eager student to make the most of
her opportunity in the School of Nursing. Perhaps, however, we sometimes
think that she just needs a change; that she will like studying for this
more practical course, and we may give her a chance. The reason for leavin-
school may be that her parents are not financially able to send her anymore;
or her parents do not themselves realize the value of education to the
girl and therefore are not willing to carry the financial burden. Another
very important reason for stopping at the sixth grade in the Kermanshah
schools is this. The only girls' secondary school in the city is a
government Normal School, and all the graduates of that school are
pledged to teach for a certain number of years after finishing the eleventh
class. If, however, we suggest that the girl go only through the ninth class
and then enter the School of Nursing, she questions: "What's the use of that?"
Those three years are wasted, for she gets no diploma at the end of the
first cycle. And so, in most cases, the applicant comes with only a sixth
class certificate.

The student applicant is also very young, often only fifteen years of age,
and the application and maturity which are so valuable for a young nurse
are not yet a part of her make-up. But at least she is eager and teachable,
and though this extreme youth is in some ways a handicap, it is not without
its good points.

-2-

Also the new applicant has in most cases studied no foreign language, for the study of English or French is not introduced into the curriculum until the seventh class. Perhaps the girl will say that she has studied English at home, but upon investigation it will be discovered that she has learned the alphabet and read the first five pages of "First Book" and she virtually knows no English.

Now Kermanshah has never had a Mission Girls' School, so ever since the beginning of the School of Nursing in 1932, the applicants have been similar to those just described, and during the entire life of the school, there have possibly not been more than five students with ninth grade education or the equivalent, so in the spring of 1943 when the writer was ready to enroll a new class, she felt a great urge to somehow carry the education to a higher level. A complete record of the vicissitudes of the two years following that decision is beyond the province of this report, but a brief summary of results to date may be of interest.

Seven s tudents hav e been enrolled since that time with the understanding that for any applicant with less than ninth grade education, the length of the nursing course will be four years instead of the usual three. The extra year is to allow time for the students to take the 7th, 8th, and 9th class (secondary school) subjects as well as the nursing course. Theoretically the student would spend at least the first six months studying only the above mentioned school subjects and take a very heavy course (10 hours a week was given) in English before getting involved in strictly nursing education. Because the seven students for the most part all entered at different times and with different levels of education the task of trying to get them sorted out into homogeneous classes has been a real one. Two of the students have since left the course, finding it to be too much of a load. Of the remaining five, two entered with only sixth class certificate and are now half way through the eighth grade work (we hope, though examination returns are still outstanding), and the last three to enter had all finished the seventh class before entering and are now going along in the eighth grade work as scheduled. One more student has been enrolled during the past year who had completed the tenth grade, and it has been a joy to have at least one who has been carrying a normal course.

The difficulties have been great. In the first place, it is difficult to find a good Iranian teacher at a price which we can afford. The girls do not consider the Persian studies an integral part of the nursing course, and do not care whether they grasp the material or not. The teacher on the other hand, refuses to fail any student in a subject, and therefore it is difficult to get work of a high standard done in these classes. A few of the courses have been taught by American colleagues and in those cases have been very satisfactory. In order to try to give the students a sense of the importance of these courses, and a realization that they must be done as a part of the nursing course, a set of final examination questions on the eighth grade subjects has been requested from Teheran. Four of those final examinations have just been completed and we are now awaiting the results. (The papers were sent to Teheran for correction also.) Just what happens if all the girls fail all the examinations, I don't know. Further comment on that matter will follow in next year's report.

Also it is difficult to find the time for all these extra studies. It had been hoped that they could be completed during the first two years, but it has now become apparent that it will take a longer time than that.

APPENDIX II

DOCUMENT CONCERNING THE HISTORY AND DEVELOPMENT OF NIOC NURSES' TRAINING PROGRAM

تاریخچه

آموزشگاه عالی پرستاری شرکت ملی نفت ایران در سال ۱۳۲۰ به منظور رفع احتیاجات پرستاری بهداری شرکت نفت در آبادان تاسیس گردید .

در آن زمان بنام آموزشگاه پرستاری خوانده میشد اولین اساسنامه آن در سال ۱۳۲۸ در ششصد و هشتاد و یکمین جلسه شورای عالی فرهنگ به تصویب رسید .

شرط ورود به آن داشتن گواهینامه سوم متوسطه بود و پس از سه سال آموزش به محصلین آن گواهینامه پرستاری داده میشد که ارزش آن معادل دیپلم کامل متوسطه بود .

با افزایش سطح معلومات در بین دختران تدریجاً عده ای از متقاضیان ورود به آموزشگاه دارای دیپلم پنجم متوسطه بودند و بدین لحاظ در سال ۱۳۳۳ هیئت مدیره آموزشگاه درخواست نمود بدارندگان دیپلم که وارد آموزشگاه میشوند و دوره سه ساله آموزشگاه را طی میکنند ارزش معلومات آنان برابر فوق دیپلم گردد .

— ۱ —

از سال ۱۳۳۴ به بعد کلیه داوطلبین این آموزشگاه باگواهینامه پنجم و عده ای نیز با دیپلم کامل متوسطه پذیرفته شدند .

در سال ۱۳۳۵ پیشنهاد اصلاح مواد ۲ و ۸ اساسنامه موجود بعمل آمد و مواد اصلاحی درنهصد و چهل و دومین جلسه شورای عالی فرهنگ مورخ ۱۳۳۶/۹/۱ بتصویب رسید و شرط ورود بآموزشگاه دارا بودن حداقل گواهینامه سال پنجم تعیین شد و ارزش گواهینامه پرستاری اینعده از فارغ التحصیلان دیپلم عالی تعیین گردید .

در سال ۱۳۳۷ اساسنامه کلیه آموزشگاههای عالی پرستاری در نهصد و چهل و هشتمین جلسه شورای عالی فرهنگ بتصویب رسید و این آموزشگاه به پیروی از تصویب نامه فوق کلیه داوطلبین را با دیپلم ششم متوسطه پذیرفته و از برنامه مصوبه پیروی نموده است و از آن پس بکلیه فارغ التحصیلان که دوره سه ساله آموزش پرستاری را به پایان رسانیده اند دانشنامه ای با ارزش معادل لیسانس اعطاء میگردد .

اولیای آموزشگاه نهایت کوشش را بعمل میآورند که دانشجویان معلوماتی را که در دوره سه ساله خود در آموزشگاه و بخشهای مختلف کسب

— ۲ —

میکنند د رسطح عالی قرارد اشته و ازهرلحاظ پرستارانی مجرب و ورزیـــده تربیت شوند .

۱- <u>هـدف :</u> عبارتست از آموزش و پرورش د انشجویان پرستاری بنحوی که پس از فراغت از تحصیل بتوانند با بکاربرد ن روشهای صحیح وعلمی احتیاجات پرستاری بهد اری شرکت ملی نفت را د رحوزه قرارد اد از نظر بهد اشتی ، د رمانی و بازتوانی رفع نمایند .

۲- <u>موسسه مسئول :</u> این آموزشگاه واحد ی از خد مات پرستـاری اد اره کل بهد اری و بهد اشت شرکت ملی نفت میباشد و بود جه آن توسط بهد اری شرکت ملی نفت تامین میگرد د .

۳- <u>اساسنامه :</u> آموزشگاه عالی پرستاری شرکت ملی نفت آباد ان تابـع اساسنامه آموزشگاههای عالی پرستاری است که د رنهصد و چهل و هشتمین جلسه شورای عالی فرهنگ مورخ ۳۷/۲/۲۸ مطـرح و بتصویب رسید ه است .

۴- <u>هیئت مد یره :</u> بمنظوربوجود آورد ن تغییرات ضروری د رخط مشی آموزشگاه و بررسی پیشرفت امر تحصیلی د انشجویان و اطلاع ازنحوه اقد امات و مسائل و مشکلات کار هیئت مد یره آموزشگاه مرکـب از

از اعضاء نامبرده زیر بوجود آمده که هر ۳ ماه یکبار تشکیل جلسه میدهند .

- رئیس اداره کل بهداری و بهداشت حوزه قرارداد
- معاون رئیس اداره کل بهداری و بهداشت حوزه قرارداد
- رئیس اداره آموزش و پرورش شهرستان آبادان
- رئیس اداره آموزش عملیات غیرصنعتی حوزه قرارداد
- رئیس اداره بهداری و بهداشت و قرنطینه شهرستان آبادان
- رئیس بیمارستانها
- رئیس درمانگاهها
- رئیس بهداشت کارکنان شرکت ملی نفت حوزه قرارداد
- رئیس امور اداری بهداری و بهداشت حوزه قرارداد
- رئیس سرویس پرستاری
- رئیس آموزشگاه عالی پرستاری

۵- <u>شرایط ورود بآموزشگاه :</u>

۱- دارابودن دیپلم کامل متوسطه رشته طبیعی یا ریاضی

۲- سن داوطلب بین ۱۸ تا ۲۵ سال

۳– موفقیت در آزمایشات هوش ، زبان انگلیسی ، فارسی و مصاحبه

٤– سلامت کامل جسمی و روانی بگواهی پزشکان بهداری شرکت ملی نفت

٥– سپردن تعهد ثبتی مبنی برانجام سه سال خدمت پس از اتمام دوره تحصیلات

٦– مجرد بودن

۷– سکونت در شبانه روزی دانشجویان در مدت سه سال تحصیل

٦– <u>تاریخ نام نویسی و امتحان ورودی :</u>

تاریخ نامنویسی ازنیمه دوم خرداد و تاریخ امتحانات ورودی هفته آخرتیرماه است . مصاحبه درمرداد ماه بعمل آمده و اعلام نتایج در آخر مرداد ماه میباشد .

۷– <u>پذیرش دانشجو</u>: این آموزشگاه درسال یك نوبت (مهر ماه) دانشجو میپذیرد تعداد پذیرفته شدگان با احتساب احتیاجات بهداریهای شرکت ملی نفت استگنجایش پذیرش هر سال ٤٠ نفر است .

۸– <u>طول دوره آموزش</u> : سه سال

۹- برنامه آموزش : دروس نظری و عملی طبق برنامه مصوبه وزارت بهداری و شورای عالی فرهنگ میباشد . برنامه تفصیلی در انتهای این راهنما بنظر میرسد .

۱۰- مدرسین : تدریس توسط مربیان آموزشگاه و پزشکان متخصص و سایرمتخصصین فنون مربوطه بعمل میآید و تجربه بالینی با کارآموزی دربخشهای مختلف تحت نظر مربیان بالینی که درکارخود تجربه و تخصص دارند عملی میگردد .

۱۱- وسائل آموزش : آموزشگاه مجهزبکلیه وسائل آموزشی مدرن آزمایشگاه وکتابخانه است .

۱۲- مقررات آموزشی و امتحانات : علاوه بر قسمتهای هفتگی پس ازخاتمه برنامه هردرس از آن ماده یك امتحان داخلی بعمل میآید .

درپایان سال سوم امتحانات نهائی رسمی با حضور نماینده هیئت مدیره آموزشگاه ، نماینده اداره آموزش و پرورش و نماینده اداره بهداری انجام میگیرد حداکثرنمره قبولی ۲۰ و حداقل آن در دروس پرستاری ۱۲ و در سایر مواد ۱۰ میباشد . چنانچه نمره امتحان دانشجو درهرماده بحد نصاب نرسد باید پس از ۳ ماه درامتحانات تجدیدی شرکت نماید .

اگر غیبت دانشجوئی در طی سه سال از ۳۱ روز تجاوزکند امتحـــان نهائی او سه ماه بتاخیر خواهد افتاد .

۱۴- تعهـد : دانشجویان پس از خاتمه تحصیل و موفقیت در امتحـان نهائی ملزم هستند با تعهد ثبتی که بمبلغ ۳۰۰٫۰۰۰ ریال سپرده اند معادل سنوات تحصیل یعنی سه سال در بهداری شرکت ملی نفت درحوزه قرارداد خدمت کنند .

۱۵- تسهیلات و رفـاه : تمام دانشجویان این آموزشگاه درشبانـــه روزیهای مجهز تحت سرپرستی مدیرداخلی شبانه روزی بطــــور رایگان زندگی کرده از تسهیلات خوابگاه ، کتابخانه ، رستوران و زمینهای ورزش استفاده میکنند . دانشجویان ملزم هستنـــد از مقررات داخلی شبانه روزی پیروی نمایند .

۱۶- کمك هزینه تحصیلی : به دانشجویان کمك هزینه تحصیلی پرداخت میگردد و مبلغ پرداخت درسالهای تحصیل متفاوت است .

۱۷- بهداشت و درمان : برای اطمینان از سلامتی جسمی قبـــل از پذیرش بآموزشگاه معاینات و آزمایشات کامل پزشکی بعمل میآید و پس از آن دانشجویان از تسهیلات بهداری شرکت ملی نفـــت

برنامه تفصیلی

<u>آناتومی وفیزیولوژی</u> – تدریس در سال اول

این درس پایه واساس سایرمباحث بوده دانشجورابا ساختمان وکار طبیعی بدن انسان آشنامیسازد وشامل قسمتهای زیراست :

ساختمان وکارسلول ، بافتهای مختلف بدن انسان ، استخوان‌بندی مفاصل وماهیچه ها ساختمان وکاردستگاههای گردش خون ، تنفس گوارش ، دفع ادرار ، اعصاب وغدد مترشحه داخلی ودستگاه تولید مثل .

<u>میکرب شناسی</u> – تدریس در سال اول

آشنائی بااصول این بحث دانشجوراقادرمیسازد این اصول‌راعملاً ضمن کاردربیمارستان ومحیط خارج ازبیمارستان بکاربندد وشامل قسمتهای زیراست :

طبقه بندی وخصوصیات موجودات میکربی ، طرق‌جلوگیری و مبارزه باانتشارمیکربها . آنتی ژن ، آنتی بادی وچگونگی پیدایش مصونیت میکربهای بیماری زاوخصوصیات آن وراهازبین بردن ومبارزه باآنها .

<u>شیمی</u> : تدریس در سال اول

علاوه برمرورشیمی آلی ومعدنی تاکید بیشترروی بیوشیمی است. این درس بدانشجوکمك میکند تامباحث فیزیولوژی ، علم الاغذیه و داروشناسی رابهتردرك کند .

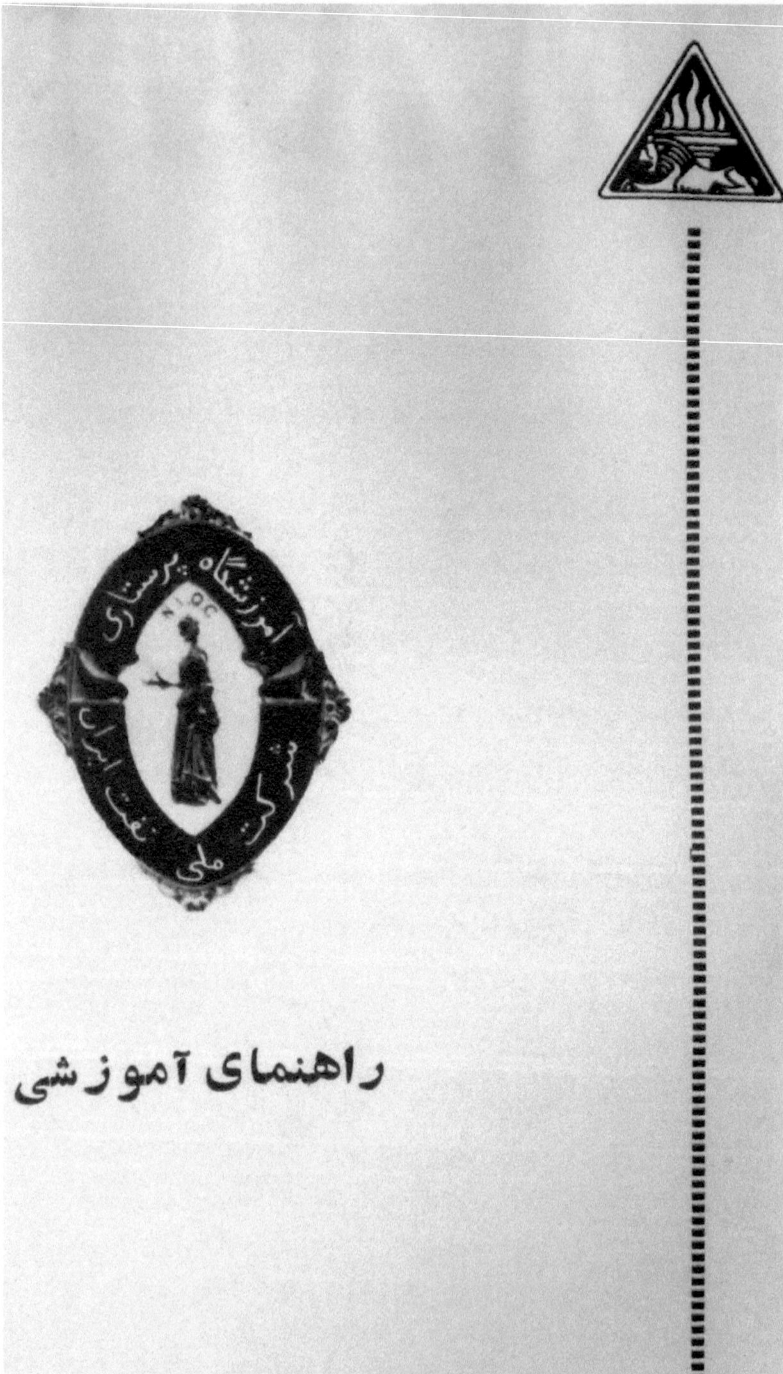
آموزشگاه پرستاری
N.I.O.C
شرکت ملی نفت ایران
راهنمای آموزشی

موضوعهای زیربتفصیل تدریس میگردند :
هیدروکربونها ، لیپید ها (چربیهای اشباع نشده) پروتئین ها
(امینواسید ها) آنزیم ها ، سوخت وساز هیدروکربونها ، چربیها
وپروتئین ها ، شیمی خون ، هورمونها ، ویتامینها .

<u>تاریخ پرستاری</u> – تدریس درسال اول

منظورآگاه ساختن دانشجووایجاد علاقه دراونسبت بگذشته وحال
حرفه ایست که برگزیده وشامل مسائل زیراست :
حرفه پرستاری درمیان ملل باستان ، نفوذ مسیحیت دردوران قدیم
انحطاط وتجدید حیات حرفه پرستاری ، نفوذ تحولات صنعتی
آغازپرستاری جدید ، پرستاری جدید درایران .

<u>اخلاق پرستاری</u> : تدریس درسال اول

هدف کمک بدانشجوست درانتخاب روشی که براساس اصول اخلاقی
ومعنوی استوارباشد چه درزندگی شخصی وچه درزندگی حرفه‌ای .
مشخصات اخلاقی یک پرستار ، سازش باشرایط شغلی وحرفه‌ای .
آشنائی باآداب ورسوم اجتماعی واحترام بآن ، پرستاربعنوان
یکفرد مسئول .

<u>روانشناسی</u> – تدریس درسال اول

درس روانشناسی بمنظورآماده ساختن دانشجوبرای درک بهتر
رفتارآدمی تدریس میگردد ومباحث زیرمورد مطالعه قرارمیگیرند :

عواملی که د ررفتارانسانی موثرند ،توارث ومحیط ،جنبه های بیولوژیکی
رفتارعواطف ورشد وبلوغ عاطفی ،شخصیت وعواملی که د رتکویـــن آن
موثـرند .
روابط انســانـی واصـول یادگیـری

<u>جامعـه شنـاسـی</u> – تدریس د رســال اول

هد ف آشناساختن د انشجوباعواملی است که علم جامعه شنـاسی را
تشکیل مید هد . آشنائی باعلم جامعه شناسی وارزش موضوعـــات
مورد بحث د رآن . عوامل اجتماعی مختلفی که د رزند گی د سته‌جمعی
تاثیرد ارند .

<u>بهد اشت فـرد ی واجتماعی</u> – تد ریس د رسال اول

هد ف آگاه نمود ن د انشجونسبت به اهمیت بهد اشت د رزنـــد گـی
فرد ی واجتماعیست ومسائل زیرمورد بحث قرارمیگیرند .
د ستورات بهد اشتی بکاربستن وطرزتعلیم آن به بیمـــاران :
بهد اشت فرد ی مراقبت ازبد ن انسان ،تغذ یه صحیح ،استـراحت
وخواب تفریح وورزش ،پوشاک مناسب ،رعایت اصول بهد اشت روانی
بهد اشت محیط : مسکن ،نور ،تهویه ،آب ،کنترل مواد غذ ائی وشیر
مبارزه باحشرات ،کنترل بیماریهای واگیروبیماریهائی که د روضـــع
اجتماع واقتصاداجتماعی موثـرند .

تغییرواصلاح رژیمغذائی درموارد بیماری تدریس میشود وشامـــــل
قسمتهای زیراست :
تفسیرتغذیه خوب وبد ،تاثیرعادات ورسوم ،عناصرمتشکله غـــذا :
پروتئین ها ،هیدروکربنها ،چربیها ، مواد معدنی ،ویتامینهـــا ،
تعادل آب والکترولیتهادربدن انرژی وسوخت وساز ،محاسبـــه
احتیاجات نیروئی ،رژیمهـــای درمانـــی .

بیماریهای داخلی وجراحـی – تدریس درسال دوم

این ماده شامل مواد اساسی پزشکی وجراحی درکارپرستاریســـت و
بدانشجومعلومات لازم وکافی درمورد علل ،درمان وپیشگیری بیماریها
رامیآموزد تابادرك بهتربتوانند تجربیات بالینی دربخشهای مختلف
بیماریهای داخلی وجراحی راکسب نماید .

داخلی – آشنائی باپیدایش وپیشرفت علمپزشکی وارتباط آنبا جراحی
– طبقه بندی بیماریها ،علل مختلف بیماری ،تشخیـــص و
درمان بیماریهابوسایل مختلف .
– بیماریها واختلالات دستگاه عصبـــی .
– بیماریهای دستگاه تنفس .
– بیماریهای دستگاه گردش خون .
– بیماریهای دستگاه ادرار .
– بیماریهای غده مترشحه داخلی واختلالات متابولیـــك .
– بیماریهای استخوان وعضـــلات .

- بیماریهای پوست .
- بیماریهای ناشی ازحالات آلرژی .
- پرستاری کلی وپرستاری مخصوص درهریك ازبیماریهای سیستمهای فوق

جراحی - آشنائی باپیدایش وپیشرفت علم جراحی

- بیماریها وحالاتیکه دررشته جراحی مورد نظرند ودرمان بروش جراحی راایجاب مینمایند .
- معاینات لازم قبل ازعمل ومعالجات بعد ازعمل جراحی جریان التیام زخمها .
- عفونت والتهاب ، اهمیت تعادل مایعات والکترولیتها
- جراحی حفره شکم
- جراحی قفسه سینه
- جراحی استخوان وشکستگی
- جراحی پستان وتومورها
- جراحی غدد مترشحه داخلی
- جراحی دستگاه ادرار
- پرستاری کلی وپرستاری مخصوص درهریك ازجراحیهای فوق

بیماریهای واگیروپرستاری مربوطه - تدریس درسال دوم

این درس برای آشناساختن دانشجوبابیماریهای واگیرمعمولی و بیماریهای گرمسیری ونحوه انتشاروطرزجلوگیری همچنین مداوا ومراقبت ازاین بیماریهاست وشامل قسمتهای زیراست :

روش انتقال بیماریهای واگیر :

بیماریهائی که باترشحات دهان وبینی منتشرمیشوند بیماریهائی که انتشارآنهاازطریق مدفوعات است ، بیماریهائی که حشرات موجب انتقال میکرب آنهاهستند ، بیماریهای آمیزشی ، بیماریهائی که ازراههای دیگرشیوع مییابند .

مراقبتهای کلی ازبیمارواگیرباتوجه به نحوه انتقال ،ضدعفونی دراحین بیماری ،ضدعفونی نهائی ،مراقبت دربیمارستان ، مراقبت درمنزل ،نقش پرستاردرجلوگیری ازبیماری وآموزش به بیمارو بستگان او ،تجربه کلینیکی دربخش بیماران واگیرکسب میگردد .

<u>روش کاردراطاق عمل وآشنائی باعلم بیهوشی</u> — تدریس درسال دوم

تدریس این ماده دانشجورابار وشهای معمول دراطاق عمل آشنا نموده . اصول ضدعفونی وعاری ازمیکرب ساختن لوازم وابزارکار اعمال جراحی رابا ویمآموزد وشناساندن اهمیت بیهوشی درجراحی ومامائی وآگاه کردن دانشجوبه اهمیت وظایف پرستاردراین زمینه مورد بحث قرارمیگیرد وشامل قسمتهای زیراست :

ضدعفونی وسائل ومحیط کاردراطاق عمل ،ادارامور اطاق عمل با رعایت اصول ضدعفونی ،کمک بجراح ،بیهوشی وراههای مختلف آن ، مراحل بیهوشی ،بروزپیش آمدهای فوری واقدامات مربوطه .

داروشناسی - تدریس درسال دوم وسوم

منظورمجهزساختن دانشجوبااطلاعات اساسی درباره اوزان ومقادیر سیستم متریك انواع مقدارمصرف وطرزتاثیرداروهاست ، همچنین آگاه ساختن دانشجوبه اهمیت مسائل اجتماعی ناشی ازبی احتیاطی درکار برد بعضی داروهاست .

این بحث شامل موضوعهای زیراست :

اوزان ومقادیر ، علائم اختصاری ، رقیق کردن محلولها مقررات و قوانین مداوا ، منابع داروئی ، داروهای ضدعفونی کننده ، سموم وتریاق ها ، داروهای انتی بیوتیك وکموترابیوتیك ، داروهای موثرومخصوص دستگاههای مختلف بدن ، اعصاب ، تنفس ، گردش خون ، گوارش ، دفع ادرار ، غدد مترشحی داخلی ، تناسلی ، پوست ، چشم ، گوش وحلق وبینی .

بیماریهای زنان وزایمان وپرستاری مربوطه - تدریس درسال سوم

هدف کمك بدانشجوبرای درك بهترمسائل مربوط به بیماریهای زنان وزایمان همچنین ساختمان وفیزیولوژی خاص بدن زن است . اهمیت مراقبتهای قبل وبعداززایمان واصول پرستاری ازنوزادان نارس بشرح زیردراین بحث گنجانده شده :

مروروره تشریح وفیزیولوژی دستگاه تولید مثل زن ، علائم واهمیت بیماریهای زنان ، معاینات وگردآوری سابقه بیماری ، عفونتها

جابجاشدگی رحم ، تومورها ، درمانهای پزشکی ، جراحی وپارادیسوم پرستاری دردوران بارداری ، پرستاری درموارد بروزعوارض مهم بارداری ، درد وزایمان ، پرستاری پس ازوضع حمل ، مراقبت از نوزاد طبیعی ونارس وعوارض نوزاد .

تجربه کلینیکی دربخشهای جراحی زنان وزایمان ونوزادان بدست میآید .

بیماریهای کودکان وپرستاری مربوطه — تدریس درسال سوم

اساس این درس بررشد ونموکودک سالم واهمیت مراقبتهای لازم از اوپایه گذاری شده ومتعاقب آن روش پیشگیری ازبیماریها وسپس بیماریهای مربوط به کودکان وروشهای مختلف پرستاری ازآنان تشریح میشود .

بهداشت کودکان ومسئولیت های پرستاردرمراقبت ازکودک سالم کودکان نارس ، نقایص مادرزادی ذکرمیگردد .

درموارد بیماری : اهمیت تعادل مایعات انجام مداوا ، تغذیه صحیح ومناسب پرستاری ، بیماریهای ناشی ازبدی تغذیه ، بیماریهای تنفسی ، قلب وگردش خون ، گوارش ، دستگاه ادراری ، اعصاب وغدد داخلی شرح داده میشود تجربه کلنیکی — دربخشهای کودکان بدست میآید .

بیماریهای چشم ، گوش ، گلوو بینی وپرستاری مربوطه — تدریس درسال سوم

دراین بحث دانشجوبا بیماریهای عضوهای نامبرده آشناشده روش

پیشگیری ومعالجه بیماریها رامیآموزد واین دانش باوکمك خواهد کرد
تابعنوان یك مربی بهداشت کمك به بازگشت سلامت بیمارنموده با و
تعلیم دهد که بسیاری ازاین بیماریها قابل پیشگیری هستند .
این بحث ابتدا باتشریح وفیزیولوژی عضوهای مربوطه شروع وسپس
به بیماریهای آن عضوها اشاره میگردد .

چشم – بیماریهای خارجی چشم ، بیماریهای غشاء ملتحمه ،
بیماریهای داخلی چشم خطاهای انکسار ، بهم خوردگی
تعادل عضلات چشم ، مراقبتهای پرستاری بیماریکه مبتلا
به عوارض چشم است وتحت اعمال جراحی چشم قرارگرفته .

گوش – بیماریهای گوش خارجی ، میانی ، داخلی ، پرستاری ازبیمار
مبتلا به عوارض گوش .

گلو – عوارض گلووحنجره ، مراقبتهای پرستاری ازبیمارمبتلا بعوارض
گلووحنجره ، خصوصا" بیماری که تحت جراحی تراکیاتومی
قرارگرفته .
بینی – بیماریها وآسیبهای وارده به بینی وپرستاری ازبیمارمبتلا به
عوارض بینی .
تجربه کلینگی دربخش بیماران چشم وبخشهای جراحی عمومی کسب
میشود .

پرستاری بهداشت همگانی — تدریس در سال سوم

تعلیم این ماده دانشجو را با اصول خدمات پرستار بهداشت همگانی و با مراجع مختلف بهداشتی که در جامعه برای کمک به افراد خانواده ها وجود دارند آشنا میسازد وشامل قسمتهای زیراست . هدف وانواع برنامه های بهداشت همگانی : اصول اساسی پرستاری بهداشت همگانی تنظیم گزارش ومدارک بهداشتی وخدمات بهداشت همگانی ونقش پرستار در خانواده ، منابع بهداشتی جامعه ، سازمانهای بین المللی .

اداره امور بخشهای بیمارستان — تدریس در سال سوم

در این درس دانشجو با اصول سرپرستی ووظایف ومسئولیتهای پرستار در مقام متصدی امور بخشهای بیمارستان آشنا شده روشهای مختلف آموزشی وارزیابی کارها را نیز با تمرین کافی میآموزد وبطورکلی شامل مباحث ذیل است .

— وظیفه پرستار مسئول در مورد اداره امور بخش
— " " " " " مراقبت از بیماران
— " " " " " آموزش کارکنان

بهداشت روانی وپرستاری در روان پزشکی — تدریس در سال سوم

این درس برای آشنا ساختن پرستاران با اصول بهداشت روانی و

پرستاری ازبیماران روانی طرح شده وشامل قسمتهای ذیل است.
رشد شخصیت ،شناخت رفتارهای انحرافی ،روابط انسانی واصول
پرستاری روانی ، طبقه بندی بیماریهای روانی ،اصول درمان و
مراقبت های پرستاری ،پرستاری درمورد معالجات مخصوص ،
مسئولیتهای پرستارروانی

موضوع	ساعات نظری	آزمایشگاه وعملی	سال تحصیلی	هفته های کارآموزی
آناتومی وفیزیولوژی	۸۰	۱۰	سال اول	
میکروب شناسی	۳۰	۱۵	"	
شیمی	۲۷	۸	"	
علم الاغذیه	۳۵	۵	"	
روانشناسی	۲۰	—	"	
جامعه شناسی	۱۵	—	"	
تاریخ واخلاق پرستاری	۲۵	—	"	
بهداشت	۳۰	۵	"	
پرستاری	۷۰	۸۰	"	
کمکهای اولیه	۱۰	۵	"	
زبان انگلیسی	۷۵	—	"	

جراحی شامل :

جراحی عمومی — سال دوم

" حفره شکم

" استخوان

" قفسه سینه

• دستگاه ادرار	۸۰	—	•	حداقل ۳۲ هفته دربخشهای جراحی درسالهای اول ، دوم یا سوم.

بیماریهای داخلی شامل :

بیماریهای اعصاب

• غدد اندوکرین

• قلب وعروق

• خون

• عفونی

• دستگاه تنفسی

• دستگاه ادرار

• دستگاه گوارش	۱۰۰	—	سال دوم	حداقل ۳۲ هفته دربخشهای داخلی درسالهای اول ، دوم یا سوم
علم بیهوشی	۸	—	•	
تکنیک اطاق عمل	۶	۲	•	حداقل ۸ هفته در اطاق عمل

— ۲۲ —

پرستاران بیماران داخلی وجراحی	۵۰	۵٤	*	
داروشناسی	٤۰	—		سال‌دوم‌وسال‌سوم
بیماریهای زنان‌وزایمان پرستاری مربوطه	۵۰	—		سال‌سوم حداقل ۸تا ۱۲ هفته درسال‌دوم وچها سوم.
بیماریهای چشم وپرستاری مربوطه	۳۰	٦	*	حداقل ۸ هفته در سال‌دوم ویاسوم
بیماریهای گوش وحلق وبینی وپرستاری مربوطه	۲۰	—		سال‌سوم
بیماریهای کودکان و پرستاری مربوطه	۳۲	۸	*	حداقل ۱۰ هفته درسال دومیاسوم
بیماریهای روانی وپرستاری مربوطه	۳۲	—	*	حداقل ۸ هفته درسال سوم
پرستاری بهداشت وتنظیم خانواده	۲٤	٦	*	
بیماریهای پوست	۱۲	—	*	
بیماریهای آمیزشی	۱۲	—	*	
اداره اموربخشها	۲۰	—	*	

III

THE BEGINNINGS OF OBSTETRICS IN IRAN

Mother and infant mortality in Iran was high until recent times due to a combination of socio-economic, cultural and religious factors, which resulted in women delivering babies at home aided by untrained traditional helpers. The unhygienic conditions in the house and people's poverty endangered the life of both mother and child, even after a successful delivery. American and British missionary hospitals offered modern and safe obstetric services, while they pioneered the introduction of pre- and postnatal care as well as of baby clinics. Their practice was the example on which the government of Iran modeled its own early programs to offer similar services and formed the basis of its public health policy in this area.

Introduction

In 1949, according to the Seven-Year Development Plan, there were no prenatal clinics, and

> Nowhere in Iran are mothers examined in advance of delivery except in the case of acute illness. ... Most babies are delivered by untrained midwives or without any assistance to the mother resulting in high maternal death from puerperal infections and hemorrhages, and high infant deaths due to neonatal tetanus and infant diarrhea. ... Also, there is a high incidence of congenital syphilis. Premature births receive as yet no attention.[1]

1. Overseas Consultants 1949, vol. 2, pp. 32-33.

The mother-and-child health situation in Iran was indeed a precarious one and the above characterization of their situation is mostly correct. I wrote 'mostly correct', because there were a few hospitals in Iran where deliveries were done by trained professionals. In Tehran, the Women's Hospital (*Marizkhaneh-ye Nesvan*, later called *Bimarestan-e Zanan*), a small one with 20 beds, became operational in 1918. The proposal for the hospital had been submitted by Dr. Amir-e A`lam on 5 May 1915. The government adopted the idea already on 20 July 1915 and a government-owned building was assigned as the premises for the hospital. Two French midwives were supposed to have been hired to train Iranian midwives, but the outbreak of the Great War made that impossible. Instead the services of Mme. Fraskina, who had been trained as a midwife in Europe and was working as such in Tehran, were engaged. When the hospital was officially opened much money was collected, but it was not enough to make the hospital functional. In 1916, there was no money to buy 50 beds and other equipment, but the Iranian government allocated 3,600 *tuman*s to pay for the staff. As a result, the hospital functioned as a gynecological out-patients' dispensary, which, as of March 1916 until 1924, was managed by Dr. `Ali Reza Bahrami Mohadhdhab al-Saltaneh. In September 1918, the then Minister of Endowments (*Owqaf*) tried to raise funds to properly equip the building and turn it into a real hospital. He was only able to acquire funds to buy six beds, where from September 1918 until March 1919 about sixty women gave birth. During that period Mme. Fraskina trained 10 Iranian girls to become mid-wives. After the end of Great War, funds became available to establish an internal medicine and surgical (obstetrics) department in the Women's Hospital, which was led by Dr. Sa`id Malek Loqman al-Mamalek. Mme Fraskina was replaced by a French female physician Dr. Dermes, who remained there until 1934. In that year Dr. Jahanshah Saleh became director of the hospital and was in charge of the obstetric department.[2] Thereafter, the hospital served as training center for the Medical School

2. Rusta'i 1385, vol. 2, p. 558; After Dr. Dermes, Drs. Pann and Serkessian worked in the hospital. Malekzadeh 1392, p. 215; Idem 1394, p. 70.

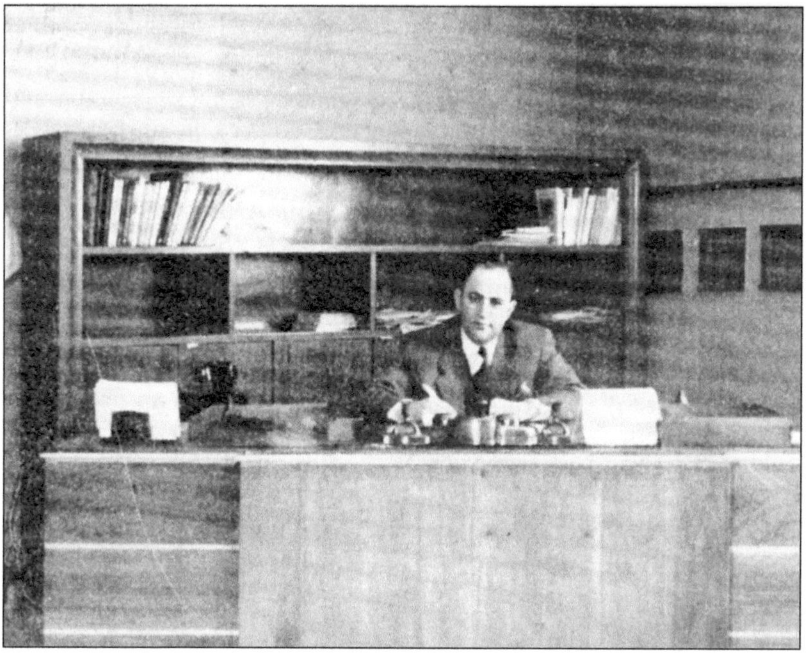

Dr. Jahanshah Saleh, dean of the Medical School of Tehran University

for Midwifes (*Madraseh-ye Qabelegi*), while women continued to be admitted to give birth. During 1923-24, of 107 in-patients, 20 suffered from malaria (14%), while of 1,342 outpatients treated, 192 suffered from malaria (18%).[3] In 1943, the hospital moved to a new building, while the old building was turned into the *Bimarestan-e Amir-e A`lam*, an otolaryngology clinic of the medical faculty.

In 1920, Nasir al-Dowleh (Ahmad Bader) founded a three-year high school program with 10 students at the Women- Teachers' School (*Dar al-mo`allemat*), which was called the Medical School for Midwifes (*Madraseh-ye Qabelegi*). In 1921, it had 13 students, who all belonged to elite families; instruction was in French. They received a training of three years that was focused on women's diseases and obstetrics. On graduating the student received a diploma. They were not physicians,

3. Gilmour 1924, p. 27. For a detailed discussion about the genesis and development of this school, see Malekzadeh 1394, pp. 66-70, 88-90, 124-85.

but more broadly trained than mid-wives.[4] Although midwifery was a subject that was taught at the *Madraseh-ye Tebb* since 1918 by Yunes Khan, it was ineffective, because the students were males and the teaching was entirely theoretical. In 1920, Masih al-Saltaneh translated a text about midwifery into Persian, but it does not seem to have been printed.[5] In the mid-1930s, Amir A`lam, the Minister of Public Health started the project of creating maternity centers (*dar al-veladah*) and schools of midwifery.[6] The *Madraseh-ye Qabelegi* was renamed the Higher School of Midwifery (*Amuzeshgah-e `ali-ye mama'i*). In 1940, the Women's hospital became part of the Faculty of Medicine of the University of Tehran. From 1949 it only accepted graduates of the Ashraf Pahlavi Nursing School and later those of other nursing schools, who, after taking the one-year program of the School, were granted the bachelor degree in midwifery.[7]

This *Nesvan* appears to have been the only Iranian hospital that provided midwifery services, although in 1931, in Bushehr, the wife of Dr. Muniri, the Quarantine and Health officer, held a French diploma in midwifery. She was hired to take charge of the *Shahdokht Maternity Hospital* for some time at 80 *tuman*s per month. In April 1931, she began a class of ten girls with an elementary school diploma training them in "midwifery and treatment of female cases."[8] However, there is no further information available on the continuation and activities of Mrs. Muniri and the maternity hospital. In addition, there were a few trained midwives, like Mme Fraskina, who were hired by wealthy patients to deliver their babies. Another initiative took place in Shiraz. In 1932, the municipality of Shiraz asked Dr. Zabih Ghorban to take charge of the *Behbudestan* and to have 30 beds available for the poor. When Dr. Ghorban's sister Keyhan graduated in nursing and midwifery

4. Gilmour 1924, p. 27. For a detailed discussion about the genesis and development of this school, see Malekzadeh 1394, pp. 66-70, 88-90, 124-85.

5. Malekzadeh 1394, pp. 70-74, 79.

6. Ebrahimnezhad 2014, p. 157.

7. Karamati 1999.

8. Administration Report 1931, p. 5; Political Diaries, vol. 9, p. 483.

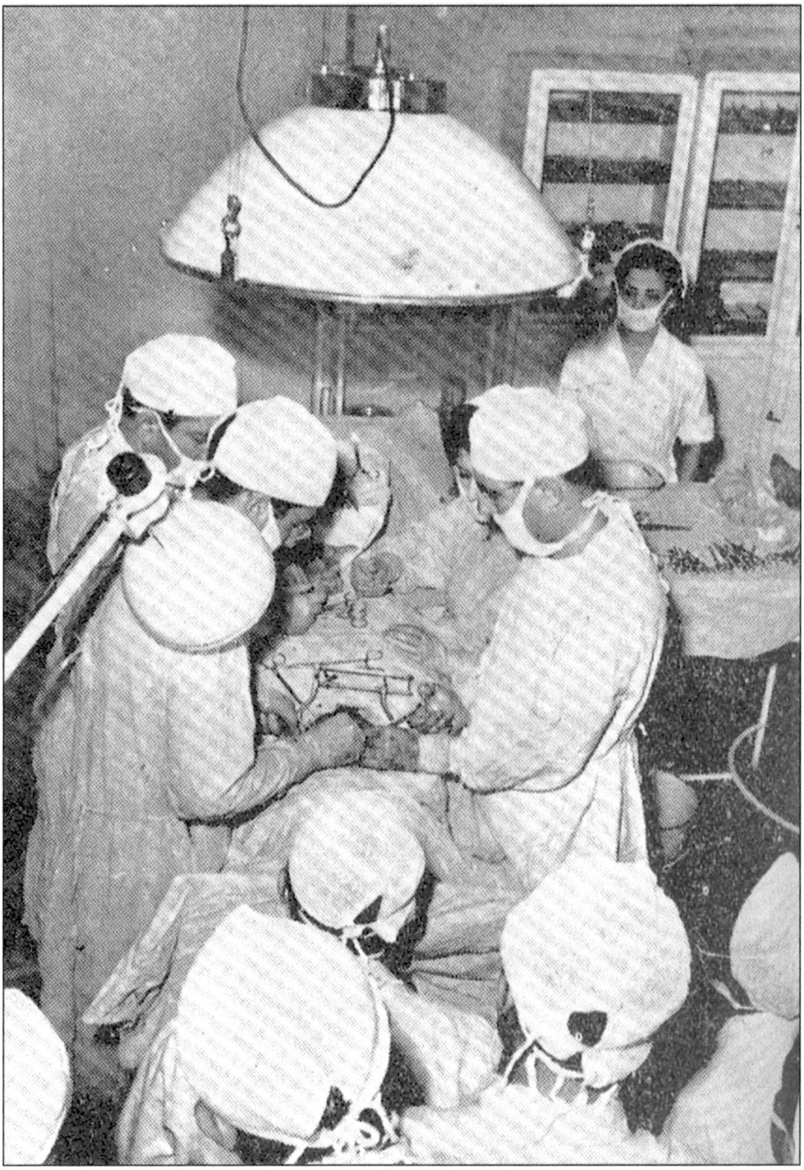

Operation at the Nesvan hospital in Tehran

from the American University of Beirut, he asked her to come and take charge of nursing at the *Behbudestan*, and train a few female staff members, whom he had convinced to volunteer for this task.[9]

As of 1920, the government in Tehran intermittently notified the various municipalities that only certified midwives were allowed to practice, but since there were hardly any graduates of the midwifery school, this notification remained a dead letter. There is the occasional action concerning single midwives, but like the above notification and many other regulations, these were merely well-intended symbolic gestures. Even the arrival of some Russian trained midwives after the October Revolution did not make a difference. That does not mean that these various rules and regulations were unnecessary or superfluous, but there was as yet neither a public health apparatus to supervise their implementation nor the practitioners (in the absence of trained graduates) to be supervised, apart from a few in Tehran. Also, under Reza Shah's reign new regulations and proposals by both government and civil society (women organizations) continued to be made after further reflection on the ills and needs concerning childbirth.[10] The result was that practically all children were still delivered with the help of traditional midwives in very unhygienic conditions leading to high a high mortality rate among newborns and mothers.

However, there were hospitals in Iran where modern prenatal and postnatal care was given, in addition to midwifery and obstetrics services. Consequently, also attention was given to premature births. This care was given by American and British missionary hospitals, which actually had very proactive obstetrics programs in place. Why the authors of the Seven-Year Plan totally ignored that experience and practice of the missionary hospitals is unknown. They only reported that "wealthy families have good care through private physicians, and the few trained midwives serve the small middle-class at Rls. 400 per

9. Ghorban 1989, p. 4.

10. On these various activities and regulations, see Malekzadeh 1394, pp. 76-88, 90-103. However, there remained a shortage of trained midwives and traditional midwives continued to work without permission to practice. Ebrahimnejad 2014, p. 140.

delivery."[11] Therefore, it is important to describe the mother-and-child practice pioneered by the missionary hospitals in Iran, on which all later mother-and-child programs were built.

Until recent times, Iran was a pre-modern society, which restricted women's social contacts outside the immediate family and in particular with men. Also, there was great reluctance to go to a hospital for medical care and it was impossible for a male physician to examine a woman. Although Dr. Polak wrote in 1861 that he had no difficulty examining Iranian women this examination probably was very limited in scope. Although, between 1854 and 1860, he performed lithomy operations on at least nine female patients, these were mostly very young girls.[12] For even in 1921, when a 30-bed missionary hospital, with room for five babies, was functioning in Tabriz, the lack of a female doctor was sorely felt, as Iranian women did not allow themselves to be examined by a male physician, even in their greatest need.[13] In Rasht, in that same year, the situation was somewhat better. Dr. Frame reported that a daughter of a chief mullah came to see him, while 10 years ago her sister chose death rather than allow him to treat her after confinement.[14]

But even women physicians felt that they had to be careful. In the 1890s, Dr. Mary Smith, who worked in the Tehran missionary hospital, feared to admit women in-patients, due to Moslem prejudice.

11. Overseas Consultants 1949, vol. 2, pp. 32-33.

12. Polak 1853, p. 219; Idem 1860, p. 679.

13. Presbyterian Church 1922, pp. 377-78; Anonymous 1922, p. 146. The same situation existed in Ahvaz where the British government had a dispensary managed by a physician. Nevertheless, it was noted that: "Midwifery practice is withheld from the practitioner by all classes, native women being usually attended by the older members of their sex. The upper classes may send for assistance when danger arises, but this is rare. Death from labour occur, and such reports reach the dispensary from time to time." IOR/L/MIL/17/15/10/1, *Military Report on S. W. Persia*, vol. 1, p. 43.

14. RG 91-19-9, Resht Medical Report 1921-22; Idem, Resht Medical Report 1919-20; Idem, "History of Resht Station," p. 3; Idem, Resht Medical Report 1932.

Although this prejudice was diminishing, she observed that a certain category of women did not even have the opportunity to visit the dispensary. Therefore, she opined that house calls were important, for "It is only by going to their homes that one can reach this class of [wealthy and influential] women, as they would never be allowed to come to the dispensary."[15] In 1906, it was reported that medical work in Tehran had increased in quantity and quality, especially for women. However, medical work for women was limited to eye cases and minor surgical ones. Women requiring major surgery were not admitted out of fear that a death might produce a severe prejudice against the missionaries' medical work.[16]

There was the additional problem that women had to first secure permission from their husband and then have to arrange for care of their children before they would be able to enter the hospital. Overtime, visits by women to the hospital became more acceptable and common. For example, in 1940, in the out-patients department of the missionary hospital in Hamadan, doctors saw more women than men, when they were able to get away long enough to see the doctor.[17] Also, apart from economic and social constraints there was much superstition to be overcome regarding childbirth. Dr. Mary Zoeckler, who worked in Malayer (Dowlatabad), reported in 1924 that she was very busy with many night calls and increased obstretical work. At that time, one of the American missionaries gave birth, which

> was one maternity case in Daulatabad where no one pawned the patient's chuddar at the nearest grocery shop for a few dates, or hung on the latch of the door to make the baby's coming easier; where the patient was allowed all the water she wanted and not made to drink a quart or so of grease so that she would get well quicker; and where no precautions at all were taken to keep the 'Aul' away. The Persians here have a great fear at such times that the aul, which belongs to the race of jinns, will come and

15. Presbyterian Church 1902, p. 221.
16. RG 91-19-11-1, Historical Sketch of Teheran Medical Work; Presbyterian Church 1907, pp. 302-03.
17. RG 91-19-27, Healing in Hamadan 1940.

> snatch out the heart and liver of the patient and then disapeear, in which case the patient will surely die. Sometinmes, instead of killing the mother the aul will substitute a jinn child for the real one. In order to keep the aul away the never for a minite leave the patient or child alone. They put an onion on an iron spit and tap the walls of the room all around, one asking "for the sake of whom" and another replying "For the sake of Mary and her son Jesus." Then the spit with the onion and some other sharp object, a sword or a pair of scissors, is put at the patient's head to frighten the Aul away. The 7th night is the most dangerous time. On that night they put a black rope all around the patient's bed and invite many guests who help to keep the patient awake till after midnight when the danger is supposed to be past.[18]

There also was opposition to the missionaries themselves and their medical care by religious leaders, and, by extension by many believers. They feared that the American missionaries would be able to lead Moslem believers astray by converting them to their infidel Christian religion. The Moslem believers mostly overcame their prejudice after having seen the advantage of the infidel medical care, but many religious leaders were holdouts. In 1929, an interesting case occurred involving the daughter of the leading *mojtahed* in Malayer, who had been very hostile to the missionary activity in his town. Against their better knowledge some relatives brought his daughter to Dr. Mary Zoeckler as a last resort, who said she needed to use forceps to deliver the child. This required the permission of the Aqa, so Dr. Zoekcler hurried to his house, where she did not get an enthusiastic reception. The *mojtahed* first wanted to cut the Qur'an (a form of divination), but one of the leading local merchants, who were sitting with the Aqa, convinced him to leave fate in the doctor's hands. After the Aqa had grudgingly given his permission, Dr. Zoeckler hurried back and wanted to start the procedure. However, somebody sneezed and thus, she had to wait until somebody else sneezed, and this happened

---

18. RG 280-1-10, Report Medical Work Daulatabad 1924. On the *Al*, see Eilers 1979. In general, see UNESCO, 1963, vol. 1, pp. 175-76.

three times. Finally, she could start and delivered a dead baby at 10 p.m. although the child's head had already been visible since 3 p.m.[19]

As a result of the absence of proper medical care for pregnant women and their newborns, infant and maternal mortality was high in Iran. Often, mothers, who came to the hospital, had only one or two living children out of eight or ten. The main cause was ignorance, both on the part of the mothers and the traditional midwives or *mamma*s. According to Dr. Adelaide Kibbe, the 'mammas' were illiterate women who never had the opportunity to learn:

> I caught one them, a popular one, with a dirty, bloody rag around a large sore on her hand; even she knew better than this, and was chagrined. None of the young women from the government's well-organized school of midwifery have come to Meshed, let alone to any of the lesser cities of Khorasan, and there is no government control of midwives.[20]

It took some time for Dr. Kibbe to develop confidence among the people. Most women still preferred home confinements with all its bad consequences (dead babies, puerperal infection, and crippled lives).[21] Of course, mistrust of the foreign doctor was a major obstacle to change that situation. According to Dr. Kibbe, a major problem was: "the teaching and training of the local midwives. Theses 'mammas' have not, of course, rushed to us eager for knowledge, but ready with dirty herbs, or sticks, or fingers, remain in the background, a sinister menace to every woman. And when a poor woman comes in, you know she is infected." Babies were brought unwashed to the clinic, were fed when they cried, joggled all day, stuffed with tea or sweets or even cucumbers, or soothed with a 'bit' of opium from the day they were born. No use to say, "Bathe your child daily," for they would have to take it to the bath, an impossible expense and those baths

---

19. RG 280-1-10, Report Medical Work Daulatabad 1928-1929.
20. RG 91-20-2, Mashad Medical Report 1932-1933. In Richardson's dictionary the term for midwifery is: *mama'i* and *dayehgari*; another term used in Persian is *qabelegi*.
21. RG 91-20-2, Mashad Medical Report 1932-1933.

are a menace in themselves. 'Give it whole cow's milk, and cereals and vitamins and eggs from seven to nine months on;' it would take a month's wages to buy these 'luxuries' for even a week for most families! Even having a nursery connected to the hospital, where the mother might be taught proper care for the child was considered as a partial solution, although that was not without difficulties either.[22]

Obstetrics Programs per City

Given these social, economic, cultural and religious obstacles it comes as little surprise that in the field of obstetrics the modern hospitals only rarely were asked to provide care. In fact, despite the presence of modern hospitals since the 1880s, obstetrics was little in demand as a medical service, for all of the above reasons. Even the presence of female physicians was not yet a sufficient factor to overcome these cultural constraints. The first hospital that started a regular obstetrics program was not in Tehran, but in Hamadan. It was happenstance, due to the wave of Assyrian refugees in 1918. It so happened that there was much obstretical work among the refugee women, which was a novelty, because Moslem women in Hamadan rarely came to a physician, and never to the hospital.[23] Since then was a growth of obgyn cases in the Hamadan Christian Hospital. As of the early 1930s, obstetrics also acquired increasingly more importance in the other Christian hospitals, when women (and their families) lost their fear of coming to a hospital for treatment.

Tehran

It was only in 1931 that obstetrical work began in Tehran under Ms Tallie and this line of work was developing well with patients from the servant's wife to the queen's sister. Ms Taillie also had a private practice for wealthy patients. The income from this activity was a

22. RG 91-20-2, Mashad Medical Report 1929-1930.
23. Presbyterian Church 1922, pp. 366-67; RG 280-1-10, Report Medical Work Hamadan 1920-21.

boon for the missionary hospital's finances.[24] Only a few years earlier, maternity work had been limited to emergencies brought after days of neglect. As of 1932, most cases were planned in advance. After Ms Taillie's departure in 1933, maternity service continued progressively. The idea of delivery in the hospital was gaining popularity among all classes. According to Dr. McDowell, credit should be given to the US-trained Dr. Abu'l-Hasan Bakhtiyar, who, as of 1931, had put the government hospital for women and the school for midwives on a sound basis. Furthermore, he was spreading the idea of the need for sound midwifery and hospitalization.[25]

In 1934-35, demand for hospital beds was increasing, especially for obstetrical services, which showed an increase of almost 50% in that year. The number of well-to-do Iranian patients increased and helped the hospital's bottom line. This ob-gyn service should be expanded, Dr. McDowell argued, because the hospital would not be treading on the toes of jealous Iranian colleagues. Also, it was a service that otherwise was inadequately given and there was an increased demand for it. Therefore, a US nurse was needed to provide oversight.[26] In 1935-36, the hospital's obstetrical department again reported a 50% increase in patients. There were 137 maternity cases, because increasingly, women realized the advantage of childbirth in the hospital as well as of prenatal care. In fact, 95% of maternity patients had received prenatal care in the dispensary. The women's dispensary was numerically embarrassing. In fact, there were too many patients and the doctors were at a loss how to reduce their number. All old patients were admitted, but only 20 new patients per morning were seen. These 20 tickets were gone before much of the morning had passed. Then the hard task was to turn the others away, which was difficult when they were sick and had come walking quite a distance, especially if they had been turned away before. However, emergencies

---

24. RG 91-19-11-1, Report Medical Work Teheran 1931-1932.
25. RG 91-19-11-1, Report Teheran Hospital 1933; Malekzadeh 1392, p. 216. For a short biography of Dr. Bakhtiar, see Azizi 2014 b, pp. 295-97.
26. RG 91-19-11-1, Report Tehran Medical Work 1934-1935.

were always admitted. As a result, there were more women in-patients than men, due to the greater number of maternity patients. The private rooms were well filled and several times the 6-bed ward was turned into a semi-private ward for maternity patients, who wanted private rooms, when there weren't any.[27]

The women's clinic continued to grow and, in fact, it was the best-known department of the hospital. For several years during spring and fall doctors had to turn away patients, because they could not properly care for them. In 1936-37, despite almost doubling the consultation fees, it still was necessary to limit admissions. Dr. McDowell and Dr. Varjavand were both very busy on the three weekly clinic days. Women's in-patient service was limited by the number of 23 beds and quite a few women were put up in the private rooms on the men's side. The maternity service was popular among the well-to-do and prenatal care was experienced as accepted routine.[28]

The obstetrical department continued to grow and was a good source of income. The hospital had to add a number of bassinettes, because several times babies had to lie on tables, on the pan of the scales and even on the window sill. The demand for obstetrical service was also growing in the city; about 1,000 were cared for in private and public institutions annually. The amount of prenatal work was difficult to assess. "The majority of the poor who are delivered at the Nesvan, Zayeshgah, etc. are abnormal cases referred to by midwives. Probably ours is the largest prenatal clinic," Dr. McDowell wrote. The missionary hospital normally didn't accept cases that had not been seen in the clinic, thus avoiding infectious cases. The doctors considered putting in a separate service for abnormal and infected cases, which, however, required the adding of additional space to this department.[29]

---

27. RG 91-19-11-1, Report Teheran Hospital 1936.

28. RG 91-19-11-1, Report Teheran Hospital 1937 (Twice there were 11 newborns in the nursery this year. The number of confinements showed an increase of 30 over 137 last year).

29. RG 91-19-11-1, Report Medical Work Teheran 1937-1938 (15 at a time is the largest number we had; in total 245 deliveries).

In 1940, the hospital employed two women doctors, one Swiss and the other Czech, who assisted in the women's dispensary and the OR (operation room) as non-paid helpers.[30] The obstetrical service developed by Dr. McDowell was very successful as indicated by the number of deliveries during the eight last eight years:

1934: 65	1935: 94	1936: 138
1937: 169	1938: 245	1939: 307
1940: 350	1941: 415	1942 ?

This was striking evidence of the rapid modernization from the women's point of view. The obstetrical service was developed under a male physician and the hospital's women physicians had never been able to develop something comparable, probably because Iranian women needed to get used to the novel idea of going to the hospital for the delivery of a baby rather than doing it the normal way, i.e. at home, with the help of a traditional midwife. What was even more remarkable was that by 1940 about half of all deliveries were attended by Dr. Varjavand, an Iranian physician. The women's out-patient department consisted of a prenatal exam, attended by a doctor and a nurse.[31] Obstetrical services continued to flourish till the closure of the hospital in 1942. Although in 1941-42, there were only 340 deliveries compared with 415 in the previous year and 350 before that, this drop was mainly due to war scarcity and the city curfew.[32]

HAMADAN

In 1918, after the start of obstetrical work among the refugee women the number of ob-gyn cases continued to grow. By 1933, the obstetrical department had expanded considerably, since the first female physician started working in the hospital. Whereas initially most women seeking

30. RG 91-19-11-1, Report American Hospital Teheran 1940-1941. The female doctors probably had been unable to get a license to practice.
31. RG 91-19-11-1, Report American Hospital Teheran, Iran1940-1941.
32. RG 91-19-11-1, Teheran Medical Report 1941-1942.

medical help were non-Moslems, in 1933 half of the women were Moslems, indicating that more women were appreciating sound medical advice. It also showed that women had greater confidence in male doctors and "increasing freedom from bigotry and oriental reserve." As a result, there were more confinements and gynecological cases than before.[33] In 1935, there were more obstetrical cases -217- than ever before, indicating women's growing confidence in doctors rather than in midwives. Several were emergencies requiring operations. Many patients came from outside Hamadan, and the hospital found itself in competition with its sister hospital in Kermanshah and vice versa.[34]

To better serve pregnant women, maternity classes were started, which lowered the reluctance to give birth in the hospital. In fact, in 1938, a total of 47 babies were born in the hospital, which was considered to be "quite an advancement, since only a short time ago we considered half of that number unusual." At the same time, it was an indication of greater freedom for Moslem women, because earlier most confinements were by non-Moslem women.[35] Although the number of obstetrical cases increased, most women still preferred "to deliver at home often by untrained and not all-too-clean midwives with post-puerperal complications."[36] With the departure of Dr. Mary Zoeckler in 1945, the number of female patients decreased; many women refused to be examined by Dr. Cohn, the male physician. However, when in 1946, the governor's wife gave birth to her child in the American hospital there was an upsurge in confinement cases. She was delivered by one of the graduate nurses with the doctor standing by outside in case of need.[37]

---

33. RG 91-19-27, Hamadan Medical Report 1933; Idem, Hamadan Medical Report 1934.
34. RG 91-19-27, Hamadan Medical Report 1934; Idem, Hamadan Medical Report 1935; Idem, Healing in the Home of Avicenna 1936.
35. RG 91-19-27, Hamadan Medical Report 1937; Idem, Hamadan Medical Report 1937-1938 (in 1938 only 28 babies were born in the hospital, all of them were difficult cases).
36. RG 91-19-27, Healing in Hamadan 1940.
37. RG 91-19-27, Hamadan Medical Report 1945-1946.

Kermanshah

With the opening of the new missionary hospital in 1932, for unknown reasons, obstretics was not as busy as the doctors had hoped. During 1932-33, there were only five ceasarians in the hospital and one in the city. Nevertheless, in that year, women patients outnumbered the men, so that sometimes empty space on the men's floor was used for women.[38] The women's ward and clinic was very important as it provided targeted and much needed quality care to women. Ceasareans were performed and general obstretics care was given. These obstretics services were a boon for the women of Kermanshah because there was no other venue, apart from some midwives who dabbled in medicine. More special attention could be given when Dr. Jenny Stead, who intermittenly was available between 1932-37, and in 1938 Dr. Mary Zoekcler, and, as of 1944, Dr. Frances Zoeckler were on call. These female physicians were in charge of the women's ward and the women's clinic.[39]

Malayer

When Dr. Mary Zoeckler returned to Malayer in January 1938, the midwife situation was very bad. The one who treated upper class women had died the year before, and her successors (three old women, and some who had no experience at all) were worse. The arrival of a trained midwife, therefore, was a boon, be it that on the negative side, such trained women tended also to present themselves as a gynecologist, which they were not. The midwife was a disappointment; she did good work, but was dissatisfied with her income and left in April

---

38. RG 91-19-28, Kermanshah Westminster Hospital 1933.

39. RG 91-19-28, Kermanshah Westminster Hospital 1933; Idem, Kermanshah Westminster Hospital 1933-1934; Idem, Kermanshah Medical Report 1937; Idem, Kermanshah Westminster Hospital 1938; Idem, Kermanshah Westminster Hospital Kermanshah 1938-39; Idem, The Westminster Hospital Bulletin. vol. 2/1. October 1939; Idem, Kermanshah Westminster Hospital 1944-45; Government of Great Britain 1945, p. 410.

1940.[40] Despite these changes, Dr. Zoeckler had plenty of work. One complaint of women was sterility, even though they already had eight children. But their reply was: "I have none left, or sometimes only one daughter, and my husband may divorce me." This situation stood in contrast with that of Hamadan and Kermanshah where missionary doctors were often called to rescue more sophisticated women from the ill-effects of self-induced abortions, or to provide contraceptive information.[41]

Mashhad

Although the male doctors in the missionary hospitals treated ob-gyn cases, even some complicated ones, these were exceptions to the rule. Even as late as 1933, "Obstetrical work in Meshed is still an almost untouched field," wrote Dr. Adelaide Kibbe.[42] In the 1930s, the number of children admitted to the hospital increased, showing that mothers had more confidence in the hospital. Obstetrical cases also increased and were taken care of by Ms Nelson R.N. or one of the Armenian nurses, and in special need the doctor was called.[43] In 1931-32, there was an increase in obstetrical cases, 60% more than the previous year, due to the presence of Dr. Adelaide Kibbe.[44] This trend continued thereafter. In 1932-33, more women than before came for their confinement- 34 of total 41 obstetrical cases; most of them had normal deliveries. Of 13 operative cases two were Cesareans; one hydrocephalic.[45] In 1934-35, there were 62 maternity cases. Dr. Kibbe's work with women was more than ever appreciated by the public and by local doctors, who sent women for examination and treatment. Maternity cases brought after having been botched by ignorant midwives were difficult ones; fetal mortality was 18%,

---

40. RG 280-1-10, Report Daulatabad Medical Work 1939-1940.
41. RG 280-1-10, Report Daulatabad Medical Work1938-1939.
42. RG 91-20-2, Mashad Medical Report 1932-1933.
43. RG 91-20-2, Mashad Medical Report 1929.
44. RG 91-19-2, Mashad Medical Report 1931-1932.
45. RG 91-20-2, Mashad Medical Report 1932-1933.

but all mothers survived.[46] When Dr. Kibbe left in October 1937 to begin working in Rasht, there was an immediate drop of obstetrical and genealogical cases. She had worked in Mashhad from 1929 to 1938, and during that period the number of obstetrical cases trebled. Dr. Cochran took over the women's wards.[47]

RASHT

In 1924, there was as yet no ob-gyn program; nevertheless, the hospital treated a case of extra-uterine pregnancy in that year.[48] In 1931, as in other American missionary hospitals, there was an increase in female patients. Obstetrics cases increased by 48% and 45% of major operations were gynecological or obstetrical. With infectious cases, abscesses, pneumonia, and influenza it was increasingly difficult to provide proper safeguards for obstetrical and clean operative cases. Therefore, Dr. Frame was very happy with a donation of $1,000 from Mrs. Meytag to add a small wing for women's patients and nurses' rooms. He intended to add seven beds, be it in small units. One unit was a small room for new born babies, who until then were kept in the operating room, when it was not used or who were parked somewhere in the hospital if it was. The same held for new mothers, who should not be in the general ward with cases of influenza, pneumonia, septic condition etc.[49]

In August 1931, Dr. Frame had eight obstetrics cases in nine days, which filled the female ward and private rooms to capacity. At that time, the addition was almost finished only lacking the final plaster coat, the woodwork was unpainted, etc., but the rooms were habitable, so the tenth patient was moved in after 10 minutes. The addition accommodated five beds and the sun parlor 3-4 patients. The addition also freed space in the main building for obstetrics and the

---

46. RG 91-20-2, Mashad Medical Report 1934-1935.
47. RG 91-20-2, Mashad Medical Report 1937-1938.
48. RG91-19-9, Resht Medical Report 1923-24.
49. RG 91-19-9, Resht Medical Report 1931; RG 91-20-8, Frame/Rasht to Speer/NY (17/02/1931).

care for babies. This was essential given the increase of obstetric cases from 33 in 1930-31 to 53 in 1931-32, and the babies to be cared for from 25 to 35. The desperate nature of these cases was indicated by 40 major operations on 53 cases. "Nevertheless, such is the resistance of the women to the mishandling of Persian midwives before admission that only four died, one of them moribund on admission." Sometimes, the women traveled many kilometers on horse or by car after many days of labor in the villages.[50]

Prenatal instruction to mothers was important in view of the increasing number of obstetric cases. This also became easier, because "More and more women are less willing to trust themselves to nature or Persian midwives." There was even the case of a marriage contract that stipulated that if the wife became pregnant "she was to have care in a private room in the American Hospital."[51] After having built a small addition to the women's wing in 1936, it was filled to overflowing with obstetrical cases.[52] Dr. Adelaide Kibbe arrived in October 1937 from Mashhad. It was a new experience for the city to have a female doctor, who was an obstetrician and a surgeon. She did a Caesarean without the help of other doctors, which amazed a British doctor working in the National Hospital in Rasht. Another surprise caused by Dr. Kibbe happened during Dr. Hoffman's illness (who replaced Frame during his furlough). One male patient left the physician's office saying he wanted a doctor not a midwife, but a former patient said he would take his chance with the female physician.[53] Due to the increase in obstetrical cases, "with one physician and several well trained midwives in the city our percentage of major operative obstetrics continues high," according to Dr. Kibbe. In 1937-38, the hospital scored a new record with more than 60 obstetric cases to deliver in the hospital. Many of them were abnormal, coming in after unsuccessful attempts by local midwives, but the number of normal

---

50. RG 91-19-9, Rest Medical Report 1932; Idem, Resht Medical Work 1932.

51. RG 91-19-9, Rest Medical Report 1933.

52. Presbyterian Church 1936, p. 151.

53. RG 91-19-9, Resht Hospital Report, 1937-38,

cases also was increasing. Out-patients and lab work showed an increase in maternity cases, especially of those coming for the free clinic, due to the financial situation of peasants. Dr. Frame had decided not to deny them admission.[54] In 1940, Dr. Frame remarked that the obstetric department was a good indicator of social and medical progress of the community, especially as this related to the life of women. Deliveries increased by 50% in that year, while 48 major operations were needed out of 128 cases. In Rasht improvement might be higher, because in 1940 there were more qualified midwives working in the city. In the villages, matters were still bad; many times, it took days before a woman was brought and doctors could only marvel at women's stamina and recovery.[55]

In 1943, there was a 9- or 10-bed maternity hospital operated by municipal taxes and supervised by a committee of prominent women, two of them midwives. It attracted a large number of the Christian hospital's free obstetrical cases, but not all and those who were able to pay anything preferred to come to the American doctor. When in June 1943 news leaked out that Dr. Kibbe-Frame was taking a vacation, immediately many people, especially women, tried to see her.[56] After the newspaper announced the proposed building of a Maternity Hospital in Rasht and Tabriz under the shah's patronage, Dr. Frame decided to further adapt this special service center and find ways to the changing medical needs of the community.[57] The above-mentioned ten-bed hospital sponsored by some leading women for obstetrical work continued to give help to many.

SHIRAZ

Initially, a building in a garden had been rented, but in 1924, with a donation of land by Hajj Mohammad Hoseyn Namazi, a maternity hospital was built. It was subsequently converted into a large general

---

54. RG 91-19-9, Resht Hospital Reports 1918-44 1937-38.
55. RG 91-19-9, Resht Hospital Report 1939-40.
56. RG 91-19-9, Resht Hospital Report 1943.
57. RG 91-19-9, Resht Hospital Report 1940-1941.

hospital with financial assistance of the IETD. The CMS hospital in Shiraz, known as *Bimarestan-e Morsalin*, established in 1924, had a male and female ward, a midwifery department plus an out-patient department.[58]

Tabriz

Because the annual medical reports have not been preserved little is known about the daily practice in the missionary hospital in Tabriz, after 1920. But a few available data show that the trend seen elsewhere in missionary hospitals also was seen in Tabriz. In 1929, it was reported that "Persian women are coming in greater numbers and the work among children has greatly increased. Follow-up work has had to be curtailed on account of the smallness of the hospital force."[59] In the 1930 and 1940s, the Tabriz hospital was full of patients and busy with baby clinics, nurses' training classes, etc.[60]

Urumiyeh

Because the old Urumiyeh missionary hospital or Galla [*qal`eh*] was situated 3 km outside the city there was little work with women and practically no maternity work, because it was hard for Moslem women to go that far.[61] Women felt afraid to go out of the city to the old hospital, where only with difficulty, friends and family were able to visit them and they were fearful to be away from them.[62] With the

58. Elgood 1951, pp. 534-535; Waterfield 1973, p. 166; Anonymous 1924, p. 182; Williams 1994, pp. 60-61; Azizi, Bahadori, and Raees-Jalali 2014 , p. 240. The move in 1922 had been facilitated by the fact that the IETD had asked the CMS to take over the medical care of its employees, on generous terms, when its own physician retired. Waterfield 1973, pp. 165-166.

59. Presbyterian Church 1929, p. 103.

60. Presbyterian Church 1947, p. 55-56.

61. RG 91-20-7, Elli/Urumiyeh to Williamson, charge d'affaires/Tehran (30/09/1930).

62. RG 91-20-7, Report Medical Work Urumia 1922-1923; Idem, Memo Jessie Lee Ellis (undated; 1925?); Idem, Famous Urumia Hospital to be

construction of the new missionary hospital within the city itself, with a maternity section, the hospital staff delivered 86 babies in 1930-31. Also, across the hall was the children's room with white attractive cribs made up with attractive counterpanes. The walls were tinted and hung with pictures. Next was the babies' room or nursery, where they were tucked in white bassinettes. These had soft coverings made by friends in the US and dainty clothes. When the babies left the hospital instead of in rags the medical staff gave going-away clothes for poor babies.[63] Because the hospital was discontinued in 1934 there was no further obstetrics care in Urumiyeh.

MATERNITY CLINICS BY CITY

In the beginning, one reason that pre- and postnatal care was not a regular service offered by the missionary hospitals was the enormous demand for other immediate medical care and their limited capacity to respond to that growing demand. With an increase in staff, partly locally trained in their own hospitals, more and more varied care could be offered. As a result, prenatal of postnatal care also became part of the service that the missionary hospitals offered.

KERMAN

In 1922, a novelty in medical care, Women's Welfare Work (WWW), was pioneered by the British Church Missionary Service (CMS) in Kerman. Later similar work was also begun by the American missionary hospitals in Mashhad and Rasht. According to Ms E. C.H. Stratton, who was in charge of WWW, the main objective of social work was "to get in touch with deformed carpet weavers so that expectant mothers may be taken to the hospital to receive medical attention they so sorely need."[64] This situation was caused by abominable working

---

rebuilt; Presbyterian Church 1926, p. 221.

63. RG 91-20-7, Cochran Memorial Hospital Report 1933.

64. Administration Report 1924, p. 32. The missionaries also had induced the governor of Kerman to get interested in the problem. On his actions

conditions of the mainly child and female labor in the carpet factories in Kerman. Conditions were such that many children and women (girls rather) often became crippled for life. Apart from having to work in subterraneous, often cave-like, badly-lit, cold, humid, unventilated areas, the workers were seated in such a way that they always were sitting stooped. This position was often conducive to "permanent deformities of the arms and legs, and irreparable damage to general health."[65] In Kerman the girl workers were often afflicted by ankylosis of the lower abdomen. When these girls became pregnant, they often died in childbirth. When a hospital was available, a craniotomy operation could be done, in up to 50 per cent of births. In the streets of Kerman the Rev. Boyland observed "one is constantly reminded of the iniquity of this child-labor by seeing deformed and stunted women, and occasionally men who are no longer able to work, as their hands are often deformed as well, and are reduced to beggary."[66]

In 1924, in all 59 confinement cases were undertaken; mostly Moslem women. As a result of this health outreach program, the British consul reported that, "the health of the carpet workers is now better than 15-20 years ago."[67] There was close cooperation between the Women's Hospital, which was under a female physician, and the WWW Center. All doubtful pre-natal cases were seen by the doctor.

---

and that of the government in Tehran, see Malekzadeh 1394, p. 75; Floor 2011, pp. 98-99.

65. Chaqueri 1978, pp. 210-12 quoting British missionaries such as Reverend Boyland (FO 248/1343). It is noteworthy that similar problems were not reported from other areas in Iran, see for example Chaqueri 1978, p. 205 reproducing a letter from the British consul at Soltanabad (FO 371/10131, f.140, f.14) and also the British consul at Tabriz, FO 371/9030, f.215 "At the commencement of the weaving of a carpet the operatives squat on the floor, as the work gradually rises from the ground they rise with it and sit cross-legged on planks. This is not considered a hardship for Persians as it is the posture they usually adopt when resting in their own homes. It they had chairs provided (or any other sort of comfortable seat) I doubt whether they would appreciate the innovation."

66. Chaqueri 1978, 210

67. Administration Report 1924, p. 32.

Two combined pre-natal and post-natal clinics were held weekly, one of which was especially for carpet weavers and children of all ages came. Pregnant women were seen and advice was given to mothers.[68] In 1928, the WWW's staff consisted of one European (Ms Stratton), one part-time European, and two trained Armenian women. WWW focused on child-welfare and maternity care, both pre- and post-natal as well as midwifery work. In 1928, the total number of visits was 3,998 and 2,055 cases were treated at the WWW center.[69]

Table 10: Women's Welfare Center Activities - CMS Kerman 1924-1935

	1924	1925	1929	1931	1932	1933	1934	1935
No. of confinements	59	97	?	76	92	89	68	75
Visits to patients' homes	-	-	3,972	1,614	1,936	2,049	1,251	1,322

Source: Administration Report 1924, p. 32; Idem 1925, p. 39; Idem 1929, p. 28; Idem 1931, p. 30; Idem 1932, p. 26; Idem 1933, p. 31; Ibid 1934, p. 35; Ibid, 1935, p. 38.

The WWW center under Ms E.M. Robinson continued strongly despite Ms Stratton's absence due to leave in October 1932, returning in December 1933.[70] In 1934, the WWW center had two senior and three junior workers; the latter had started midwifery training. Two workers passed the CMS doctor's examination (equivalent to CMB = Central Midwives Board) in September 1934 and another was to retake it in January 1935. The hospital claimed that the result of WWW's activities was that the number of abnormal midwifery cases among weavers was decreasing; partly due to improved weaving conditions and partly because the native midwives were "afraid to perform the awful deeds which they formerly performed. Public opinion had also been raised as a fruit of the years of midwifery and welfare work

68. Administration Report 1925, p. 39.
69. Administration Report 1928, p. 32.
70. Administration Report 1933, p. 31.

by the C.M.S. workers."[71] In 1935, Ms Robertson was in charge of the WWW center in town assisted by three Iranian midwives. They continued their standard program of regular prenatal instruction and further teaching during convalescence.[72] In 1936, the level of WWW's activities dropped, because Ms Robinson went on furlough in April, while Ms Stratton only returned in October.[73] In the following period Ms Stratton remained in charge of WWW until mid-1945 when she went on furlough. On 6 June, Ms Woodruff arrived to relieve her.[74]

Mashhad

The CMS hospital in Kerman was not the only one to offer mother-and-child care. To reduce infant and maternity mortality, Dr. Adelaide Kibbe had considered starting a program of pre-natal care in Mashhad, which, she wrote, is "almost unthought-of and untranslatable into Persian." Most mothers came only once, usually in the 9th month and only returned when they were in labor. In 1931-32, she had been able to persuade a few to come for regular pre-natal care and everyone was satisfied. She reported that: "A leaflet in Persian on pre-natal care, adapted to Persian customs, is in preparation: a first step toward ironing out eclampsia and preventing unnecessary suffering and death."[75] The new Shah Reza Hospital in Mashhad forced the Christian hospital to develop new projects, such as well babies clinics and pre-natal instruction clinic.[76] The establishment of baby clinics, or under-five clinics, was a real necessity given high infant mortality. According to Dr. Hoffman:

71. Administration Report 1934, pp. 34-35, 45.
72. Administration Report 1935, p. 38.
73. Administration Report 1936, p. 26.
74. Administration Report 1945, p. 4.
75. RG 91-20-2, Mashad Medical Report 1932-1933.
76. RG 91-20-2, Mashad Medical Report 1935-1936 (In 1935, the Shah Reza hospital had two German doctors, one of whom was a gynecologist and who was the hospital's superintendent at the same time).

When a baby is born, if the weather is very warm, he may be washed; but if cold he is sure not to be, for fear he will take cold. He is wrapped in "old clothes," and his head tied up tightly in a couple of handkerchiefs and a cute little cap. Persian houses are not heated in winter [but use is made of a *korsi*].[77] The room is cold, and "opening up" a baby, as they call it, is a thing to be avoided. When a mother wraps her baby up, she first spreads out her five or six shawls, then lie Mr. baby on them, straightens out his legs and holds his knees tight together while she folds in his legs, lapping over the shawls first from one side then from the other, and then pins his hands down to his sides and wraps them in, too: when the package is smoothly folded, she ties it up with a long ribbon or sash, and the baby is easily handled, for he is not in a position to raise much objection. After a baby has learnt to walk, his head is still tied up closely with a cap and two or even three handkerchiefs, only his face, from eyebrow to chin, being exposed; he wears from two to five short coats- and frequently nothing else. I wonder that the babies do not all die, running about as they do in their bare feet in winter; as a matter of fact, most of them do, for the infant mortality is appalling; probably less than 30% of all babies born here reaching the age of three. I asked a woman when she had taken her baby, of three months, to the bath; she said, "Oh, I have not taken him to the bath yet; his skin is not yet finished peeling!" Babies born in the winter are commonly kept till the summer to be taken to the bath, and then go with their mothers to the filthy public bath, where the water is simply replaced as it is used up, all the bathers using a common tank. There is no possibility for a bath in the homes, for aside from the poverty of the people and cold houses in the winter, less than the proper amount of water is ceremoniously unclean to your carefully guided Mussulman. Of course diseases are very common among the children. A large percentage contract the terribly common trachoma (granulated eye-lid), and favus (scabby head) very early in life. Most of them must sooner or later have small-pox; the common expression used in asking about small-pox is, "Has

77. For an explanation of what a *korsi* is, see Willem Floor, "Korsi," *Encyclopedia Iranica*.

> he brought out small-pox yet?" - the idea apparently being that everyone has the disease in his system, and when once it has come he becomes free of it. Besides these diseases, the other diseases of childhood common in America are found here.[78]

Hamadan

In Hamadan, as of 1938-39, to better reach and sensitize young mothers there was a well-attended baby clinic one afternoon per week at the downtown Kababian dispensary.[79] This initiative was the outcome of the realization of the medical staff of the American missionary hospital that it should do more preventive work, in particular concerning endemic diseases, VD, and infant mortality. To that end some health literature was distributed. Dr. Lichtwardt "made some health talks, shown some health movies, but very little has been done here and elsewhere to make laymen and doctors health-conscious."[80] Other preventive activities included a complete physical exam, including urine analysis and blood pressure readings, of all Mission staff, pupils of the Avicenna boy's middle school and the girls of Faith Hubbard hostel, and of many AIOC employees. Typhoid and smallpox vaccinations were given to many, and health literature was distributed in the dispensaries.[81]

Kermanshah

As of 1940, Mrs. Packard R.N. conducted a baby clinic (feeding problems, weight loss, slow development, digestive troubles). For this the hospital wanted a special room with equipment. Here women of all layers of society intermingled, rich and poor, European and Iranian.

---

78. RG 231-1-2, NN (Hoffman) to Friends, Meshed, March 1918. "A new born child was not washed until it was taken to the public bath after several weeks or even months. Tetanus from infected cords carried off many new-borns." RG 231-1-6, Hoffman, Pioneering in Meshed, p. 28.
79. RG 91-19-27, Christian Healing in Hamadan 1939.
80. RG 91-19-27, Christian Healing in Hamadan 1939.
81. RG 91-19-27, Hamadan Medical Report 1937.

The clinic was continued after she and her husband retired in 1943.[82] The clinic was the Mecca for women with women's diseases. The only alternative were some midwives who dabbled in medicine. In 1945, there were only two male doctors, but they wrote that if they had a female doctor more women would come.[83]

TABRIZ

In 1929, a new program was started, i.e. a weekly clinic for mothers and babies.[84] This baby clinic was very useful, not only in curing, but also in preventing disease. No further information is available on the functioning of this clinic over the next 20 years. However, it must have been continued. For, in 1949, a new center was opened in Charandab, where poor children were given their 3-R's and where baby and eye clinics were held weekly, be that it was doused with social evangelism. Here Dr. Laura Müller conducted her Baby Clinic with 40-50 mothers each week.[85]

TEHRAN

In 1942 the Iran Presbyterian Mission was forced to close one of its larger hospitals, the one in Tehran. Thereafter it was used by the US Army.[86] After WW II, the Tehran hospital remained closed, due to lack of physicians, although the US Army had repaired and improved it. However, to reopen the hospital two new physicians were needed, who the Iran Mission was unable to attract. Therefore, the Tehran hospital remained permanently closed.[87]

---

82. RG 91-19-28, Kermanshah Westminster Hospital 1940.
83. RG 91-19-28, Kermanshah Westminster Hospital 1944-45.
84. Presbyterian Church 1930, p. 164.
85. Presbyterian Church 1950, pp. 44, 46; Idem 1952, p. 67.
86. Presbyterian Church 1945, p. 69.
87. Presbyterian Church 1946, p. 55; Idem 1947, pp. 55-56; Idem 1949, p. 67.

However, its Baby Clinic continued. This clinic always had been quasi-independent from the hospital, although supervised by its medical staff. Of course, children had been treated by the hospital since its inception, but usually not many came to the dispensary for treatment. This started to change in 1933, when it was noted that there were more children patients than usual that year. Dr. Blair highlighted some of the cases:

> One morning in the clinic I saw a two month's old baby with a severe acute mastoiditis. I advised immediate operation which the parents refused. They took the kiddie to several Persian physicians all of whom apparently gave the same advice. The next evening they brought the baby about ten o'clock at night – operation and convalescence uneventful. In April a premature Persian boy was born weighing three pounds two ounces. Two mothers already in the hospital, one Armenian and one Persian, nursed her for the first three days. The father insisted that she stay in the hospital until her mother had learned the routine of our method of care. When last seen in the clinic she was growing and developing normally. A similar case last year died of neglect soon after leaving the hospital.[88]

It was in particular Dr. `Ali Asgharzadeh, a Russian woman physician and pediatrician, who freely donated three mornings per week to the dispensary for children. In 1934/35, 1,214 children under the age of 12 were treated, about half were under three. Although there was a great need for pediatric care, the medical staff was firm in its belief that this care should be complemented by instruction to the mothers so as to prevent more common ailments. Therefore, Dr. `Ali Asgharzadeh wrote and printed simple instructions for mothers and she wanted to develop more preventive medical activities.[89]

Because pediatric care was something of a novelty, no particular space had been planned for it in the hospital. In fact, since 1933, the children's clinic was held in a corner of Dr. McDowell's office.

---

88. RG 91-19-11-1, Report Teheran Hospital 1933.

89. RG 91-19-11-1, Report Tehran Medical Work 1934-1935.

Therefore, in 1936, the children's clinic moved into separate quarters and took on a new life. It left the women's dispensary quieter and more orderly, and enabled a more adequate examination. Work in the new space began on 1 October 1936 and during 1936/37, as many as 1,180 patients were seen. Apart from preventive and curative care, the children's dispensary could not exist without providing for those who needed hospital care. Until 1936 they were placed with older patients, which was unsatisfactory. Dr. McDowell found a room in the old Women's Court that was used as a kitchen store. The stores were moved, the room was cleaned and used as a children's ward. Six small iron beds, linoleum on the floor, some pictures on the wall made the place bright. Being separate from the hospital was an advantage and disadvantage. Although the children were freer and could be let outside, it was difficult to have proper nursing, but that was all the room there was. It was Dr. Asgharzadeh, who made the children's work possible as she gave so much of her time and skill to it. Thanks were also due to Ms Sahiyeh, who helped getting drugs to patients, who were too poor to pay. Cod liver oil helped malnourished children over the winter months, and as of 1936 quinine was also given, which helped against malaria.[90]

In 1937, a further change was made by cutting off the east end of the women's waiting room to make a children's clinic, where Dr. `Ali Asgharzadeh and Mrs. McDowell, a trained nurse and two medical students, were fully occupied all morning. A beginning was made at a children's ward in part of the old women's hospital that was not abolished in 1930, when the new hospital was built. This building was condemned as unsafe and in 1929 a two-story building was built primarily for children, financed by an Iranian lady. Until the Nurses Home was built, the doctors had no choice, but to use the proper children's building to house the nurses.[91] In 1937/38, the children's clinic was busier than ever. There was a great need for this kind of medical care, since child mortality was a major problem in Iran. At that time, there was only one government Children's Hospital, "and for

90. RG 91-19-11-1, Report Teheran Hospital 1936.

91. RG 91-19-11-1, Report Teheran Hospital 1937.

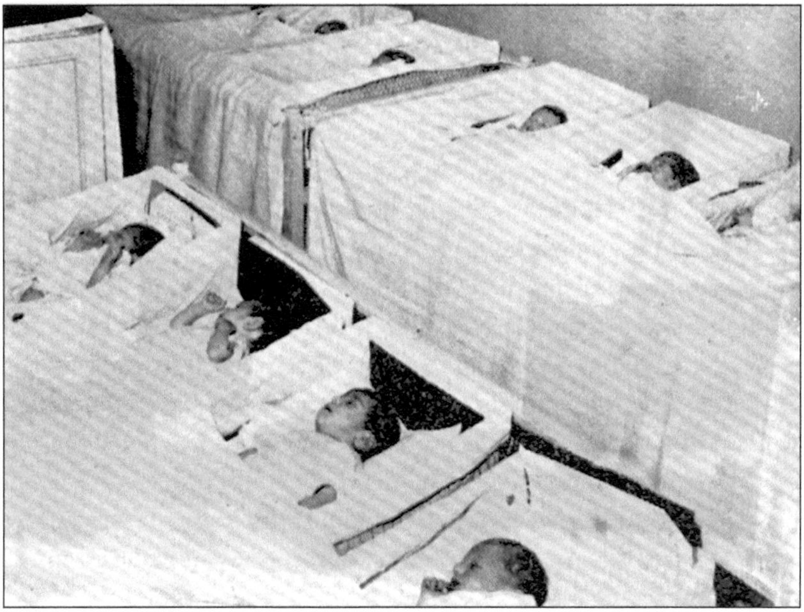

Newborns at the Vaziri Hospital

some reason it is so hedged by restrictions that it is not being utilized." Despite the wish to act, given the high need, the American Hospital was faced with the high cost for this activity, which caused it financial problems. This was because most children seen were from poor and middle-class households and were unable to pay the actual cost. Also, most children came in badly nourished. "The most therapeutic measure is a liberal supply of milk, eggs and vegetables." Therefore, it was astounding what good rest, feeding and cod liver oil was able to do in one month to a child.[92] Consequently, the children health centers were popular. One held among friends in a missionary's house was visited by 1,500 mothers and children during 1939-40. Also, "local gifts were received such as clothing and other gifts made by friends, cod liver oil, an Iranian doctor provided diphtheria prophylactic and the Iranian woman doctor on the staff added several hours a week to her responsibilities."[93]

92. RG 91-19-11-1, Report Medical Work Teheran 1937-1938.

93. Presbyterian Church 1940, p. 64.

The children's ward was the cheeriest and best furnished spot in the whole hospital, according to Dr. McDowell. Mrs. J. D. Payne took over when Mrs. McDowell left, in addition to the clinic for so-called well babies that she had held for long in the city (see below). When Mrs. Payne left on furlough in the spring of 1941, Ms Jane Doolittle took over. In 1941, the hospital had more surgical cases, in particular, tonsillectomies, empyemas, bone cases, and TB spines. Therefore, young adults were admitted when there was no room in the men or women's departments.[94] The three mornings per week children's clinic continued to be in charge of Dr. Asgharzadeh assisted by Ms Doolittle. The latter's help was important as translator and social worker. In 1941, the clinic began with prenatal work and then during the week, while the mother was there, the staff continued to teach her. Then these mothers were urged to take their children regularly to the children's clinic for supervision, feeding advice and preventive inoculations. The clinic's staff realized that they needed more and better literature along these lines.[95]

In 1941, to address this great need for mother-and-child care, the *Bongah-e hemayat-e madaran va kudakan* (Institute for the protection of mothers and infants), an institute founded by Reza Shah in December 1940, commissioned a maternity hospital with twenty beds and a number of clinics in Tehran. Later another maternity hospital with fifty beds was opened, as well as a nursing home and two clinics in different parts of the city.[96] These newly established maternity hospitals were in addition to the already existing government Women's Hospital (*Nesvan*) and the Maternity Clinic (*Zayeshgah*).

THE HEALTH CENTER

Elite families had access to good pediatric medical care and advice. In fact, at the request of the publisher of the *Salnameh-ye Pars*, Dr.

---

94. RG 91-19-11-1, Report Teheran Hospital 1940-1941.

95. RG 91-19-11-1, Teheran Medical Report 1941-1942.

96. Encyclopedia Iranica1989; see also Malekzadeh 1392, pp. 231-37; Idem 1394, pp. 186-90.

Rastegar, a pediatrician practicing in Tehran, wrote a long note to acquaint mothers with the growth and 'growing pains' of babies. The note is filled with advice what to do and when and emphasized the importance of breast-feeding, hygiene and weighing. However useful the information of the note was, the vast majority of Iranians could not read, let alone buy this booklet. Also, much of the advice (e.g., a separate room for the baby) was perhaps relevant for mothers of wealthy families, but totally at odds with the means and living conditions of the majority of Iranian mothers.[97]

Tehran

Therefore, it was very fortunate that the Health Center for so-called well babies was opened on 25 August 1936 on the arrival of the baby scales, when Ms Payne invited 16 friends with their children, as a mother's club. It was held in Ms Payne's house in Khiyaban-e Paris. Dr. Marianne Leppman, a German doctor examined them; she had offered her services for the year. Two graduate nurses, both midwives with foreign training, helped. It was clear that an extra room was needed and for the next Center day a waiting room was prepared. Thereafter no invitations were sent but Ms Payne relied on word-of-mouth. It was decided to ask a small fee of 10 *shahi*s to avoid large groups coming, who only would come out of curiosity with no intention to apply the advice. This fee was collected the first six months, after which it was raised to 2 rials per child. Half a dozen families were taken gratis. The record system was copied from the successful program of the self-supporting Health Center in the American University of Beirut. One-third of the blanks used to date were hand-ruled until funds sufficient for printing were at hand, which was done immediately once funds were available. Only the cross-section paper needed for the graphs of the weight of small infants still was lacking. A block notebook donated by a college professor made it possible to make graphs of all babies. The furniture was painted white and looked neat. "A cheap linoleum blackboard is a help in amusing the youngsters

97. Rastegar 1312.

of school age and a decided advantage when one is teaching private pupils." There were also toys, and colored blocks for babies.

In 1936-37, there were 40 Health Center days with a total 97 families; 365 adults accompanied the infants or an average of 9.1/day. The total number of children seen was 286 or 7.1 per day, or higher than was expected. Based on the Kerman and Beirut experience the medical staff had thought that on many days no one would come, but that happened only once on a holiday. Ms Payne paid one nurse 15 rials per afternoon, who had years of experience in the Kerman Health Clinic. The second nurse (Shams ol-Bahar Hejazi) did not want weekly pay, she wanted an American book on nursing, which the hospital paid for; she attended the clinic 35 of 40 times. She also worked as anesthetist at the Women's Hospital. The first nurse was absent two periods when she was night nurse at the US hospital. She received 45 rials for her services. The Presbyterian mission felt that she should have donated her services, but Ms Payne thought it is wise to have an experienced help in the beginning. She had doubts about the second nurse as well as about the doctor, who did not come eight times. Each time she warned her one day before, and arranged another doctor each time. These were paid 2 *tuma*ns for 2 hours of service. On one extra Health day, one doctor donated his time for typhoid inoculations.

The medical supplies were simple; a thermometer, a hypodermic needle, a tongue depressor, a nasal speculum, cotton and alcohol, a basin for sterilization and a primus. An enamel wash basin bucket and stand, soap dish, towel rack complete the outfit.

Table 11: Receipts of the Health Center over 9 months (ending 30 June 1937):[98]

From the Mission (scales, measuring rod, table, steps)	1252.50
From individual missionaries	150
From friends	845.55
From health center fees	370.50
From books sold	105.50

98. RG 91-19-17, Jane Payne, Health Center for Children.

From private English lessons	3253.90
Total	5977.95

The Hospital nor its staff helped in the Center, because they had neither the time nor the inclination to do so. Also, Drs. Bussdicker and Blair opined that in the then reigning anti-foreign political atmosphere of 1938 a licensed Iranian pediatrician should be in charge of the center, and therefore, they did not want to officially be involved with the Center. That did not mean that they did not support the idea and the need for the Center, which they did, because they also argued that many such Centers should be opened in a big city like Tehran, given the high and preventable infant mortality.[99] In November 1938, it was decided to move the Center from Ms Payne's basement to a room to ensure a normal growth and in a more a suitable site, to which end a room was prepared in the Mission Compound. It was also decided to raise the fee to 5 rials per child after the change of location and charge 1 *tuman* for any special service. Also, Dr. Varjavand was found willing to be involved and that Dr. Leppman, who still had not been able to obtain a license, would formally work under his supervision.[100] The baby health center continued to be conducted by Mrs. Payne. During her 1941 furlough Mrs. Fischer and later Mrs. Dr. Muller took over, until her return in May 1942. Two women doctors, `Ali Asgharzadeh and Leppmann assisted. In the winter of 1941/42, all pupils of the *Mehr* School were given a physical. Many children were vaccinated and still more weighed and given feeding and other advice. By then, the center occupied several rooms in the Central compound.[101]

After the closure of the American missionary hospital in September 1942, the baby welfare center, as it was then called, continued in Tehran, where in 1947 Ms Payne opened a second center in the poorest part in the south of town, due to a gift from the Shah; she also wrote a book

99. RG 91-19-17, Memo Bussdicker-Blair, 14 May 1938.

100. RG 91-19-17, Circular letter concerning the Health Center, 11 November 1938.

101. RG 91-19-11-1, Teheran Medical Report 1941-1942.

on “Child Care.”[102] This meant that henceforth there were two child welfare centers in Tehran- a baby clinic and a recently opened clinic among the very poor. In the latter, Moslem doctors were contributing; even though they knew that Christian evangelism was stressed there.[103] The Iran Bethel Center for Women and Girls in Tehran held a clinic, which looked after 1,241 poor families. It also organized other activities such as sewing, literacy, bible study, hygiene, and a nursery. This Child Welfare Center in a better section of the city was self-supporting and continued even when the political agitation was at its height (1950-53). The Clinic of Hope in the slums of S. Tehran, near the brick kilns, was served by volunteer doctors, in addition to a regular part-time doctor and a nurse. Its program expanded beyond the limits of a small rented one-story house. A piece of land was purchased for a modest two storey building to house not only the medical clinic but also sewing and literacy classes.[104]

RASHT

Baby clinics had been one of Dr. Frame’s latent plans; he made a feeble start during the famine years (1917-18), but it was crowded out by other demands on his time. Mothers who delivered in the hospital were invited to return with their babies for supervision, but nothing general was done. In 1933, one of the missionary teachers, Mrs. Wright wanted that the 10th class in baby care (of the Girls School) be given a course in baby care. Because this might have some application in hospital work, Dr. Frame organized a baby clinic; one for children with malnutrition and another for well babies. There was great interest among the nurses and many such babies were seen. The growth of the clinic was hampered by the outbreak of a whooping cough epidemic in Rasht making it necessary to select cases with care. Closely related

102. Presbyterian Church 1948, p. 53.

103. Presbyterian Church 1950, p. 44.

104. Presbyterian Church 1951, p. 57; Idem 1952, p. 50; Idem 1954, pp. 54-55; Idem 1955, p. 54. On the workers of the brick-kilns and their living conditions, see Willem Floor, “The brick-workers of south Tehran: a striking record (1953-1979),” in *International Review of Social History* 48 (2003), pp. 427-55.

was the effort to offer prenatal instruction to mothers, where babies were regularly weighed and women learned about feeding and care. This was important in view of the increasing number of obstetric cases (see above).[105]

Baby clinics were held Monday and Wednesday afternoon and were very popular. Many well-to-do parents attended for the regular weighing of babies and the special instruction. Poorer women were perhaps more grateful and tried within their means to carry out the instructions, but too many were unable to afford to buy fresh milk and provide special food for supplemental feeding. Fortunately, lactic acid milk (*mast*/yoghurt or *dugh*/butter milk) was a common household article and protein milk could also be obtained, both were less expensive than fresh milk. It was by word of mouth that mothers learnt about the clinic. Many (67 out of 143) heard about it at the out-patient department. The school girls who helped in part of their course in child care spread the word; people also read about it on the back of the prescriptions.[106] The baby clinic by Mrs. Wright with graduates of the missionary Girls School indeed filled a need as shown by increased number of new cases and the many return visits. In 1934-35, 229 babies registered compared with 143 in the previous year; there were 636 return visits and the previous year 540.[107]

In 1935, the baby clinics were taken over by Mrs. Brinkman with the help of two graduates from the Girls School. This was a great help to the mothers and Dr. Frame as the clinic required much time. The change in babies was sometimes remarkable through a change in their feeding schedule or type of food. Sometimes house calls were made, but mothers were reluctant, possibly because of the condition of their house.[108] Interest in the baby clinic continued to grow. During March-June 1937 there were almost 500 visits. The largest single attendance was 26 in one afternoon, 41 different babies in one week. The total

---

105. RG 91-19-9, Rest Medical Report 1933: Idem, Resht Medical Work 1932.
106. RG 91-19-9, Resht Medical Report 1934.
107. RG 91-19-9, Resht Medical Report 1934-35.
108. RG 91-19-9, Resht Medical Report 1935-36.

number of active clients was 60-70. The mothers who had been helped encouraged friends to come. There were three categories of babies:

I. Babies of up-to-date mothers able to give their babies the best care;

II. Babies from homes with limited means. The mother being unable to nurse adequately, having difficulty in weaning the child to proper diet, etc. Many were too poor to buy cow milk, which was expensive and not too reliable. The hospital was unable to offer free milk or even an orange, but those who needed it were given free cod liver oil. It was a challenge to provide adequate diets within the parents' means and the limitations of the local markets.

III. Babies that were undernourished and for whom homecare had proven to be inadequate. Some babies were admitted to the hospital, others refused out of fear of the family even when it was free. Also, the hospital was not really geared for this problem, as it was mainly a surgical establishment and the limited number of nurses had neither the time nor training to care for special cases.[109]

The baby clinic was run as a social service rather than as a public health project. Many were well babies referred to by the maternity section or by friends. A large part was referred by other dispensaries, because of feeding problems. The Christian hospital's own dispensaries were overcrowded and "to refer the babies to their family doctors means referring them to men who know and care little about modern feeding of children. Opium is too often their answer for diarrhea or colic." In 1937-38, about 150 babies enrolled for 1538 recorded visits. Also, there was informal consultation after hours.[110] By 1938, it became clear that the baby clinics were very popular, but it was beyond the Christian hospital's ability to handle all. It had a cross-section of society of mothers, who all wanted an easy way to care for their children and

109. RG 91-19-9, Resht Medical Report 1936-37.
110. RG 91-19-9, Resht Hospital Report 1937-38.

were prepared to make sacrifices. Poor women often were unable to give better feeding, in which case the hospital provided them with free drugs and cod liver oil as part of its free service; for extra feeding it depended on gifts. In the meeting room there was a box for gifts, in which also warm winter clothing was given.[111]

Every Monday and Wednesday afternoon, while surgery was done upstairs, Mrs. Browning received babies for weighing and general nutrition advice in the women's dressing room. In 1940-41, there were 719 visits, on average 7-20 per clinic day. The doctors wanted to extend and improve the Baby Clinic Social Service to include maternal welfare, prenatal and otherwise and to re-arrange Ms Benz's house, so that in addition to the big room then used for women's meetings and nurses' classes, there would be three rooms for Baby Clinic Work to include demonstrations and special instruction to women as to cooking of simple but necessary baby food; making of clothes, baby bath demonstrations, minor treatments, health talks, etc. The Frames believed that mothers would feel more at home there than in the hospital. Dr. Kribbe-Frame was on hand one afternoon per week. Mrs. Browning and Ms Benz did the Clinics. Baby Clinics had always been more a branch of dispensary work for poor patients; those able to pay being in the minority. Baby Clinics were always in the hands of a married lady of the mission not directly working in the hospital. The baby clinic remained open even when the hospital was temporarily closed after Dr. Frame's death. The hospital contributed quarters, equipment, linen, wood, laundry, etc. Free cod liver oil and drugs were given to many of the poor patients. "Gifts and contributions, such as the teaching salary of Mrs. Browning this past year, as a rule, has been expanded on providing supplementary food etc., which, after investigation, was found to be beyond the purchasing power of the family."[112]

Babies were from all classes of society; often both parents came and seemed to understand the value of proper feeding and accepted

---

111. RG 91-19-9, Resht Hospital Report 1938-39.

112. RG 91-19-9, Resht Hospital Report 1940-1941; Idem, Resht Medical Report 1941- 1942.

advice, and that this was often preventive for situations that lead to disease. They agreed that feeding a baby cucumber and expect an instant cure with a 'suzan' (injection) of bowel trouble was just not common sense. Many doctors in the city referred their patients to the Christian hospital for prenatal care and also encouraged them to come for post-natal care. Poor women were the saddest as they were under the influence of older women, who were steeped in superstition and old customs that were detrimental to the child and were too poor to buy proper food or milk; "about 80% of these [babies] are opium fed, for it is cheaper to quiet with opium a hungry crying baby than to buy milk or other food and prepare it." A large number of babies had scabies, because they could not afford soap to bathe the baby or properly wash its clothes. "In this climate, babies should be fed cod liver oil a good part of the year. However, as soon as the baby got a cold, the cod liver was stopped and when it died it was blamed on the cod liver oil, not on the real disease that the child had."

With kudos the Presbyterian Board concluded that Rasht had pioneered in the development of a child welfare program. A home visitor, a practical nurse-evangelist, did steady follow-up work.[113] Ms Gertrude E. Benz went twice per month to the government foundling home to weigh babies and checked on progress made; the girl in charge was a former nurse of the Christian hospital and she put her experience to good use.[114] The baby center represented the Hospital Social Services Center (HSSC) and was in charge of Mrs. Browning for four months, but in October 1944 Ms Benz returned and took over. The baby clinic was held two afternoons per week, but the mothers came at odd times to Ms Benz's home or asked her to visit them to discuss their babies. Dr. Mohammad Kar came one hour per week to see babies, who were in need of doctor's treatment.[115] The HSSC was centered in the Baby Clinic two afternoons per week, but moved from the hospital into a suite of three rooms formerly part of Ms Benz's residence. It was more commodious and convenient and with

113. Presbyterian Church 1944, p. 75.

114. RG 91-20-8, Resht Hospital Social Service Center 1944-1945.

115. RG 91-20-8, Resht Hospital Social Service Center 1944-1945.

a full-time nurse, Khanom Mowlud, the clinic was able to help more than before. She was able to carry on alone, when Mrs. Browning was on vacation. Dr. Kar came 1 hour per week on Wednesday.

From among the educated mothers some 20 formed a club in November 1943 with a Nurbakhsh school graduate as president,[116] which met every week for study, cooking, handwork and a social hour. Its purpose was self-improvement and helping others. Three of these mothers were on the Board of Managers of the Municipal Free Maternity Hospital (10 beds) which was very well run. They urged mothers to go there for check-ups, while the Christian hospital encouraged them to go there for confinement.

In the city Foundling Home, babies picked up from the street were in a pitiful condition, syphilitic and starving. Its budget was insufficient and politics too evident, but the graduate nurse in charge, who had been trained and had worked for the Christian hospital, did her utmost to make things better. From the other clinic mothers, with the equivalent of 6th-9th grade education, 50 wanted to form a second club. Almost every home of the clinic's 350 babies was visited regularly. The reports were placed in the individual files so when the mothers came, the responsible person knew the home conditions, whether there was illness, the father out-of-work, etc. When babies were brought to the clinic it was found that about two-third were doped with opium once or twice daily. "Some have survived through their second year on opium, castor oil, tea, pillau, cucumbers, and skimpy breasts." When babies did not gain weight, Dr. Kar usually discovered worms or syphilis. The cash for milk to prevent starvation ("now the best man's wages scarcely buys the raw rice for a family of four") went to 12 babies this season. When mothers didn't cooperate, the clinic stopped the help with milk. "People sometimes sold all they owned to buy milk for the baby and when the father was out of work the mother sold her two good teeth; then we helped and fortunately the father found a job again."[117]

---

116. The Nurbakhsh school in Rasht had been established and was managed by American missionaries.

117. RG 91-20-8, Resht Hospital Social Service Center 1942-43 (Total

Apart from the Christian hospital, the National Philanthropical Hospital (*bimarestan-e kheyriyeh-ye melli*) had reserved one room with three beds for sick women and maternity cases until its closure in 1928. Dr. Petros Tashchiyan, assisted by Ms Taku'i, took care of these female patients. On 16 December 1940, the maternity ward in the Pur Sina Hospital was closed, after the creation of the *Bongah-e hemayat-e madaran va kudakan*, which established a 10-bed maternity unit. This ten-bed hospital for obstetrical work was sponsored by some of the leading women of Rasht. The Pur Sina Hospital offered surgical services until the August 1941 invasion of Iran, when this hospital was taken over by the Soviet Army. However, the ten-bed maternity hospital continued to give help to many. A Russian midwife did much of the work, but in 1945 one of the Christian hospital's nurses joined their staff. The missionary doctors hoped that 'this civic project, financed by special taxes on cinema, tea, etc. will continue in this needy field."[118] The local maternity hospital cared for many cases, while two new private hospitals have been opened, with over 20 beds each.[119]

DISCUSSION

Given that Iran until recent times was a country that had no real medical infrastructure, childbirth and related events was and remained in the hands of traditional midwives. Modern medical services were hardly available, even in the mid-20th century, while the majority of the population, even when they had access to those services, still felt great reluctance to avail themselves of them. Also, the fact that female physicians and trained midwives were rare also constituted an obstacle

---

number of babies born in the hospital: 350. The number of new babies this year: 153. Total baby visits to the clinic: 1,184; average daily visits 12). RG 91-19-9, Resht Hospital Report 1944.

118. Ta`eb 1384, pp. 24-29, 224-29 (with names of the staff of the old and new maternity clinic as well as of the leading sponsoring women); Malekzadeh 1392, p. 256; RG 91-20-8, Resht Hospital Report 1944-45.

119. RG 231-1-5, Personal Report 1949 and Resht Hospital Report.

for women seeking modern medical help. Thus, it was unsurprising that modern mother-and-child care was slow in becoming available to women. The more so since the demand on the fledgling modern medical institutions for a host of other important medical problems was high, their capacity was low. Also, traditional providers of medical services (*hakim*s, *mama*s, *`attar*s) were still the ones that the majority of the population still turned to for their medical problems.

The government of Iran recognized the importance of pre- and postnatal programs. In fact, the Ministry of Health was responsible for "the health of mothers and children" and had to establish "prenatal and postnatal clinics, the development of well baby clinics, promotion of the health of school children, and assistance in preventing the spread of disease among all of these groups." After WW II, with the Red Lion and Sun Society, the Ministry had developed such a program in Tehran serving 250 well babies. The program encouraged breast feeding and distributed dried milk. Babies were examined and mothers received instructions in infant care. Wassermann tests (for syphilis) were given when they came to the clinic, but the tests were done after the birth of the baby. The program was staffed by a few professional and volunteers, and served a group in which the head of the family earned about Rls. 12,000 a year. The cost of the service was about Rls. 2,000 per family. Some mothers had a daily caloric intake of less than 1,000 kcal. The authors the Seven-Year Development Plan considered that "this well baby clinic is a good beginning, but does not exist elsewhere in Iran."[120] This, as we have seen above, was clearly untrue, and, for reasons unknown, the team's consultants had not properly done their data collection.

This does not mean that the authors of the Report were wrong. After all, due to the lack of medical, public health and sanitation facilities and services in most of the country, the available health statistics still showed how bad the situation was. However, the authors

120. Overseas Consultants 1949. vol. 2, p. 32. They also were unaware that allegedly some maternity clinics had been established in a few major cities in the 1940s and that is was even planned to establish such centers in rural areas, see Malekzadeh 1394, p. 105.

of the Seven-Year Plan should have been aware of the 20-year old experience of the missionary hospitals, where delivery mechanisms, attitudes, and means had been field tested. The same situation existed in many other developing countries at the time, countries where the team members had previous experience. Thus, they should have known that field- and mean-tested methods are very important. Perhaps the team discounted the experience gained locally, because, as yet, it had failed to make a significant impact on infant mortality in Iran, which was still very high.[121] "Dr. R. Leslie Cherry, head of the health division in 1954 and 1955, believed that fifty per cent of Iranian babies die in their first year. Of those who live one year he thought fifty per cent would die before the age of six. The infant mortality rate may be even higher."[122] The Report also noted that there was no profession of public health nursing or home visitors, and thus, it recommended that training facilities be established to develop such public health nursing capacity. The need for such a service was highlighted by the fact that, although most babies were breastfed, which the Baby Clinics advised, most of them were infected with intestinal diseases through lack of sanitary precautions.[123]

The situation of child birth was still a major medical nightmare. A Point-Four advisor reported that "Old crones of the village become midwives without any knowledge or sanitation or training in their calling. They employ folk ways and folk medicines, the leaves, seeds, roots of plants that grow in the deserts of hills."[124] In one village there were no children, because "all the babies there died of the 'stiff disease.' This sounded like tetanus. The investigation the nurse ordered showed that the two village midwives, for reasons best known to themselves, were using cow dung to staunch the flow of blood

---

121. For steps taken by the government after 1950, see Malekzadeh 1394, pp. 106-22.

122. Warne 1956, p. 140.

123. Overseas Consultants 1949, vol. 2, pp. 32-33.

124. Warne 1956, p. 140; see also Reza'i 1398, which is an interview with a traditional midwife, who tells how she became one and how she still works.

after severing the umbilical cord." An Iranian visiting health trainer showed the midwives "how to sterilize a scissor over a candle flame and gave them other elementary instructions." Thereafter babies were born again and remained alive in the village, and the health visitor was honored at a public celebration.[125]

Unfortunately, as this situation was normal, it made perfect sense that the Report recommended that, in addition to more trained midwives, the quality of midwifery needed to be raised by increasing cleanliness and technique.[126] In 1960, the Institute of Midwifery in Tehran graduated about 30 nurse-midwives per year and the Behyar Midwifery School of the Red Lion and Sun Society Maternity Hospital in Shiraz trained about 12 *behyar*-midwives per year.[127] At that time, it was also reported that there were five (non-missionary managed) Mother and Child Centers, which had an attendance of more than 1,700 a month.[128] Thus, whether it were state or missionary hospitals that provided modern ob-gyn services, their number and capacity was too small as yet to make a difference in the way children were delivered in Iran. Therefore, the contribution of the missionary hospitals was not that they changed or supplanted the traditional system of child birth at home, but, like in other areas of hospital care, that they established a modern alternative with clear standards and protocols as well as trained a nucleus of local professionals that would form the basis of the current modern ob-gyn system practiced in Iran.

---

125. Warne 1956, pp. 141-42.

126. Overseas Consultants 1949, vol. 2, pp. 32-33. On the various steps undertaken by the government to train more midwives, see Malekzadeh 1394, p. 105-21.

127. US Army 1963 pp. 154-55.

128. CARE 1961, p. 2 (In Iran, assisted by local personnel, direct 25 medical institutions, such as a hospital in Teheran, health centers in Teheran and the provinces, school clinics In Teheran and the provinces, and a sanitation division in Teheran. About 6,000 persons a month receive medical aid in these institutions.)

IV

AMERICAN MISSIONARY HOSPITALS: A ROLE MODEL

The American missionary physicians tried to be of service not only to their patients, but also to their medical colleagues and their profession. They did so in various ways and by various means, and in particular by avoiding unnecessary and unwanted competition and conflict with their Iranian colleagues. More positively, they focused on introducing (i) medical treatments, (ii) surgical techniques, (iii) technical means, (iv) information-sharing and (v) on other services that were new, in short supply, useful, and supportive to patients, colleagues and the country.[1] Apart from being innovative and supportive in the medical or surgical field, the American missionaries also offered technical services that initially were standard elsewhere, but often unavailable in government hospitals. These technical services included the use and maintenance of the X-ray machine as well as the use of a medical laboratory. None of the American hospitals had a totally adequate laboratory, but among the Iranian government and private practitioners there often were no lab facilities available whatsoever. Finally, the missionary medical staff was not trying to compete with their Iranian colleagues, but sought collaboration and exchange of information in a cordial and collegial atmosphere.

MEDICAL

In the medical field the American missionary physicians tried to be up-to-date, innovative and introduce new methods of treatment or draw attention to neglected endemic diseases, which were easy treatable,

1. Khakestar 1395, p. 182.

or focus on treatment of neglected groups such as lepers, which is discussed in a separate chapter. Here I want to highlight the role of the missionary physicians in acquainting their Iranian colleagues with (i) the latest treatment methods of a very common skin disease (favus), (ii) the best practice of treatment of TB patients, including the latest surgery techniques, as well as with (iii) the detection and treatment of intestinal parasites such as hookworm.

FAVUS OR RINGWORM.

Many children were afflicted with *kachal* (کچل) – ringworm (dermatophytosis) or favus of the scalp.[2] Favus or scabby head lasts for years and makes most of their hair fall out very early in life.[3] Therefore, it was one of the most common and tenacious diseases in Iran. For example, favus in Gilan's humid climate was very prevalent, especially among the poor who could not afford soap.[4] In the 1920s, either irradiation with an X-ray machine or the use of thallium acetate were the available treatments for ringworm. In the early 20th century the use of thallium acetate to treat ringworm was rejected, but later studies established the treatment on a sound basis.[5] The use of thallium was considered safe, if the drug was properly administered. However, if this was not the case, as was the case in Iran, then physicians felt that "a disastrous overdosage is a possibility which could not be ruled out if the method came into general use."[6]

Due to the lack of an X-ray machine, Dr. Frame (Rasht) was unable to use it for this scalp disease of which many children suffered.[7] Even if he would have had an X-ray machine treatment might not have been as

2. RG 231-1-6, Hoffman, Pioneering in Meshed, p. 79.
3. RG 231-1-2, NN [Hoffman] to Friends, Meshed, March 1918.
4. RG91-19-9, Medical Report, Resht Station, 1921-22; Idem, Report Medical Work 1919-20.
5. Ingram 1932, pp. 8-10.
6. Shanks 1931, p. 121.
7. RG91-19-9, Resht Medical Report 1921-22 ; Idem, Resht Medical Report 1919-20.

good as expected, because it required an expert operator in superficial therapy.[8] The US physicians had acquired a reputation for treating favus or sore head, the despair of many mothers. Many children, who came to the dispensary "are utterly miserable and ashamed of their scalps, a mass of dirty, itching, smelly crusts, and they look so nice and clean after epilation, with heads as bald as dice". The US doctors also had been in despair until they began using thallium, taken by mouth, which made the hair fall out that allowed them to get to the infection at the roots. X-ray epilation was quite beyond the range of possibility of the American hospital in Mashhad, but the very small risk of using thallium was justified by the generally satisfactory results. The hospital pharmacist was very careful, because of the danger in using thallium (a deadly poison) carelessly. About half of the children were cured, the rest much improved. The hospital only did epilation when the hair was long enough to make it easy, and, of course, the child had to be in good health. Also, a responsible person had to commit to carry out the daily epilation, scrubbing and medication.[9] The treatment required persistence and patience of mothers. However, what Frame found in Rasht was disappointing: there were 489 new cases and only 1,231 return visits. If mothers had done the treatment properly, this number should have been three times higher, he wrote.[10]

In 1936, favus became a major problem in Iran, when modern head dress was imposed on both men and women. In the past it did not matter so much, the turban and *chador* covered the scalp. Thereafter, it was a stigma of inferiority and its poor victims cried for relief.[11] Moreover, "children with evident favus … are forbidden to attend school until their disease has been cured."[12] Consequently, favus work was a large part of lab work, because children had to have clean scalps before they were allowed to attend their classes.[13] In 1936, Dr. Katzenstein, the

8. Ingram 1932, p. 9.
9. RG 91-20-2, Mashad Medical Report 1932-1933.
10. RG 91-19-9, Resht Medical Report 1933.
11. RG 91-20-2, Mashad Medical Report 1935-1936.
12. RG 91-20-2, Mashad Medical Report 1931-1932.
13. RG 91-19-9, Resht Medical Report 1935-36.

German radiologist at the Shah Reza Hospital at Mashhad, cautiously began epilation with the X-ray, working on some of the many cases of the orphanage. The X-ray department of this hospital was the only one with the right and sufficient equipment to do so. The government was helping "by doing away with the old-fashioned public baths where all go into the same tank of water, which is rarely changed. Shower-baths are now being installed."[14]

Because of the good results with the thallium treatment it became very popular. Nevertheless, Dr. Mary Zoeckler in Malayer had not wanted to use the treatment, because she lacked the proper scales to weigh the patients. However, because after 1936 the cap or *charqad* could no longer cover the bald spots and children with favus were sent away from school the treatment was in great demand. Also, the public baths were closed until showers had been installed, so that the almost universal favus scourge might finally belong to the past.[15] As a result, whether in Malayer or elsewhere, favus treatment was a major part of the dispensary's work. In Malayer, the year 1940-41 was a busy one with 5,154 patients, of which 861 were favus cases. Many of the latter came from outlying districts, because in the city it had almost been eradicated.[16] In 1941-42, more than 600 favus cases were treated in Malayer, which, to Dr. Zoeckler's experience, seemed to present an inexhaustible supply.[17] In Rasht, Dr. Frame had a similar experience. During 1940-41, a total of 2,438 lab exams were done, besides 2,200 men's dressings and 1,581 favus treatments.[18]

Continuing the thallium treatment was not only a challenge for illiterate mothers, but also for medical staffers. In 1945, Ms Nicholson R.N. reported, "Rather apologetically, an orderly from the Government

---

14. RG 91-20-2, Mashad Medical Report 1935-1936.
15. RG 280-1-10, Report Daulatabad Medical Work 1938 [-1939]. In the UK, the dosage, irrespective of age, was 1/8 grain per 2.25 lb. of body weight. Firth 1927, p. 1097.
16. RG 280-1-10, Report Daulatabad Medical Work 1940-1941.
17. RG 280-1-10, Report Daulatabad Medical Work 1941-1942.
18. RG 91-19-9, Resht Hospital Report 1940-1941 (in 1939-40, a total of 3,017 favus cases were seen).

Hospital [in Rasht] brought his two sons today. At the other hospital many things had been tried, but in the end, this sort of scalp infection always comes to us for the Thalamine Acetate treatment."[19] The chief of the Health Department of Hamadan sent cases of favus and other cases that he thought the Christian hospital could better handle.[20] In the absence of a better alternative thallium acetate remained the treatment of choice until better and safer treatments came available.

Tuberculosis

Tuberculosis, which, according to Dr. Polak (1852) and Dr. Baker (1885), hardly occurred in Iran, and which Dr. Schlimmer (1874) did not even list in his *Terminologie*, had become quite prevalent by the end of the Qajar regime, if not before that time. It not only prevailed in densely populated Tehran, but also in the villages and among the nomads. In Tehran it was the leading cause of death in the 1920s. Dr. Neligan ascribed its spread to bad hygienic housing conditions, the use of wadded quilts, which were shared in an unwashed state, bad health condition of the people, and late diagnosis.[21] The missionary hospitals only in the late 1920s and the early 1930s began paying attention to tuberculosis. Probably, this was because there were so many other medical problems that they had to deal with. Apart from sun-therapy the American physicians, in particular in Rasht and Mashhad, also performed pneumo-thorax operations.[22]

It would seem that the first missionary hospital that began regular treatment of TB patients was that in Hamadan. Despite Hamadan's altitude there were many pulmonary and bone TB patients. In fact, most chronic cases seen were tubercular. Therefore, the American

---

19. RG 91-20-8, Resht Hospital Report 1944-45.

20. RG 91-19-27, Healing in the Home of Avicenna 1936.

21. Floor 2004, p. 25; Polak 1852, 742; Neligan 1926, part II, pp. 693; Gilmour 1924, pp. 65-66; Rice 1923, p. 256 ("in particular tubercular bone trouble is common"); *Tarbiyat* 1377, Index q.v. *Sel.*

22. This experience is not reported by Abbasi-Dezfouli et al. 2014, pp. 201-02 and totally ignores the experience gained by the American missionary physicians.

hospital began to pay more attention to the treatment of this disease. On his return from furlough in 1928, Dr. Joseph W. Cook introduced the Rollier sun treatment in treating surgical TB patients with good results. TB inpatients were placed on the veranda of the hospital and in shelters to benefit from the open air and sunshine treatment.[23] The number of TB patients was increasing, because it appeared that the hospital had acquired the reputation of being able to treat these cases. Almost every day a new case showed up. Most of them were from outside the Hamadan district, including a hopeless TB patient from faraway Baluchistan. Also, more TB patients from the south were coming using the new road via Khorramshahr. Although the climate of Hamadan was good for TB treatment, the Christian hospital had only place for two or three patients at a time, and each case required at least 6 months' hospitalization. Therefore, many patients had to be sent away for whom they could do nothing. The hospital had a portable X-ray machine, which was great for the diagnosis in these cases. Unfortunately, its capacity was too limited for adequate diagnosis service, especially for fluoroscopy, for which a new and better one was needed.[24] In 1939, a large covered veranda was constructed on the south side of the men's hospital to accommodate patients with pulmonary TB, so that the hospital was able to accommodate at least four men there. It was the intention to screen it and eventually insulate it with glass for the long cold winters, if and when funds would become available.[25]

Probably the second American hospital to begin treating TB patients was Rasht. It also introduced the most advanced treatment in the country. TB was very prevalent in Gilan, both 'surgical' and

---

23. RG 91-19-27, Hamadan Medical Report 1933; Idem, Hamadan Medical Report 1939; Presbyterian Church 1932, p. 169. Dr. Auguste Rollier, was the most famous heliotherapist of his day. At his peak, he operated 36 clinics with over 1,000 beds in Leysin, Switzerland. Anonymous 1954; Billings 1957.
24. RG 91-19-27, Hamadan Medical Report 1934; Idem, Hamadan Medical Report 1937.
25. RG 91-19-27, Hamadan Medical Report 1940.

pulmonary. In fact, there were more TB cases than Frame had thought. The damp climate and uncertain weather "make it difficult to arrange for outdoor treatment. Any permanent hospital must have sun parlors for men and women."[26] Dr. Brinkman, who arrived in 1931, had a great interest and familiarity with the newer chest surgery.[27] This encouraged the doctors to operate on a number of tubercular cases, which, in early 1932, led to the creation of the TB Unit.[28] In 1932, a beginning was made for an outside shelter for TB patients, which in, 1934, was enlarged.[29] The TB Unit was successful therapeutically and certainly financially, but not a flourishing establishment. During this time the doctors of the Christian hospital showed that TB could be arrested even in Rasht with its bad climate. This gave some hope, because until then a TB diagnosis meant relocation to the plateau for the patient "and thereby simply change the location of his grave, or he could remain and first 'cough up' his last 'shahi' for injections and later cough out his existence." By June 1937, three patients had been discharged, who were greatly improved, while three others were under treatment. The discharged cases returned bi-weekly for follow-up exams. Also, the doctors used the time in the hospital to educate them on their disease and to have them better understand their treatment. It was impossible for the hospital to keep patients until their complete recovery, because there was no room and the patient's poor financial situation, since the treatment lasted long. At the hospital patients received an initial treatment and then they were sent home to continue treatment there.

---

26. RG91-19-9, Resht Hospital Report 1919-20.
27. In the late 19th and early 20th centuries sanatoria developed for the treatment of patients with tuberculosis. The repose provided there was supplemented with pulmonary collapse procedures designed to rest infected parts of lungs and to close cavities. As of the late 19th century artificial pneumo-thorax as a procedure for lower lobe cavities became widely used. Although it is considered a useful therapy there is uncertainty about its efficacy. Daniel 2006.
28. RG 91-19-9, Resht Hospital Report 1932; Idem, Resht Hospital Work 1932.
29. RG 91-19-9, Resht Hospital Work 1932.

The TB clinic was popular, although people expected too much from it. Often, people came too late, could not afford the long supervision treatment, got discouraged, and heard that some other doctor guaranteed a cure in shorter time. During a short stay in the hospital the patient was taught how to care for himself. Frame had several cases that checked the disease, but never completely cured ones. Dr. Brinkman gave lantern talks on TB that was curable, but told the audience that patients had to come early.[30] Fracture cases were slow to discharge and hindered the admission of ordinary patients, who needed operations. Therefore, Frame had an outdoor shelter made as an experiment for tubercular cases. They found that a few of them, who came early enough, had the money and patience to carry out proper treatment. Therefore, the doctors mainly diagnosed the disease and offered suitable cases, who would live at home, pneumo-thorax treatment. The shelter was occasionally used for those who were unable return to their village until their treatment was finished.[31]

Each Thursday afternoon there was a regular clinic for fluoroscopy and pneumo-thorax treatment for a few TB patients, which helped them by arresting the disease.[32] In the beginning of the TB unit, Dr. Brinkman offered constructive help to a small number of TB patients, but he soon found that hospitalization for them was not feasible. Gradually, with Dr. Mohammad Kar's help in giving treatments, a pneumo-thorax clinic was developed by the end of 1942. Brinkman conducted this clinic two afternoons each week. During 1942-43, 496 pneumo-thorax treatments were given. More and more TB patients were seen in the dispensary and no other physician in Gilan had the equipment or was capable of giving this treatment.[33] Even after Dr. Brinkman had left, the Rasht hospital continued to treat TB patients. Two afternoons per week were used for giving pneumo-thorax treatment. Some patients were induced to go to the government Shahabad sanatorium north of Tehran. There, allegedly 40-50% of patients came from the Rasht

30. RG 91-19-9, Resht Hospital Report 1934.
31. RG91-20-8, Resht Hospital Report 1936-37.
32. RG 91-19-9, Resht Hospital Report 1939-40.
33. RG 91-19-9, Resht Hospital Report 1943.

district.[34] Many returned from there to continue their treatment with the Christian hospital, which also collaborated with the health department in tuberculin testing in the local orphanage. The hospital's staff took 100 of the healthiest looking children, 6 to 14 years, and found that 48% were positive with the first test and 10 more with the stronger dilution, a total of 58% positive! It was concluded that it was safe to say that over 60% of these orphans were tuberculin positive.[35]

At about the same time as in Rasht, other missionary hospitals offered regular treatment for TB patients. The CMS hospital in Kerman reported that there was much tuberculosis of every variety in the city. "The Tubercular Ward in each of the two Mission Hospitals is always full, mainly of bone cases. These patients receive daily sun-treatment all the year round, which, combined with Cod Liver Oil, good food and constant 'scraping', produces slow, but good results in most cases."[36]

Another encouraging development took place in the American missionary hospital in Mashhad, where, in 1930, Dr. Hoffman observed that no anti-TB work had been started, while there was no hospital care for these cases. He further stressed the need to do more work for TB in prevention, segregation and treatment.[37] In 1933, Dr. Hoffman further noticed that TB seemed to be on the increase. "Presently more than half the patients in the hospital wards are there for various forms of bone, joint and gland tuberculosis, and even in our limited laboratory, over 100 positive sputa were picked up in the year." That in itself was bad enough, but what was more worrisome, was that each of these sufferers were "a greater menace to people in Mashhad than the 140 lepers!" Therefore, the US physicians gave leaflets to patients with the disease, including the one written by the late Dr. Cook (d. 1934) and printed by the Presbyterian Iran Mission. The

---

34. RG 91-20-8, Resht Hospital Report 1944-45. The Shahabad center, a TB sanatorium was established in Tehran in 1937. Azizi and Azizi 2010, p. 356, n. 38; see also Azizi and Bahadori 2014, p. 358, which article does not mention the American missionary experience.
35. RG 231-1-5, Personal Report 1949 and Resht Hospital Report.
36. Administration Report 1934, pp. 44-45.
37. RG 91-20-2, Mashad Medical Report 1929-1930.

doctors also instructed the patients what to do about their sputum and general hygiene. Dr. Hoffman rhetorically asked: "Does no one else care about this?"[38] This question was also somewhat a cry for help, because in 1936 he wrote that still nothing was done about anti-TB work, although "new possibilities appear in social, antivenereal [sic] education with the unveiling of women."[39] Although the US doctors treated many TB patients in their hospital, they really preferred not to have them there, because even after improvement, "the short time we can keep them these poor folks return to their old haunts and insufficient food."[40]

Unfortunately, most sufferers of TB came too late to get an X-ray at the well-equipped Shah Reza Hospital and had bilateral involvement that were too late for treatment. Some came "waving their axe" (photo;عکس) thinking that they should get well from this and didn't need further treatment.[41] The American physicians referred many patients to Dr. Katzenstein, the German radiologist at the Shah Reza Hospital and his diagnoses helped them, because X-ray interpretation took time and expense and they were handicapped by unsatisfactory interpretation of the films and the inability to do their own fluoroscopy exam. Therefore, they admitted more patients with pulmonary TB for a few weeks "to begin treatment by pneumothers [sic] or more often a phrenicectomy, because villagers are unable to return for proper refills and follow-up with pneumo-thorax treatment." Several benefited from this, however, Frame opined: "this city needs a TB sanatorium."[42] Dr. Katzenstein was cordial, but was permitted to do very little free work. Charges were steep at the Shah Reza Hospital, so that after X-ray work, patients often had no money left for treatment. Many thought that the 'lightning' (X-ray) machine would cure them.[43]

---

38. RG 91-20-2, Mashad Medical Report 1932-1933.
39. RG 91-20-2, Mashad Medical Report 1935-1936.
40. RG 91-20-2, Mashad Medical Report 1936-1937.
41. RG 91-20-2, Mashad Medical Report 1935-1936.
42. RG 91-20-2, Mashad Medical Report 1937-1938.
43. RG 231-1-6, Hoffman, Pioneering in Meshed, p. 119,

Fortunately, there was a positive change in 1942, when in Mashhad an anti-TB society was started. For a while, it tried, in a half-hearted manner, to run a small section in the free City Hospital and a TB hospital. However, thereafter it just petered out and stopped altogether in 1945. This happened despite the great need for anti-TB activities, because the disease was widely prevalent. Because the US hospital had only an inadequate X-ray machine and no radiologist (which it would like to get), it had to rely on the Shah Reza hospital. This government hospital had five X-ray machines. In 1945, they had a dozen or so under treatment, who benefited from this. Those who could afford it were sent to Tehran where something was done. However, what Mashhad really needed was a TB sanatorium. Dr. Hoffman concluded that, apart from at the Christian hospital, there was still no one who treated TB in Khorasan.[44]

Hookworm

Part of the missionary hospital's educational work was that its physicians tried to make local physicians understand the seriousness of certain diseases in the community. One of these diseases was hookworm, which was very prevalent in Iran, because people who live in warm climates in areas with poor hygiene and sanitation are more at risk of developing hookworm infections. If left untreated hookworm infection causes anemia and nutritional deficiency, especially when people are not well-fed or suffer from malaria, a condition from which many people suffered in the past.

Gilan was one of the areas where hookworm was a major problem. At the end of the 1930s, Dr. Morton observed that: "In the low land around Resht, hookworms reduced the vitality of thousands."[45] Before coming to Rasht in 1948, Dr. Hoffman, who had worked in Mashhad for 30 years, was told by a leading Tehran doctor that mortality from surgery would be 5% higher in Rasht than in Mashhad, "because of people's debilitated state of health." There was much hookworm

44. RG 91-20-2, Mashad Medical Report 1944-45.

45. Morton 1940, p. 215.

and more rickets than on the plateau; also, more tape worm; general vitamin deficiency, due to lack of sunshine and the watery nature of fruit and vegetables. "It is often necessary to keep patients needing surgery a week or so longer, to get rid of their parasites and malaria, before operating."[46]

Initially, Dr. Frame (Rasht) had not realized how important hookworm infection was in Gilan.[47] However, once he became aware of its importance, he, with the help of Sayyed `Ali, his lab technician, tried to examine every case coming to the hospital. Of 11 cases in one week eight had hookworm. The hospital's lab found the same with out-patients.[48] In one year (1931), the hospital found that 40% of in-patients were affected. As a treatment, Frame probably prescribed Epsom salts (magnesium sulphate) to reduce protective mucus, followed by thymol to kill the worms as treatment. Although Frame did not report his method of treatment, Epsom salts and thymol had been used in the southern USA to almost eradicate the problem.[49] Therefore, Frame showed the success of his treatment in many clinics. But it was only after a few years that pharmacies carried the remedies and some of the doctors only occasionally diagnosed and treated such cases.[50] Frame's drive to get more attention for hookworm was finally bearing fruit, for more attention was paid to it in 1929. However, the Christian hospital's drug room in Rasht was the only place with the proper remedies. Not all cases reacted promptly, but the results were so good that people expected miracles in case of other ailments.[51]

---

46. RG 231-1-5, Personal Report 1949 and Hospital Report R.E. Hoffman, Rasht.
47. The population of Gilan was not only infected by the hookworm. In the Caspian littoral the tapeworm (Taenia lata; *hobb al-qar`*, *kadudaneh*) had infected almost the entire population, according to Häntzsche, as reported by Polak 1865, vol. 2, pp. 315-16.
48. RG 91-19-9, Resht Medical Report 1924-25.
49. Ferrel 1914, p. 15.
50. RG 91-19-9, Resht Medical Report 1931.
51. RG 91-19-9, Resht Medical Report 1929.

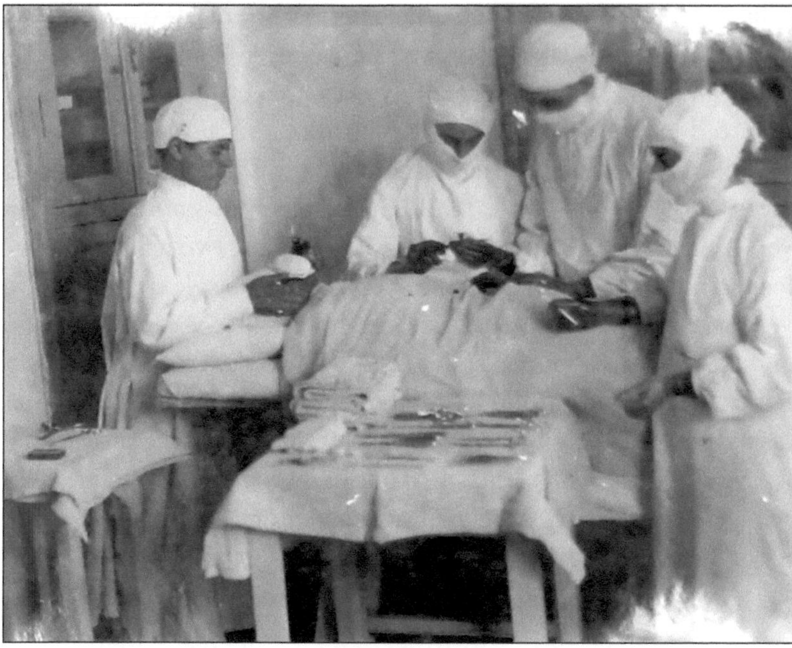

Dr. Lichtwardt operating assisted by three Iranian assistants.
Mashhad, 1922

Surgery

Even as late as the 1940s most Iranians preferred to visit their Galenic medicine trained Iranian doctor (if they could afford one) or, more likely, have recourse to folk medicine, rather than go to a hospital, whether it was an Iranian government hospital or a foreign one. However, in one respect modern physicians had an advantage over traditional healers and that was their skill in surgery. Dr. Polak opened the door for operations, which, because of the high success rate were considered to be miraculous. Also, he and Fochetti introduced general anesthesia into Iran in 1852 through the use of ether and later also of chloroform.[52]

This first path to surgery was widened and paved by British and American physicians, both missionaries and those belonging to the

52. *Vaqaye`-ye Ettefaqiyeh* 1373-74, vol. 1, p. 591 (no. 99. 12 Rabi` I 1269/24 December 1852); Polak 1857, p. 937.

Indian Medical Service (in the Persian Gulf ports British consular hospitals). The only city that offered surgery in an Iranian hospital was in Tehran in the *Dowlat* Hospital. However, even then professionals preferred to work in the American hospital, because it provided a nurturing environment and any contribution was not only appreciated, but put to very good use. In 1928, for example, its surgical facilities were used by three Iranian, one British doctor and two US missionary doctors, who were in the city for a short period. Outside surgeons were welcomed by the American physicians. In fact, they wrote: "There are an increasing number of Persian Drs. whose character and training justify trusting part of the hospital's reputation to them."[53] Despite its capacity the Tehran hospital was sometimes overwhelmed by the demand for surgery, in particular, if one of its doctors was on furlough. Fortunately, Dr. Davies of the British Legation and Dr. Mo`aven helped out in the missionary hospital on many occasions.[54]

In 1933, Dr. Hoffman (who came from Mashhad to substitute for a colleague on furlough) wrote to his family that, "I have done more abdominal operations that I ever did before in the same length of time. I have also done in all seven thyroids, - and so far I have not heard of anyone else in Persia doing them except one Englishman in Isfahan. And all patients have recovered."[55] The American hospital performed a large variety of operations. In 1928, for example there was an 11-year old boy from Varamin, who had been wounded by a boar a few years earlier. After his wounds had been healed by the village barber and old women he developed

53. RG 91-19-11-1, Teheran Hospital Report 1928. In that year, the American hospital had its first case of a patient flown in by plane (also a first one for Iran). It concerned the older brother of a *Majles* deputy, who had swallowed his false teeth. He was flown in by a Junkers plane from a place 400 miles away. The American physicians "removed the partial plate. Esaghophoscopy was unsuccessful, and we got it out thru an incision on the neck. In spite of the serious infection, which had already developed, he recovered satisfactorily."

54. RG 91-19-11-1, Tehran Report Medical Work 1931-1932.

55. RG 231-1-2, Hoffman to family. 04/01/1933.

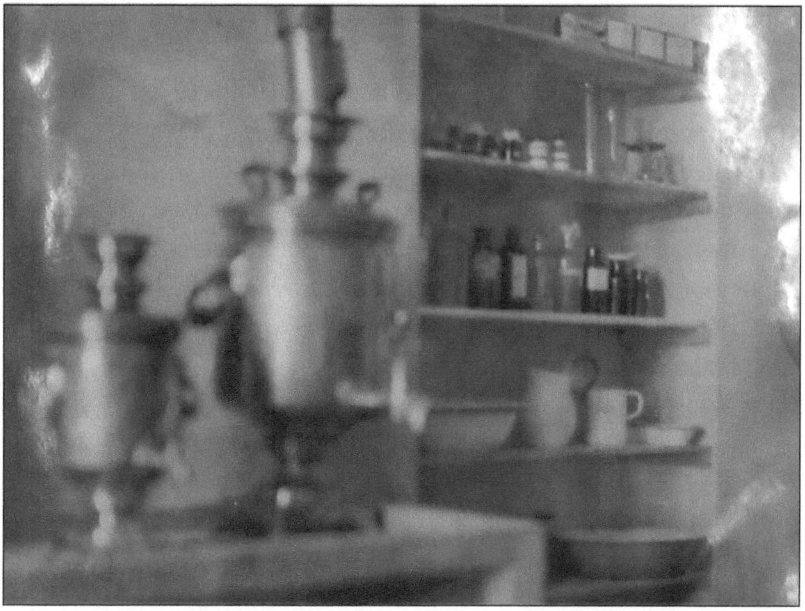

The sterilizing room and autoclave, Mashhad American Hospital, 1920s

> a lumbar hernia, a ventral hernia, and a fecal fistula. Last summer, begging along the Teheran-Isfahan road, he was picked up by the wife of a government official and brought to us. After surviving four major operations –an exploratory laparotomy, repair of lumbar hernia, entero enterostomy, and a ventral herniaplasty – he left the hospital. … Now, instead of a repulsive cripple, he is leading the normal life of a school-boy - for his benefactress also gave him an education.[56]

How great the reputation of the Tehran hospital was may further be clear from the following case. In 1932, Dr. Hoffman and Dr. Blair had a consultation of 12 doctors, who had been called in the case of Mrs. Dadgar, the wife of the *Majles* president. Immediate operation was needed as it was a ruptured ectopic. The only places where this operation was possible were: (i) the Russian hospital, which was the Bolshevik propaganda center, thus this was not possible for the

56. RG 91-19-11-1, Teheran Hospital Report 1928.

political bigwig, (ii) a private hospital run by a Persian doctor educated by the missionary college in Tehran and (iii) the American hospital. The family decided to bring her to the American hospital in Tehran. "It was agreed that no other hospital in all Teheran was safe!" The family decided to bring her to the American hospital in Tehran. Thus, the American doctors felt that surgically they still had the comparative advantage, even in Tehran, "which has more doctors per thousand population than has the USA! But in the provinces, there is only one doctor to 15,000 people and our hospitals are still the only places where laparotomies may be done safely."[57]

Therefore, outside Tehran, the situation was problematic for patients who needed surgery. In Khorasan, "The Mission's American Hospital was the only place where surgery was done; there were no Persian surgeons."[58] This was no exaggeration. In October 1918, Dr. Hoffman reported that, "Yesterday at the Shrine Hospital the new Persian doctor amputated a man's leg, who died shortly afterward. This was the new doctor's first operation in Mashhad and the third amputation done there, each by a different doctor, and all the patients died; a mortality of 100%! It is good for us, but to-day I had 161 patients more than we can properly can handle with current staff."[59] In fact, even as late as 1936, there was only one other surgeon in the whole of Khorasan.[60]

In Rasht, the missionary hospital's strong point and comparative advantage was surgery, because there was hardly any one else in Gilan who did so. Nevertheless, people were still reluctant to come to the hospital for surgery. Dr. Frame submitted that he needed to avoid risky desperate cases, so as not to scare away less desperate ones.[61] For a long time the American hospital was the only in Rasht one doing surgery. One of the local doctors told Frame: "This too

57. RG 231-1-2, Hoffman/Tehran to McClanahan, 01/12/1932.

58. RG 231-1-6, Hoffman, Pioneering in Meshed, p. 31

59. RG 231-1-2, Hoffman to Speer, October 1918.

60. RG 231-1-6, Mashad Medical Report 1935-1936; Idem, Mashad Medical Report 1944-45.

61. RG91-19-9, Resht Medical Report 1924-25.

is your doing for if you had not taught the villagers that hernia can be cured by operations they would not now be coming to us in such large numbers."[62] Dr. Adelaide Kibbe arrived in October 1937. It was a new experience for the city to have a female doctor, who was an obstetrician and a surgeon. She did a Caesarean without the help of other doctors, which amazed a British doctor working in the National hospital.[63] In 1948, Dr. Kibbe wrote that, "There is a fairly nice Iranian hospital, but no one there is doing surgery. The Russian hospital does no charity work."[64]

In 1937, although there were many Iranian doctors in Hamadan, but practically only one (a former assistant in the missionary hospital) was qualified for surgery. He was the head of the local health department and chief of the government hospital, where many of the poor were treated.[65] Also, the local municipal hospital had hardly any real surgical capacity, and then only minor operations were carried out there. In fact, the health department asked the Christian Hospital to do their surgery for them.[66] Between 1942 and 1946, Dr. Cohn worked as chief surgeon and as director of the men's ward. He became very popular and in 1943, there was even a waiting list for surgical patients. The year 1943-44 was a peculiar surgery year, because it was 'appendicitis year.' This used to be rare and operations were even rarer, but in this

---

62. RG 91-19-9, Resht Medical Report 1930.
63. RG 91-19-9, Resht Hospital Report, 1937-38.
64. RG 231-1-5, Hoffman/Rasht to Friends, 12/09/1948; RG 231-1-5, Personal Report 1949 and Resht Hospital Report (Mrs. Hoffman fell ill in December 1948 and Dr. Hoffman had her transferred to the Hospital of the National Bank in Tehran, where the nurses were mostly from the US mission hospitals. Dr. Raji, an eminent Tehrani surgeon, trained in Europe, attended Mrs. Hoffman, who had cancer and died on 4 February 1949).
65. RG 91-19-27, Hamadan Medical Report 1937.
66. RG 91-19-27, Hamadan Medical Report 1935; Idem, Christian Healing in Hamadan 1939.

year a record of 110 were done, on one day even seven of them.[67] Also, even in 1940, neither the small government hospital with a minimum of equipment nor the local municipal hospital was doing any surgery. They had no surgeon and, therefore, the health department continued to ask the Christian hospital to do their surgery for them. In spite of this and the two free government dispensaries the work of the missionary doctors was increasing.[68]

Apart from being the only action in town, the missionary hospitals also often pioneered new possibilities for operation and introduced new techniques. For example, even though the American hospital was the only medical institution where surgeries were performed in Hamadan, with the only-X-ray machine and with a functioning lab, its physicians tried to keep up with modern techniques and practice. As of 1933, they used less chloroform and did more spinal and local anesthesia as well as experimenting with sodium amytal and also using 'twilight sleep' in obstetrical cases.[69] The addition of a new operating room in Urumiyeh after 1906 made abdominal surgery possible.[70] Dr. Edward Blair (1925-36) developed a nose and throat specialty, in addition to general medical work in Tehran.[71] In 1931/32, Dr. Vassei did much of the operating in the Tehran hospital, and he adopted the new method in cataract operation of peripheral iridoctomy.[72] In 1936-37, there was an increase in stomach and thyroid surgery and a decrease in industrial and accident surgery, while Dr. Vassei broke all records for the number of cataract surgery.[73] In Rasht, Dr. Brinkman had training in TB work and genital-urinary diseases. Therefore, his experience with the cystoscope opened the field of urology in the hospital, so that they were able to operate on long standing cases of

---

67. RG 280-1-10, Hamadan Medical Report 1943-1944.
68. RG 91-19-27, Christian Healing in Hamadan for the year ending June 30, 1939; Idem, Healing in Hamadan. for the year ending June 30, 1940.
69. RG 91-19-27, Hamadan Medical Report 1933.
70. Speer 1911, chapter 16; Wilson 1896, pp. 267, 275; Presbyterian Church 1920, p. 237; Idem 1894, p. 188; Idem 1920, p. 326.
71. Presbyterian Church 1930, p. 187.
72. RG 91-19-11-1, Report Medical Work Tehran 1931-1932.
73. RG 91-19-11-1, Report Teheran American Hospital 1937.

kidney stones and other cases. Also, his familiarity with the newer chest surgery encouraged them to operate a number of tubercular cases (see above).[74]

Due to an increase of equipment, the American doctors were able to do more. However, they also had to be inventive to get the tools they needed, but that were not available. For example, a set of Thomas splints was made by a local iron maker, so that broken arms and legs could be splinted without delay.[75] Having seen other patients being relieved by surgery, more patients also demanded that intervention. The use of local and spinal anesthesia made that operations were more popular than when done under general anesthesia.[76] Conditions in the OR also improved. Dr. Hoffman wrote in 1946, "The sepsis in the OR is reliable, post-op care can be relied upon, dressings are done without cross-infection, and over-worked doctors are relieved of much worry."[77]

There remained two main problems. Even in the 1920s, there was still a reluctance to have an operation, and therefore, people came late, "partly due to fatalism, partly due to lack of confidence in doctors in general, mainly due to their ignorance of the urgency of the symptoms."[78] Moreover, the patients' problems often were made worse by the quacks they went to see first, before going to the dispensary.[79] Fortunately, this reluctance faded away over the next two decades. In fact, the increase in the number of operations was due to a change in patients' attitude. The second major problem was the continued lack of trained Iranian surgeons, even in Tehran. In the summer of 1936, three students of the University of Tehran worked with the Christian Hospital in Mashhad for credit in surgery, for there was a shortage of

---

74. RG 91-19-9, Rest Medical Report 1932; Idem, Resht Medical Work 1932.
75. RG 231-1-6, Hoffman, Pioneering in Meshed, p. 71.
76. RG 231-1-6, Mashad Medical Report 1929.
77. RG 231-1-6, Mashad Medical Report 1945-1946.
78. Presbyterian Church 1921, p. 337-38.
79. RG 91-20-2, Mashad Medical Report 1930-31.

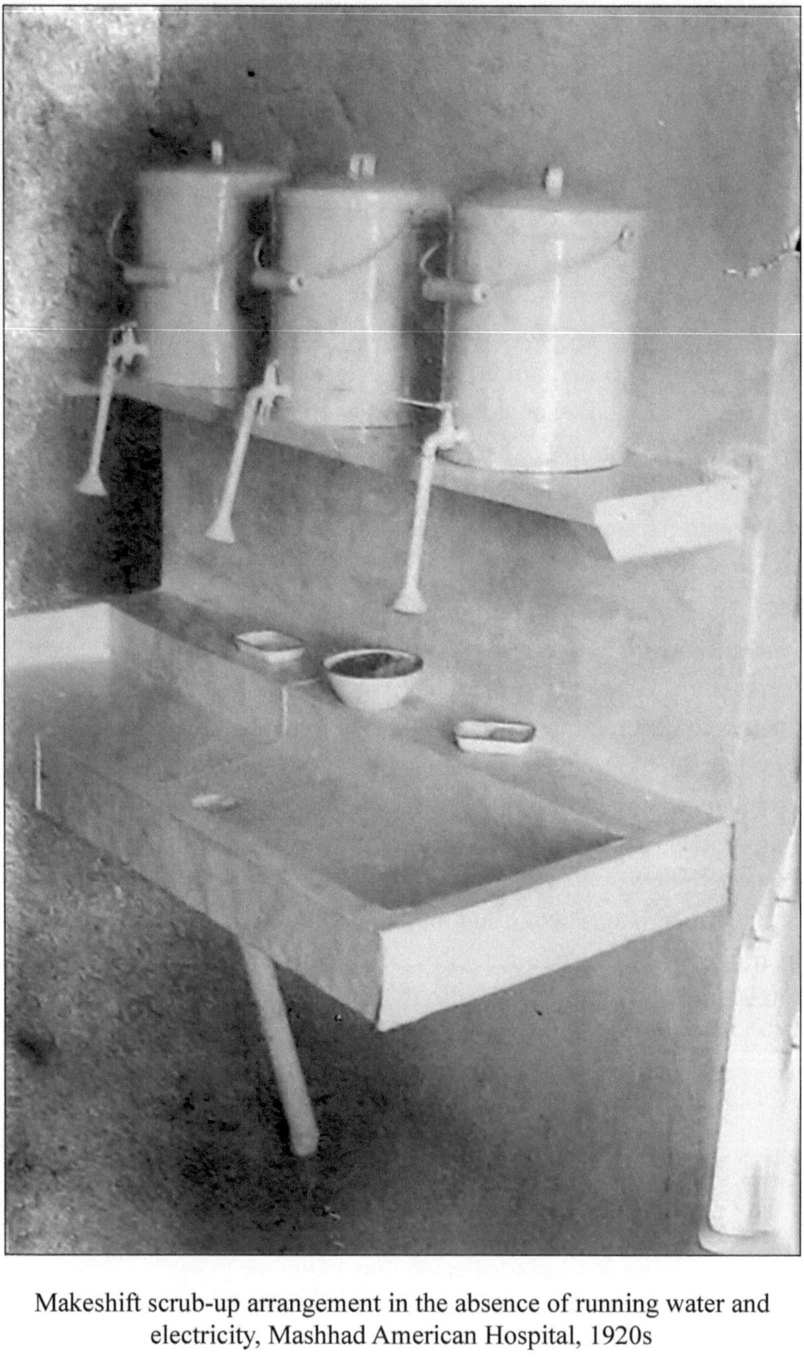

Makeshift scrub-up arrangement in the absence of running water and electricity, Mashhad American Hospital, 1920s

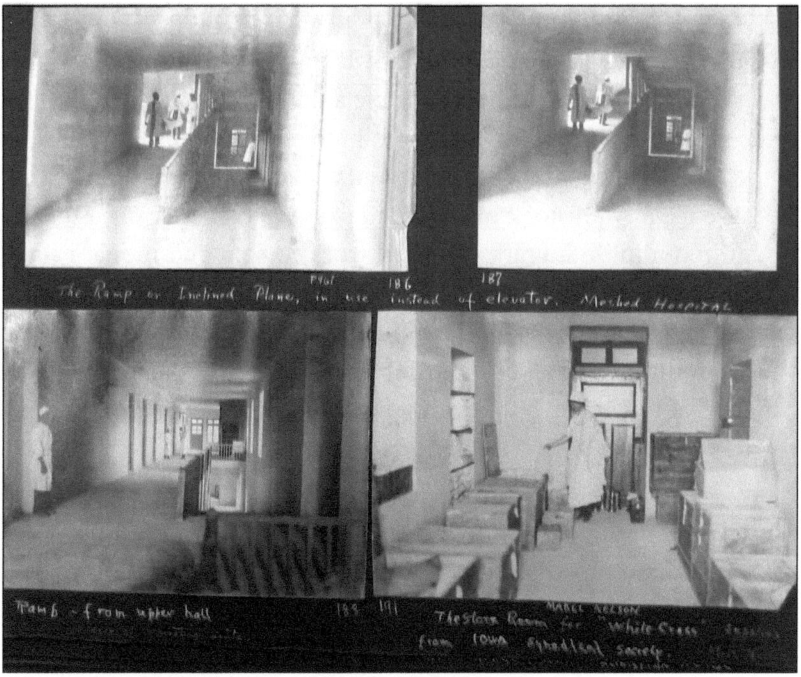

Lacking an elevator the American hospital in Mashhad used inclined ramps to facilitate transport of patients, 1920s

surgeons in Tehran.[80] This remained a persistent problem, for in 1945-46, Dr. Hakim-A`la worked for nine months in Mashhad and assisted in the OR, because surgical training in Tehran university was sketchy. He took over most tonsillectomies, pneumo-thorax refills, tuberculous glands, removal of small tumors and other minor operations.[81] As result, the expertise of the American missionary medical staff was recognized and used by outsiders. Many patients were referred to the American doctors by physicians in other cities (Isfahan, Shiraz, Hamadan, Kermanshah, Kerman, Tabriz, Rasht, Mashhad), because only the best care was found in the capital and had prestige and travel was easy.[82] Even four years before the Hamadan hospital was closed, the newest technology was introduced. "We did skin grafts, because

---

80. RG 231-1-6, Hoffman, Pioneering in Meshed, p. 123.
81. RG 91-20-2, Mashad Medical Report 1945-1946.
82. RG 91-19-11-1, Report American Hospital Teheran 1940-1941.

we had a new skin grafting machine flown 2 months ago from the US; who here can do this kind of plastic work?"[83]

Not only the OR, but also the sterilizing and dress preparation room were two of the busiest places in the hospital. In Kermanshah in the mid-1930s, a graduate nurse and a student nurse worked there. Because usually all stock of sterilized gauze and goods was used and it required nimble fingers and hard work to fold and prepare linen for the sterilizer. On 12 May 1938, the hospital used a new electric steam dressing sterilizer for the first time, a gift from the Westminster church in Buffalo. The kerosene one blackened the room and tried the patience of the nurse, but nevertheless was kept as back up.[84]

TECHNOLOGY

The American physicians also introduced new technologies and techniques and shared these as well as their experience with Iranian colleagues. In this chapter I draw attention to the fact that the American physicians were early users of the X-ray machine, while they also had their own labs to improve their diagnosis and treatments. Some even sent slides of lab tests to the American University of Beirut for examination. There were, of course, other modern techniques that the American missionary physicians introduced in particular those in the field of anesthesia and surgery (see above).

X-RAY

The X-ray is the oldest form of medical imaging and is used for diagnosis and treatment. X-ray machines were central to hospital diagnosis by the 1930s. In Iran, screening for TB and other medical problems, for example, took place with a portable X-ray machine, which was invented in 1919.

83. RG 91-19-27, Dr. Homer Rice to Ms Frances Gray 05/06/1956.
84. RG 91-19-28, Kermanshah Medical Report 1938.

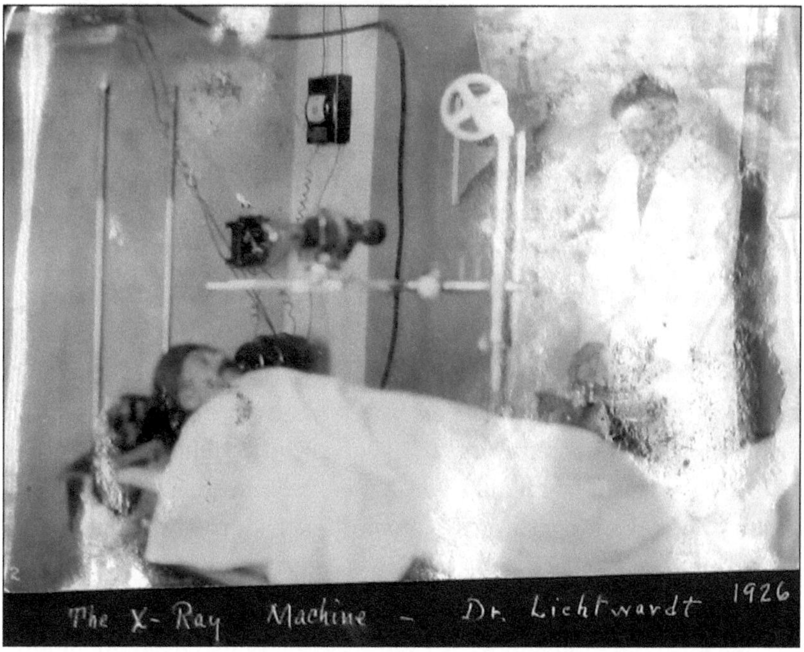

The X-ray machine of the Mashhad American Hospital with Dr. Lichtwardt, 1926

It appears that the first X-ray machine in Iran was brought by the British Army and was used in its hospital in Mashhad. For in August 1920, Dr. Hoffman wrote: "They even have a complete dental outfit and X-ray which we may get very cheap."[85] He did not get it, although it is not known what happened to it. The second X-ray machine in Iran was almost also supplied by the British government in 1922, when Dr. Scott and Dr. Neligan were managing the *Dowlat* Hospital in Tehran (1921-23). As part of the arrangement with the government of Iran, Great Britain would finance the establishment of an X-ray department at the hospital. Because the arrangement fell through the X-ray machine never came, at least there is no report of its presence in the hospital.[86] However, the AIOC hospital in Abadan had X-ray equipment from the early 1920s and throughout its continued existence.[87]

85. RG 231-1-2, Hoffman to brother, 05/08/1920.
86. RG 91-19-11-1, Notes on medical work of Teheran station Jan. 1922.
87. Williamson 1927, pp. 128-132; Gilmour 1924, p. 39; IOR/L/

Thus, it would seem that the British were the ones who first introduced this new technology to Iran. However, it was not used in the British CMS hospitals or the British consular hospitals, because it was still an expensive piece of equipment and required some training in operating, maintaining, and interpreting the photos. These facts as well as the US missionary physicians' use of X-ray are not reported in a recent article on the development of radiology in Iran.[88]

In 1920, Dr. Frame in Rasht wrote that having an X-ray machine, especially in the case of patients with bullet wounds, would make things simpler and even save lives, of which he cited various examples.[89] In 1920, the Presbyterian Board had set aside $2,000 for an X-ray machine, but it appears not to have been bought and sent.[90] For in 1921, the Rasht hospital had an X-ray machine financed out of the Sunday School Xmas offering, but unfortunately the wrong tubes were sent. This was a setback, the more so, because an adjacent cinema had offered free electricity. Fortunately, the Tehran missionary hospital needed this type of machine, so Frame gave it to that hospital, hoping that a friend would bring a new one.[91]

In 1923, returning from home leave, Frame brought a portable X-ray machine, which was installed at the end of the year. However, there were some problems with the X-ray equipment, although a Russian electrician claimed he could get the needed items locally. After several months he abandoned the plan, but a Russian engineer got it installed and it was working in May, and the first photo was made on 29 May 1925.[92] For a long time, Frame had problems in using the city

---

MIL/17/15/24, 'Military Report on The Anglo-Iranian Oil Company's (South Iranian) Oilfield Area', p. 49.

88. Vessal, Rad, Alizadeh, and Jalal-Shokouhi 2014, pp. 157-58.

89. RG 91-19-9, Report Medical Work 1919-20; Presbyterian Church 1921, pp. 332-34.

90. RG 91-19-9, Resht Medical Work 1932.

91. RG 91-19-9, Medical Report Resht 1921-22; Idem, Report Medical Work 1919-20; Idem, "History of Resht Station," p. 3; Idem, Resht Medical Work 1932.

92. RG 91-19-9, "History of Resht Station," p. 3; Idem, Resht Medical

current, which was changed just after he had made the adaptation. This proved to be inadequate and then a rival appeared with an X-ray apparatus in the city until he went bankrupt. Slowly the hospital was able to acquire parts of good quality, added homemade accessories such as a viewing box, a sliding cassette carrier and even an upright fluoroscope. With Dr. Frame's knack for tinkering with technical instruments, he thought that he might even make a horizontal fluoroscope, but his expertise fell short to make a Bucky Diaphragm, which had "to wait a gift from a fairy." In 1930, the X-ray machine developed problems and was replaced. The city power line was rehabilitated and gave adequate service, but it was only available at night. As a result, the hospital was able to offer comprehensive diagnostic service, which was increasingly appreciated, both by patients and local physicians.[93] Until then Frame's portable X-ray was the only one in town, but from then on, there was a much larger one available. Despite all this there were calls for more and better service than Frame was able to provide. He also added to his own X-ray equipment. Its reputation meant more work, because he received demands for complex cases beyond the abilities of his machine. Therefore, he needed a larger fluoroscope, a Bucky Diaphragm, and a regular X-ray table for better diagnosis.[94] Because it was the only X-ray apparatus in Rasht other doctors sent their patents to the American hospital. This meant extra income and allowed the hospital to order additional pieces of apparatus. Having the X-ray machine also meant more major surgeries, which increased by 6% and minor ones by >100%, because of increasing cystoscopies, pneumo-thoracies, etc.[95] The increased income due to the use of the X-ray machine by local physicians allowed the American hospital to buy a Potter-Bucky Diaphragm, which increased the quality of its work. As of that time, the equipment was as complete as Frame needed with

---

Report 1924-25.

93. RG 91-19-9, Resht Medical Report 1930; Idem, Resht Medical Report 1933.

94. RG 91-19-9, Resht Medical Report 1930; Idem, Rest Medical Report 1931.

95. RG 91-19-9, Resht Medical Report 1934.

his limited experience in this field. The fluoroscope, apart from the tube and screen, was made locally. He took 95 radiographs and did 336 fluoroscopies, of which 65 were of the gastro-intestinal tract and about 230 of the chest, mostly follow-ups of TB exams.[96] The X-ray machine was not only sufficient for his present needs, but its income continued to rise, because its use was increasingly appreciated by local doctors. Moreover, as of May 1936, the local power company offered a 24 hours service. This was an enormous improvement, because until then the X-ray could only be used at night. It was also cheaper than with the auto-generator, which had been installed in 1930. Although the hospital used only 20 kW at cost of 60 rials, it made fixed technique possible ensuring better radiographs. In 1935-36, Dr. Frame took 120 radiographs and did 537 radioscopies.[97]

At first, in Rasht probably a hospital generator was used, although this is not reported. However, in 1936, Dr. Frame reports that electric lighting was new in the hospital, although the lights were off in the early hours of the morning until hospital works started at 8 a.m. This made the X-ray machine more available; it helped the doctors operating on dark days, enabled them to use infra-red or other heat appliances, and it tempted them to buy electric fans, irons and instrument sterilizers. The power company tempted the hospital with still further conveniences such as driers, water heaters, etc., but the electricity rate was still so high that the hospital could not afford that kind of service. The X-ray unit was more used, and although much of the accessory equipment was of local construction it was sufficient for the hospital's needs. The chief problem was the time required and the lack of special training on the part of the doctors. Since Brinkman's departure, Frame tried to set aside 11-12 o'clock for fluoroscopy. Picture taking did not cause much delay, because he had trained an assistant to get the machine

---

96. RG 91-19-9, Resht Medical Report 1934-35.

97. RG 91-19-9, Resht Medical Report 1935-36; RG91-20-8, Resht Medical Report 1936-37 (Frame trained Hanifeh Nikzad to operate the X-ray machine).

ready and develop pictures. Many outside doctors referred patients for an X-ray and many had heard about the new means of diagnosis.[98]

> In former days we were often puzzled to satisfy the villager who expected us to make a complete diagnosis by feeling the pulse without any cooperation on his part. Now many present themselves saying: "I am ill. Please make a complete examination with the X-ray and tell me is my trouble." Again, the patient is unwilling to cooperate and fails entirely to realize the technical difficulties and the expense of making a complete X-ray study of the body without any symptoms as a guide.[99]

The availability of the X-ray machine was a great help to the physicians. In 1937, the doctors of the Rasht hospital were surprised by the large number of 'acute abdomens' they saw. They explained that as an indication of people becoming more conscious of the value of hospital treatment. Also on the increase were accidents due to cars, heavy construction works, factories, etc. Foreign companies especially sent their fracture cases to the missionary hospital, because of the new laws as to workmen's compensation. Some of these cases came from 300 km distance. These cases were problematic, because without a portable X-ray it was not possible to examine patients in bed. The hospital's home-made Balkan frames were often not adequate to a particular case. Sometimes adhesive did not arrive on time from abroad. Therefore, it took much ingenuity by doctors and nurses to keep these patients in good condition.[100]

The X-ray machine remained in high demand in Rasht and became so popular that not only patients had unrealistic expectations of its capabilities so did local doctors, who sometimes expected an exam that was outside the province of X-ray diagnosis. Unfortunately, in 1938, the machine developed a problem and Dr. Frame fell ill and he was

---

98. RG 91-19-9, Resht Medical Report 1935-36; Idem, Resht Medical Report 1936-37.

99. RG 91-19-9, Resht Medical Report 1935-36; Idem, Resht Medical Report 1936-37.

100. RG91-20-8, Resht Medical Report 1936-37.

unable to identify the problem or repair it.[101] The out-patient service was greatly handicapped by the breakdown of the X-ray machine. With the help of the makers, the problem was identified. New parts were ordered, but it took a year (transport, customs waiting time) before it arrived in the hospital and was able to perform again.[102] Everybody was happy that the X-ray unit, the only one in the province, was back and working again. Consequently, it was in great demand, because this X-ray unit was closer than the one in Tehran and worked year-round. Therefore, every physician in Rasht and in the province relied on it. "Many times the tall, blond Russian Consul doctor will bring an auto full of people from Pahlavi for X-ray. He knows no Persian or English, his patients usually speak nothing but Russian, so one of our three Russian speaking nurses must be on hand." However, the electricity in Rasht was a varying current and also due to normal wear it could easily stop working. Moreover, Dr. Frame was the only one who could repair the X-ray machine. In the spring of 1940, it refused to work. After a few days of experimentation, Dr. Frame was able to find the cause and make it work again.[103]

Usually, on Tuesday afternoons, many waited for pictures of gastro-intestinal fluoroscopy. Thursday afternoons an increasing number of young men and women with TB came for a fluoroscope check-up and pneumo-thorax. More than 300 fluoroscopy and 283 pneumo-thoraces were made in 1940-41. The medical staff realized that they should do more, but their other tasks forced them to limit this to one afternoon only. In fact, in 1941-42 they were able to increase the number of pictures and fluoroscopies. Moreover, Dr. Frame taught the hospital's record clerks and pharmacist to take satisfactory pictures, which relieved Dr. Frame of that extra work.[104] In 1944, Dr. Frame-

---

101. RG 91-19-9, Resht Hospital Report, 1937-38.

102. RG 91-19-9, Resht Hospital Report 1938-39.

103. RG 91-19-9, Resht Hospital Report 1939-40; Idem, Resht Hospital Report 1940-1941.

104. RG 91-19-9, Resht Hospital Report 1940-1941; Idem, Medical Report Resht Hospital, 1941- 1942.

Kibbe wrote: the X-ray machine and tubes are on their last legs and the whole instrument is outmoded and too small. [105]

Some time during the mid-1940s the X-ray machine of the American hospital in Rasht stopped working and could neither be repaired nor replaced, which handicapped the doctors' diagnostic capabilities.[106] In the fall of 1944, the Russians opened a 20-bed hospital that had "a workable fluoroscopy and some therapeutic lamps for which the new-rich are glad to pay good prices. All their charges are very high."[107] The X-ray situation in Rasht had improved by 1948, because there was an Iranian hospital that had an X-ray, but it had nobody who could operate it. The American hospital sent some patients to the Russian hospital for examination, but the physician was not happy with the indifferent results. Also, the Russians did not do any charity work.[108] Therefore, the new physician of the American hospital in Rasht, Dr. Rolla Hoffman (formerly working in Mashhad) asked the Presbyterian Board for a small portable X-ray for bedside work,[109] even though a regular X-ray machine was already expected that same year. In 1949, he reported that the X-ray machine was installed. It was a new Picker 'Century' model X-ray that finally arrived in February after two years and in a somewhat damaged condition. With the help from Mr. Wallace and Dr. John Frame Jr. from Hamadan it was fixed. He further noted that "the only other X-ray here is the Russian hospital's rather antiquated outfit, whose range of work is limited and beyond the reach of most people as it is not free at the Russian hospital."[110]

Although Rasht seems to have been the first, Mashhad was the second American missionary hospital to get an X-ray machine. When Dr. Lichtwardt returned from furlough in 1927 he brought an electric

---

105. RG 91-19-9, Resht Hospital Report 1944.

106. RG 231-1-5, Hoffman/Rasht to Friends, 12/09/1948.

107. RG 91-20-8, Resht Hospital Report 1944-45.

108. RG 231-1-5, Hoffman/Rasht to Friends, 12/09/1948.

109. RG 231-1-5, Memo Medical Needs Rasht Hospital undated, probably 1948.

110. RG 231-1-5, Personal Report Hoffman 1949 and Resht Hospital Report.

generator with a storage battery of 110 volts and a small X-ray machine. The Rev. Charles Murray, one of the evangelists of the Mashhad mission, erected a tower for the windmill that ran the generator. In this way, the hospital had electric lights during evening only; after 9 p.m. kerosene lamps and Dietz lanterns were used. Then they found a kerosene engine to run the generator. Later they bought power from a commercial local company and had lights until midnight. The use of the X-ray was limited to the evenings.[111] The Mashhad hospital's small electric generator supplied the electricity for the X-ray machine and for part of the year to the building. But it was too small to get satisfactory lighting for the hospital and the residencies and supply adequate current to the X-ray machine and therefore, they needed a larger generator. Unfortunately, not one of the 7-8 electric lighting companies of the city was near the hospital. Moreover, these plants were small, unreliable and expensive, and only supplied from sunset to about 11 p.m. To be able to do that as well as to maintain work and enable the physicians to employ better helpers the hospital needed an extra $5,000/year.[112] The physicians in Mashhad wrote that the X-ray machine was a great asset, especially for bone work, but it was too small for abdominal work, except in case of very thin people, because as yet, the hospital did not have an upright fluoroscope or Bucky Diaphragm. [113] In 1931-32, the electric-light plant was overhauled, while their amateurish wiring was taken out and the building was rewired. Also, new storage batteries were installed and, as a result, the X-ray and lights were working better. Although better, it was not what the physicians needed, because the machine's capacity was much too small. Therefore, Hoffman repeated that the hospital needed a bigger dynamo, and new supplies such as a diathermy outfit and a Bucky Diaphragm for the X-ray machine.[114]

---

111. RG 231-1-6, Hoffman, Pioneering in Meshed, p. 63.

112. RG 91-20-2, Mashad Medical Report 1929-1930. For the electricity situation in Mashhad, see Hamed and Habibi 1376.

113. RG 91-20-2, Mashad Medical Report 1929-1930.

114. RG 91-20-2, Mashad Medical Report 1931-1932.

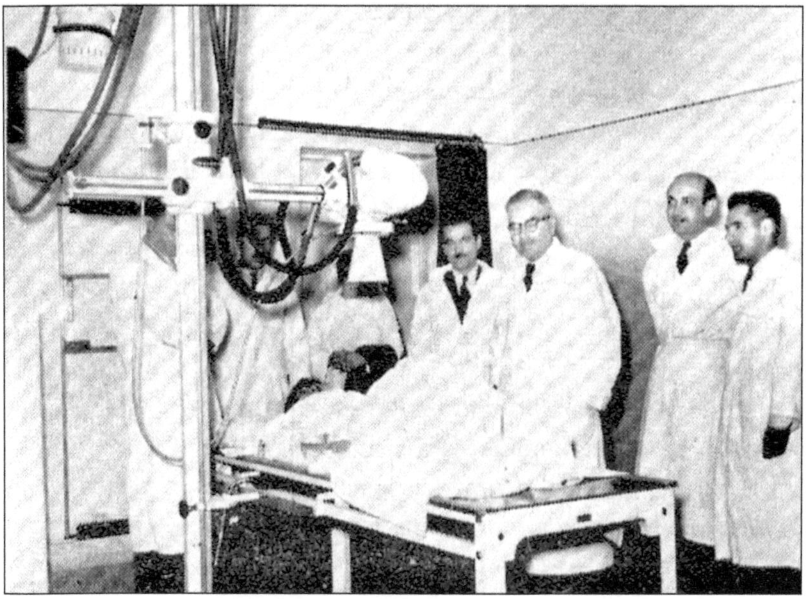

Radiology Department, Ibn Sina Hospital

In 1935, the newly built Shah Reza Hospital in Mashhad had two German physicians, one of whom, Dr. Katzenstein, was a radiologist with five X-ray machines plus diathermy, ultra-violet lights and other equipment. A German technician helped with the X-ray work. Consequently, Dr. Hoffman wrote: "the X-ray department at Shah Reza has no more enthusiastic patrons than ourselves, because ours is inadequate. For the first time a specialist in Mashad is better equipped than us; we send patients for X-rays for examination of chest, stomach, spine or bones, receiving an expert opinion and diagnosis in English." The very poor were served free by securing a certificate of poverty from their local police station.[115] Unfortunately, in 1937, Dr. Katzenstein, the young and enthusiastic German X-ray man and their fine X-ray equipment was idle. Dr. Katzenstein had suddenly disappeared, but showed up 10 years later in Germany, returning from Russian prisons. The German technician still made plain films as requested and these were of some help. However, the charges were very high and beyond

115. RG 91-20-2, Mashad Medical Report 1935-1936.

that of most patients. Therefore, the missionary physicians felt that they had to treat them for free after they had spent about all their money for a plain X-ray film. A few of the poor they sent got a free X-ray.[116] In 1945/46, there was only one local technician in the Shah Reza Hospital to 'take pictures' with its several X-ray machines, which were German, and therefore, more and more difficult to maintain. "Sometimes there are no films, often they are disappointing and there is big delay and large expense."[117]

The Tehran hospital finally also received an X-ray machine.[118] For years the medical staff had stressed the need for an X-ray machine, a requirement secondary only to a second storey over the central wing of the current building to have more clinic and patient rooms.[119] When in 1930, the X-ray unit was installed the doctors were able to diagnose 48 duodenal gastric ulcers. This they considered to be a great new development. Another development was Dr. Hoffman's work for bone and joint TB in children, based on his experience in Mashhad. In 1932, there were five such cases undergoing the long but hopeful treatment, because, if not treated they died or became crippled.[120] In 1933-34, the X-ray machine continued to be used regularly; over 100 pictures were taken, and 239 fluoroscopy exams done; 63 of the chest,

---

116. RG 91-20-2, Mashad Medical Report 1936-1937; RG 231-1-6, Hoffman, Pioneering in Meshed, p. 119.
117. RG 91-20-2, Mashad Medical Report 1945-1946 ("A man with a compound fracture of the thigh was sent from our hospital, more than a mile, for a 'picture.' The film showed the wrong part of the femur, missing the fracture. He was taken a second time and refused, with the explanation that a picture could not be taken with his Thomas splint on, and we would send a nurse a long to remove it. So we send him to the new Russian doctor, who made a satisfactory examination and a film, with the splint on. We really look forward to securing a really good X-ray equipment of our own.")
118. It is neither clear what happened to the X-ray tubes that Dr. Frame sent to Tehran in 1921 nor since when that hospital had an X-ray machine.
119. RG 91-19-11-1, Teheran Hospital Report 1928.
120. RG 91-19-11-1, Tehran Report Medical Work 1931-1932.

160 of gastro-intestinal tract and 15 for fracture or foreign bodies.[121] In 1934-45, a total of 239 fluoroscopy exams were made, more than of them half gastro-intestinal tract. The doctors also began microscopic exams of many tumors removed at operations. They also did a few sections for outside doctors. Although no pathological work was done in Tehran, Dr. McDowell hoped to stimulate an interest in this field, one of the fundamentals of modern medicine.[122] In 1940-41, the reasonably good X-ray machine had not been much used, because of lack of time and there was no technician to operate it. Those needing X-rays were sent outside, "if they can pay the stiff prices," because in Tehran at that time there were half a dozen good radiologists. One of them was Dr. Habib Adle, trained in Paris, who offered to train one of the Christian hospital's helpers, Agha Shahi, as to the technical part. After a few months he was able to make routine exposures of fractures and other bone cases. As a result, his service was increasingly becoming valuable, which also meant more income for the hospital. In 1941-42, X-ray service remained very limited due to scarcity of films and the failure of the Presbyterian Board to fill the January 1940 hospital's order.[123]

Also, in 1928, the Hamadan hospital finally acquired an X-ray machine, be it that it was a portable one, which was great for the diagnosis in these cases. Unfortunately, its capacity was too limited for adequate diagnosis service, especially for fluoroscopy, for which a new and better one was needed.[124] In December 1947, a new X-ray unit arrived. Until that time the hospital had used the old portable X-ray unit.[125] This new machine was very essential, because it was

---

121. RG 91-19-11-1, Report Medical Work, Teheran 1934.

122. RG 91-19-11-1, Report Tehran Medical Work 1934-1935.

123. RG 91-19-11-1, Report Hospital, Teheran 1940-1941; Idem, Teheran Medical Report 1941-1942. On Dr. Habib Adle's experience with the X-ray machine, see Vessal, Rad, Alizadeh, and Jalal-Shokouji 2014, p. 158.

124. RG 91-19-27, Hamadan Medical Report 1934; Idem, Hamadan Medical Report 1937.

125. RG 91-19-27, Hamadan Medical Report 1939 (a gift of $3,000 for

the only one in Hamadan. Already, in 1939 it was strongly felt that a modern X-ray machine was needed to improve the diagnostic capability of the medical staff. In 1944, the cost and possibility of giving Hamadan a new X-ray machine were discussed in New York. The new X-ray unit as well as ordered lab supplies only arrived at the end of 1946.[126] As a result, the Hamadan hospital had the best X-ray machine and the only radiologist of all American hospitals in Iran! The new X-ray machine was still the only one in city and local doctors referred their patients to the Christian hospital. During five months of operation (February-June 1947), 123 fluoroscopies were made and 156 radiographs, earning 34,400 rials. Although the start-up costs were rather high, it was hoped that the X-ray unit's payback time would be two years. Also, two Iranian assistants had already learnt how to operate it and develop films, while another one was in training.[127] The long-awaited lab supplies were also a boon, because now the hospital was really well-equipped to do all kinds of tests. Moreover, it was decided to add blood typing for transfusions and sedimentation tests to the lab's arsenal. It was further intended to start bacteriological work soon. One orderly was made lab assistant. Dr. Frame Jr., who had arrived in December 1947, started a course in physiological chemistry for the X-ray and lab workers.[128] In 1947-48, some of the operations the physicians would have been unable to do without the new X-ray machine.[129]

The lack of an X-ray machine remained a problem for the Kermanshah hospital. Patients had to travel 160 km or more to have one taken and treated by X-ray. Although instrument-wise the hospital was almost fully equipped, the doctors really hoped to get an X-ray in the near future.[130] In 1936, the doctors still could complain that theirs

---

the purchase of an X-ray machine, etc. in 1928).

126. RG 91-19-27, Hamadan Medical Report 1939; Idem, Medical Report Hamadan 1941; Idem, Hamadan Medical Report 1946-1947; RG 280-1-10, Hamadan Medical Work 1947-1948.

127. RG 280-1-10, Hamadan Medical Work. 1947-1948.

128. RG 280-1-10, Hamadan Medical Work. 1947-1948.

129. RG 280-1-10, Hamadan Medical Work. 1947-1948.

130. RG 91-19-28, Kermanshah Medical Report 1933-1934.

was the only US hospital in Iran that had no X-ray, which they really needed for better diagnosis and treatment. Fortunately, in 1937 they were promised one and, therefore, renovations were made to be able to receive the X-ray machine.[131] On 12 May 1938, the steam dressing sterilizer was used for the first time and on 20 May the first X-ray photo was taken. It and the electric generator were slightly damaged on arrival and needed repairs. On 21 May, the first treatment with the Diathermy was given.[132] The X-ray and Diathermy Department demanded more time from the doctors and, therefore, was mostly done in afternoons. It was the only apparatus in the province and, consequently, demand for its use was high, because people thought that it could be used to diagnose and treat any disease or pathological condition.[133] Much diathermy treatment was done in the out-patient clinic to the benefit of many patients.[134] The Westminster Hospital collaborated with the staff of the state hospital in the area of the use of its X-ray machine and its superior facilities in obstretics and surgery.[135]

Laboratory Facilities

A laboratory is essential in a modern hospital. The US missionary physicians were quite aware of this, but the means to do so were not always there. However, that did not mean that they did not establish simple laboratories, whose capabilities over time were further developed and extended. For example, for many years there was not even an autoclave in the surgery of the Urumiyeh hospital, the oldest

131. RG 91-19-28, Kermanshah Medical Report 1936; Idem, Kermanshah Medical Report 1937.

132. RG 91-19-28, The Westminster Hospital Bulletin. vol. 1/2. May 1938; Idem, Kermanshah Medical Report 1938-39 (The money for the X-ray machine, physio-therapy department and power plant was a gift from Mr. Muncie from Indiana).

133. RG 91-19-28, Kermanshah Medical Report 1938.

134. RG 91-19-28, Kermanshah Medical Report 1940.

135. RG 91-19-28, Kermanshah Medical Report 1940. The arrival of this civil state hospital was already expected in 1932, see RG 91-19-28, Packhard to Speer, 30/07/1932.

American hospital, and lab work was quite sketchy.[136] However, with the development of its medical school it also acquired a medical lab. Therefore, it is erroneous when Bahadori states that "Tissue examination facilities were not available for ordinary Iranian patients," as is clear from what follows. It is also erroneous when he writes that "the first medicine laboratory … was established in 1936 in Tehran," which likewise is shown hereunder to be in error.[137] Not only the American hospitals had a lab, but so did the British CMS hospitals.[138] Sometimes hospital lost their lab facilities, such as in the case of Tabriz and Urumiyeh, where due to the invasion of Turkish troops in 1918, followed by plundering, the hospitals lost all their equipment. In 1919, the Tabriz hospital still did not have lab equipment, which had all been taken by the withdrawing Turkish troops.[139] It took about a decade before the Urumiyeh hospital was almost back to 'normal' again, for they still lacked adequate lab equipment. They really needed it, because even as late as 1931 neither government nor private lab facilities existed in Urumiyeh.[140]

RASHT

In the early years (1910-17) of the Rasht hospital, Dr. Frame did his own lab exams and he offered better lab methods for diagnosis.[141] Because Iranian doctors increasingly sent specimens to him for exams,

---

136. RG 91-20-7, Last annual report of the Cochran Memorial Hospital, Rezaieh 1934.
137. Bahadori 2014, p. 144.
138. Administration Report 1934, p. 34 (For example, at the hospital in Kerman: "The Pathological Examinations are also increasing in usefulness and number. Dr. Pigott has started the Kahn test for Syphilis since her return from furlough, and finds it an extremely useful aid in diagnosis."
139. Presbyterian Church 1920, p. 331-32; Idem 1921, p. 346; Speer 1920, p. 69.
140. RG 91-20-7, Hugo Muller, Rezaieh to Cady Allen, Hamadan, 22/06/1931.
141. Presbyterian Church 1917, p. 300.

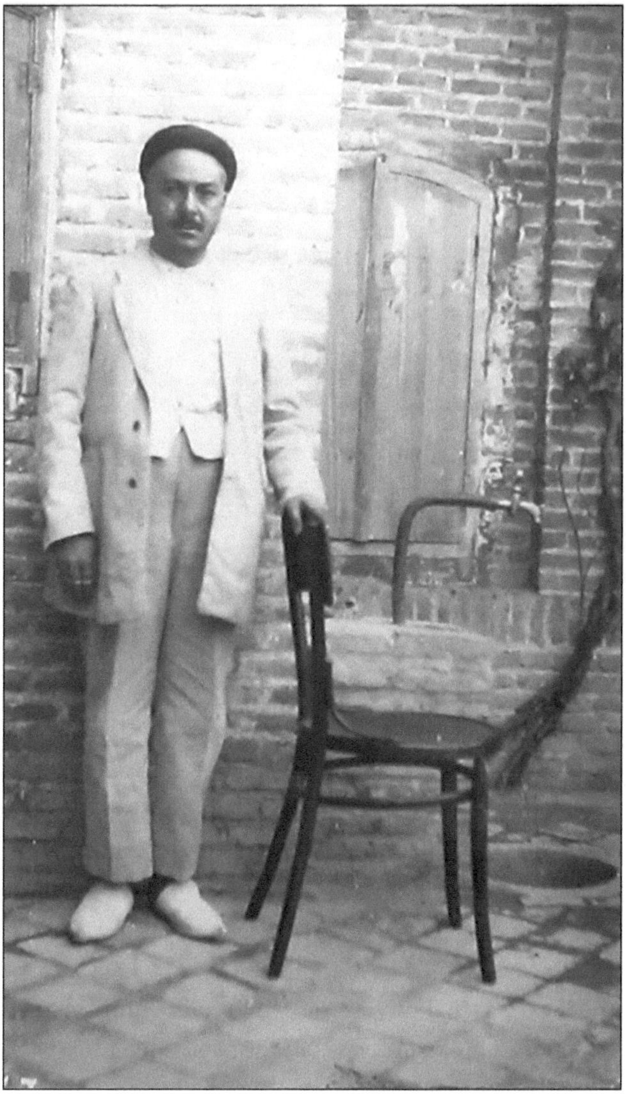

Dr. Boqrat al-Molk, physician-in-chief of the Mashhad police department and prison ca. 1920

he needed somebody who could do the routine work. Another option for local physicians was a young physician from Istanbul, who recently had come to Rasht with full lab equipment. He maintained that he was able to do all kinds of exams. Nevertheless, he wanted an agreement

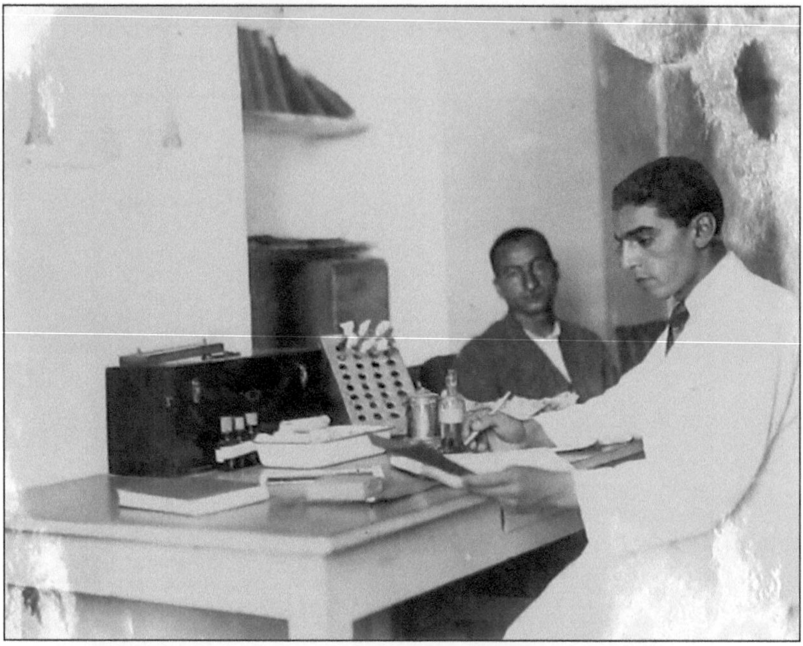

Ajdari, the Iranian lab technician of the Mashhad American Hospital

with the American hospital by which Frame would oversee his work to be able to endorse it to others.[142] In 1921, Dr. Frame reluctantly had accepted to train Sayyed `Ali, a simple village boy, who showed an aptitude for the lab and who was better than any former assistant. He found that without him he would have been greatly handicapped. Sayyed `Ali's most noteworthy assistance was in studying hookworm prevalence. An Iranian physician trained in Europe in lab work congratulated Frame on having such a competent and enthusiastic pupil. In 1924-25, Frame trained another apprentice for the lab.[143] The quality of the hospital's lab work attracted the attention of the better-class doctors in Rasht. Local physicians often asked for lab exams on TB, hookworm and leprosy and would use it more if the hospital lab would be able to meet their demands. Improvement in lab service gave better diagnosis. The assistant made progress despite Frame's

142. RG 91-19-9, Resht Medical Report 1921-22.

143. RG91-19-9, Resht Medical Report 1924-25.

lack of time to train him. Medical work had so much increased that he had taken an understudy.[144]

Dr. Bussdicker, who had come to Rasht to relieve Frame in 1927, did the lab work himself from September and, on his return in 1928, Frame continued that practice. At that time, he thought that he had found another helper, who might be a good lab man.[145] This arrangement apparently worked out, because Frame reported because his regular lab man had to do his 4-months military service, his understudy had taken over under the supervision of the hospital's druggist, the previous lab tech (i.e. Sayyed `Ali). The lab was important for both the American hospital and doctors in the city, who asked the hospital to do lab work for their private patients. Favus work was a large part of lab work, because children had to have clean scalps before they were allowed to attend their classes.[146] According to Frame, the lab might have been the busiest part of the hospital. The man in charge did 3,000 diverse exams, vaccinated 317 children with 885 return visits; treated 215 children for favus with 2,900 return visits and did 2,196 dressings or treatments. He also made agreements with in-patients, reported deaths and births to the government and kept the hospital's accounts. In 1938, Frame got a blood urea outfit and equipment for the Kline test for syphilis, but he decided not to use it until the lab would be a quieter place for such delicate work.[147]

In November 1942, Dr. Mohammad Kar, a German-French schooled Christian Iranian physician, with a German wife and two small children came on a one-year contract to work part-time, especially in the mornings in the out-patient clinic. Because Dr. Kar and his wife were basically lab people, they immediately suggested taking responsibility for that. The hospital kept Bahram Chahri, who had been an assistant for the last 10 years, but he thought his prestige was lessened and left. As of January 1943, the Kars took over the lab, adding a few

144. RG 91-19-9, Resht Medical Report 1931; Idem, Resht Medical 1929.

145. RG 91-19-9, Resht Medical Report 1927-1928.

146. RG 91-19-9, Resht Medical Report 1935-1936.

147. RG 91-19-9, Resht Hospital Report 1937-1938.

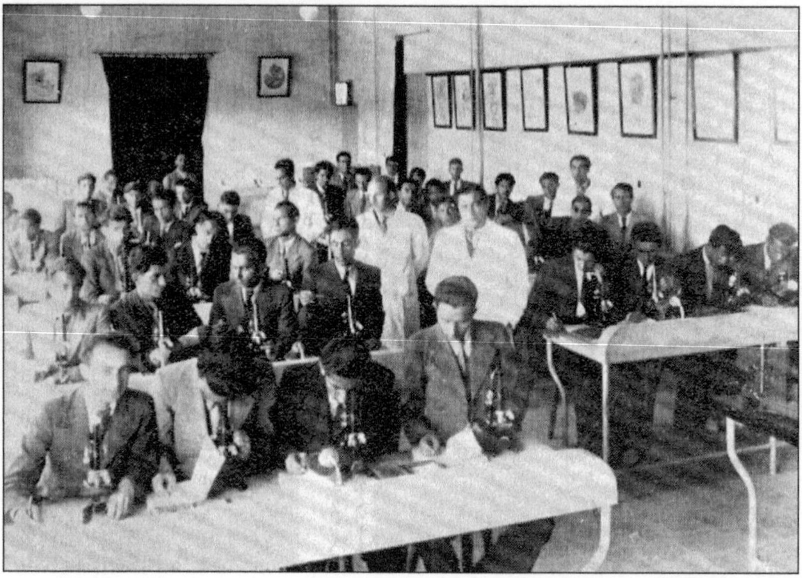

Dr. Mostafa Habibi during pathology practical teaching at the University of Tehran School of Medicine

supplies, agreeing to do all routine exams for bed patients, charging for tests such as Widal, Weil-Felix, etc. (the Wasserman test had not started yet). All out-patient exams were charged a reasonable fee; the hospital paid for free patients, just as they did for drugs. In return for their service, the Kars had at their disposal a lab room with equipment, furniture, heat, telephone, cleaning service, some autoclaving and all outside and city work, which income, until then had come to the hospital. This was an important development, because there still was no other reliable lab in Rasht. Also, the quality of lab work distinctly improved due to the Kars. Bahram Chahri had been able to do simple lab procedures, but he did not have the scientific background to appreciate the importance of what he was doing or the possibilities of more delicate and varied tests. In the past, Dr. Frame had taught him all he knew and supervised him, at least to the degree that he did not incline to drift into conscious slackness, but after Frame's death he was not supervised, and other work such as men's dressing, favus treatment, vaccination of large number of babies, etc. crowded out and diverted his attention from the more painstaking lab work.[148] The laboratory continued to do outside work as it had time and equipment. Urine and feces of all hospitalized patients were routinely examined; sputum, blood and other special tests only at doctor's orders. Dr. Frame was firmly convinced that without a lab they could not work. During 1940-41, a total of 2,438 lab exams were done, besides 2,200 men's dressings and 1,581 favus treatments.[149]

Mashhad

In Mashhad, in the 1920s, Dr. Hofmann and Dr. Lichtwardt established a small lab in their hospital, where simple tests could be done. In the absence of any trained lab technician, they had to do most of their own lab work.[150] In fact, this simple lab was the best one in the entire city of Mashhad. Therefore, the US hospital lab was used by Iranian doctors as well, who sent patients and specimens for examination. Common exams desired were: blood smear for malaria, sputum for TB bacillus, urine, complete exams and stools for ova and amoeba. As yet no serological tests were done. These exams were similar to the standard lab routine for the hospital's own patients, which also included the occasional blood count. However, the doctors realized that they needed more and better lab work, which meant having a trained lab tech, which they did not have. To improve their lab capacity and competency Dr. Hoffman and Dr. Lichtwardt gave a few lessons in urine work to male nurses. Dr. Ranjit, an Indian physician, did the sputum. In 1930, during the first six months, 20 positives were found.[151] Unfortunately, in 1933, the young boy who had been trained to do

148. RG 91-19-9, Resht Hospital Report 1943.

149. RG 91-19-9, Resht Hospital Report 1940-1941 (in 1939-40, a total of 3,017 cases were seen).

150. RG 231-1-2, Hoffman to Friends 10/03/1930.

151. RG 91-20-2, Mashad Medical Report 1929-1930; Idem, Mashad Medical Report 1935-1936.

most of the lab work was drafted to do 2-year military service, so they had to train somebody else.[152]

In 1935, the missionary hospital in Mashhad got competition from the lab of the newly built Shah Reza Hospital, which was under an Iranian doctor, educated in France and with a French wife. He began by requiring all staff to have a Wassermann test and dismissed all those with a positive result. This gave the lab a bad reputation; there were protests and the policy was reversed. The dismissed staff was not only retained but received free treatment. The health department asked reports of the work done and here our record system was very helpful. Also, certificates of births and deaths were required.[153]

In August 1936, the lab of the missionary hospital was improved by the addition of the Kline test; for three years the hospital had sent an increasing number of surgical pathology specimens for diagnosis to Prof. Sayhun, the pathologist of the American University in Beirut and he was happy to do so. Masih Aqa, an Iranian medical student working in the Beirut lab found out that the slides for his examination were all from Mashhad and he became so interested that he came for a summer to work in the Mashhad hospital. He set up its newly acquired equipment for the Kline test and taught Gholam Reza Ajdari the technique to use it. The latter had to do his military service in March 1937, but a second boy Kasmai learned the technique from him and with some supervision from Dr. Kibbe he regularly carried out the tests. At first, only 20 blood exams were taken per week, but later 60 per week. The result was that more of those with the disease received systematic treatment over periods of months. Because of the high cost of medicines, general poverty, failure of doctors to realize and urge the necessity of regular treatment as well as their inability to diagnose the disease in absence of any serological work, very few patients continued treatment for more than a few weeks. The doctors gave patients a statement of their diagnosis and the amount of treatment received when they left Mashhad for their home town. The hospital

152. RG 91-20-2, Mashad Medical Report 1932-1933.

153. RG 231-1-6, Hoffman, Pioneering in Meshed, p. 120.

purchased arsenical wholesale in large tubes from the US, where it was cheaper than in Europe to help the poor. Also, the doctors made our own bismuth mixture for injection using local cheap poppy-seed oil as a vehicle, one of the blandest oils available. In this way they were able to demand from the poor very low prices, only 4-5 rials (20-25 c) per visit, which covered most of the cost of medicines.[154]

In 1938, the Christian hospital continued to use the Kline-test for serological diagnosis of syphilis, and purchased necarsphenamine wholesale in large tubes and had its pharmacist made bismuth in oil for injections. As a result, syphilis patients came in larger numbers, attended faithfully and scores of patients benefited from it over the months. The doctors followed the routine of giving both necarsphenamine and bismuth injections at the single weekly visit. They also permitted an assistant to do routine treatment for periods of some weeks, as long as no complications arose. In such cases fees were charged in accordance with the patient's ability to pay, often only five rials down to even one rial (=ca. 6 c). But if a patient failed to attend the clinic for a whole month the charge was automatically doubled or more. Out of town patients were given a note for their doctor when they went home to guide him in future treatment. Many of the local profession learnt to evaluate the Kline test and often sent their patients to the hospital, which was a help to them and a source of income for the hospital.[155] In 1940, Dr. Walter Norem joined the Mashhad hospital with his wife, a highly trained lab technician, who improved the lab and trained Tooba Rezai to be a technician.[156] Because in 1941, the hospital lost two assistants, the doctors and the lab tech had to do their job as well.[157]

---

154. RG 91-20-2, Mashad Medical Report 1936-1937; RG 231-1-6, Hoffman, Pioneering in Meshed, p. 123
155. RG 91-20-2, Mashad Medical Report 1937-1938 (Mrs. Norem also helped in the lab and she trained the two Iranian technicians); RG 91-20-2, Mashad Medical Report 1940-1941.
156. RG 91-20-2, Mashad Medical Report 1942-1943.
157. RG 91-20-2, Mashad Medical Report 1940-1941.

The lab technician did the general run of exams, and the druggist carefully and promptly filled the prescriptions, using as far as possible stock formulas to save his and the doctor's time. In total, there were some 15 workers in the dispensary from 7 a.m. till 4-5 p.m.[158] The lab tech examined blood for malaria and relapsing fever, of which there was an epidemic in 1945-46; counting blood cells and taking specimens for serological tests to be done the next day.[159]

KERMANSHAH

Until the opening of the new hospital in Kermanshah in 1932, the lab only existed of a table in the corner of the Drug Room. Equipment was very meager, consisting of a urine analysis apparatus and a microscope. After 1932, there was a large room on the second floor of the new hospital with a proper lab table, the gift of a local Jewish merchant. Churches in the USA also contributed equipment. Every patient had urine analysis and, when needed, many malaria blood smears were done, while a few sputum and other analyses were also made. The hospital acquired some apparatus to do blood chemistry tests. In 1933, there was no lab assistant who knew English, which made training difficult. During the time that he worked in the hospital, Dr. Rustam Sarfeh also helped in the lab. Once a week, since 1 January 1934, the lab did the Kahn test for syphilis. Mirza Yonan did most of the tests, but not yet the microscopical work; nevertheless, he saved the doctors much time.[160]

HAMADAN

The Hamadan missionary hospital had no lab. What changed was the hiring of a new lab assistant in 1944, who had worked for years as lab technician for the AIOC in Abadan, who returned to his home

158. RG 91-20-2, Mashad Medical Report 1942-1943 (Ali Soheyl, the business manager bargained and collected the fees.)

159. RG 91-20-2, Mashad Medical Report 1945-1946.

160. RG 91-19-28, Kermanshah Hospital Report 1933;Idem, Kermanshah Hospital Report 1933-1934.

town of Hamadan. Although the hospital didn't have all the necessary equipment his work was an asset.[161] In 1947, the long-awaited lab supplies arrived, so that the hospital was really well-equipped to do all kinds of tests. Moreover, it was decided to add blood typing for transfusions, and sedimentation tests to the lab's arsenal. It was further intended to soon start bacteriological work. One orderly was made lab assistant. Dr. Frame Jr. started a course in physiological chemistry for the X-ray and lab workers.[162]

Tehran

The Tehran hospital seems not to always have had a lab. When Dr. Hoffman from Mashhad did backstopping in 1940, he reopened a lab of sorts, run by a doctor of the military hospital. This was very convenient, although any profits went to the doctor not to the hospital. However, Hoffman stressed that if the Tehran hospital was to continue it needed to have its own lab, but there was no change in the lab situation thereafter. Because the outside army doctor was only available three mornings per week, Hoffman flagged the need for the hospital to have its own pharmacy. The more so, because the pharmacy had to do some dispensing of medicines as prices in outside pharmacies have sky-rocketed and especially sulfonamide drugs were very scarce.[163] If the hospital would be continued then one of the doctors should have experience in lab work, including serology, also a lab technician with adequate lab equipment for serological tests, blood chemistry and all other ordinary tests; the hospital also should develop a school for X-ray and lab technicians.[164]

---

161. RG 280-1-10, Hamadan Medical Work 1943-1944.
162. RG 280-1-10, Hamadan Medical Work 1947.
163. RG 91-19-11-1, Teheran Medical Report 1940-1941; Idem, Teheran Medical Report, 1941-1942.
164. RG 91-19-11-1, Teheran Medical Report 1942-1943.

COLLABORATION

Often representatives of the central or local government asked the American physicians to render certain services. The type of service was varied in nature ranging from medical, surgical to research and educational. As to the latter, in a previous chapter the role of American missionary nurses was highlighted with regard to the establishment and managing the government schools of nurses. Dr. Blair inaugurated the first year of the Gross Anatomy course at the Tehran medical school. Dr. Blair continued teaching in the Anatomy Department at the Medical School until his departure in 1938, which the School very much regretted.[165] In Tehran, Dr. McDowell served some years on the National Board of Medical Examiners. In 1935 he spent several days examining graduates of the medical college. Dr. McDowell also served on a committee for reviewing the government course for the schools of nursing, aided by inputs from Ms Fulton.[166] Similar requests were made from American doctors at the local level such as in Rasht and Hamadan. During the typhoid epidemic in spring 1927, Dr. McDowell and Dr. Bahrami of the Pasteur Institute collaborated and isolated the bacterial cause, a distinct species from any known bacterial cause of typhoid.[167]

In Hamadan, there were good relations with local government organizations. In 1915, Dr. Funk served as sanitary adviser to the Municipal Council.[168] Relations with the local health department and the local municipal hospital remained good. The latter had no surgeon and in 1939 the health department asked the Christian Hospital to do their surgery for them[169] In Rasht, Dr. Frame collaborated with government or government sponsored activities. In 1920, the Sanitary

---

165. RG 91-19-11-1, Report Tehran Medical Work 1934-1935.
166. RG 91-19-11-1, Teheran Medical Report 1936; Idem, Teheran Medical Report 1937-1938; RG 231-1-2, Hoffman, no date (probably 1938).
167. Presbyterian Church 1928, p. 188.
168. Presbyterian Church 1916, p. 295.
169. RG 91-19-27, Christian Healing in Hamadan 1939.

Council in Tehran wanted to resume public vaccinations after the defeat of the Jangalis. For two years, Frame had been chairman of the Gilan section. The province was still too disturbed, but he established two stations in Rasht and Lahejan. The governor of Gilan asked Frame to undertake a permanent hospital for the police force, but he had to refuse, because he was going on home leave.[170] In the mid-1930s, the chief of the Health Department of Hamadan sent cases of favus and other cases that he thought the Christian hospital could better handle.[171] In the spring of 1952, service to the lepers by the American hospital in Tabriz was re-established (after a 45 year hiatus). This was made easier, because with the new road it took only 40 minutes of travel by car, when it was dry. These visits were made at the request of the Department of Health, which asked the American doctors to supervise the use of sulfone drugs. The Minister of Health himself, `Ali Asghar Hekmat, gave Dr. Stewart 100,000 rials, a substantial supply of sulfone drugs and a government jeep. As a result, there was a statistically significant improvement in only six months.[172]

Relations with former students of the medical school were excellent. In 1913, for example, many outside calls were consultations for former students, which helped making the hospital self-sufficient.[173] But over time, other local Iranian physicians referred their patients to the Christian hospital for surgery, lab work and X-ray diagnosis. (see above). The American Hospital in Tehran also had good relations with some practicing doctors, who were graduates from its hospital. In fact, some had been trained only by missionary doctors. Several others had graduated from the Iranian medical school, while at the same time had been working as interns in the Christian hospital and getting much practical work experience. Many asked the American doctors for consultation or sent them patients. Also, they usually called them

---

170. RG 91-19-9, Resht Medical Report 1919-20.
171. RG 91-19-27, Healing in the Home of Avicenna 1936.
172. Presbyterian Church 1951, p. 67. There was a fire in the Tabriz hospital, for the detailed repair bill, see RG161/3/51. For the history of treatment of lepers in Iran, see the next chapter in this book.
173. Presbyterian Church 1914, p. 329.

when they were sick. In 1932, the hospital employed one graduate of the Iranian medical college, who worked half time in hospital as a staff member and half time in his own practice. He did more surgical work (cataracts, hernias, small tumors, tonsillectomies, etc.) than the American doctors and saved them much time. At that time, the missionary physicians had no regular contacts with government doctors or Russian ones, who were not well trained in their opinion.[174]

Dr. Frame (Rasht) realized the importance of having good relations with the local government, the local medical establishment and with the community at large. That meant that he wanted to create an environment in which the American hospital and its staff was seen not as a threat or obstacle, but rather as a complementary asset that served the community to improve its welfare.

> It is not our purpose to compete with local physicians but rather to complement and supplement their efforts; by doing what they cannot do. Therefore, our first step was to discuss with city physicians how the hospital could cooperate with them and not prove a rival. We gave them a circular pointing out what benefits we could offer. The doctors asked that I would not do private practice in the city and confine myself to surgery and specialized work for which the hospital is fitted. I said I did not want to do private practice on condition that I was assured that poor people would not be neglected in times of emergency, such as child birth and to ensure that I would not do private work I suggested that they send me as many paying surgery cases as possible, because then I could not complain of lack of work or income. Their response was satisfactory. A few still wait too long before sending surgical cases. I only do consultations in the city and even in the office increasingly my work is surgical, eye and gynecological a considerable part referred to by city doctors.[175]

---

174. RG 231-1-5, Hoffman/Tehran to Dr. McClanahan/Cairo (31/07/1932).

175. RG 91-19-9, Resht Medical Report 1924-25.

Dr. Frame was successful in creating a cooperative attitude among local doctors toward the hospital. These called him for consultation and referred cases to his hospital.[176] Dr. Blair (Tehran) argued that the missionary doctors needed to nurture friendship with Iran and this meant that they had to identify themselves "with Iranian interests, sometimes to the apparent detriment of our own."[177] Therefore, Frame and his American colleagues did not consider the arrival of new Iranian hospitals as competition, but as a welcome complement. That did not mean that he was not critical of some of the government's activities, but he accepted those as the 'cost of learning' and whole-heartedly gave his help to those 'rival' hospitals, whenever he was asked to.

> Persians really try to develop their country to their own concepts, sometimes overestimating their conception of needs and anti-foreign in attitude, but on the whole a commendable attitude. Some years ago, the merchants submitted to some special taxes for philanthropic purposes. There is friction between them and the municipality. They have now an orphanage, a 'national' hospital, an alms house and a clinic for medical control of prostitution. The national hospital is in charge of an old acquaintance- not always a friendly one-trained in Geneva. He called on me regularly for surgical consultations and has sent me patients and we have sent some patients to him and have operated several times in his hospital as they have no surgical equipment. A few years ago I had the same relationship with the military hospital but the past year they have made efforts to handle all their own work. None of their doctors had surgical training, probably because a Persian doctor, my only local rival in surgery, was trying to get an appointment to this hospital. Recently two of their officers called on me and told that their surgical efforts had not been very successful blaming it mainly on their lack of a sterilizer. I offered to sterilize for them all their material they needed. They thanked

176. RG 91-19-9, Resht Medical Report 1929.

177. RG 91-19-11-1, Report Tehran Medical Work 1934-1935.

> me and said they also liked to have some personal help from me. Since then I have been doing major operations there.[178]

Frame refused treatment in homes, but in his hospital held frequently clinics for interested doctors; the size of the meeting varying according to the subject. In response, doctors sent more cases for special study, lab, X-rays or physical exam and sometimes even for treatment in the out-patient department.[179] Frame liked the consultations most. Local doctors were not good consultants, he opined, "too often advising dilatory tactics where haste is important and then urging last minute operations after hope has gone." This was important, because of the possibility of emergency operations.[180] Frame also advised the National Hospital to include sun parlors to treat cases of bone disease.[181]

Dr. Frame observed that in 1931, although the National Hospital had increased its beds, while financial considerations led many to go there, "there is still great prejudice in favor of our hospital, because of better service and nursing we offer."[182] And this came to the heart of the matter. Frame wanted the Christian hospital to be non-competitive, but to be better, in particular in those fields where it provided treatment that the others could not offer. This required continuous adjustment and learning to remain at the leading edge, and the missionary doctors did so with success. Given "the steady development of government health and general Persian medical services the permanence and need of Mission hospital work depends largely upon our ability to keep ahead of these programs and continue some contribution which the Persians are not yet making and thus continue pioneers in new lines of medical activity."[183]

---

178. RG91-19-9, Resht Medical Report 1924-25.
179. RG 91-19-9, Resht Medical Report 1930.
180. RG 91-19-9, Rest Medical Report 1932.
181. RG 91-19-9, Resht Medical Report 1930.
182. RG 91-19-9, Resht Medical Report 1933.
183. RG 91-19-9, Resht Medical Report 1933. This working ethos was much appreciated by Iranian physicians, see Ta`eb 1384, pp. 46-47, 57-58.

The Medical Society

The availability of data for American hospitals varies and for some, information is lacking for many years of their operation. With this proviso, it would seem that Dr. John Frame in Rasht was the first to form a discussion group of local physicians. Dr. Frame realized how hard it was for Iranian doctors to keep up with modern developments. Therefore, in 1920, he invited them to the hospital for two conferences. Some 10-15 came and discussed hookworm, malaria, and dysentery. As to hookworm few of them recognized it. Frame explained how to diagnose and treat it. Later they told him that they also found it in their practice.[184] As of 1923, there was a consulting group of physicians who met on Friday afternoon, consisting of an Armenian, a Greek and a Tartar physician trained in Baltimore, Istanbul and Berlin respectively.[185] With some other doctors, the best in the city, Frame held a 'consultation clinic' as described above. They met one afternoon per week to discuss special cases, charging the patient a small consultation fee and fee for the lab exam. Patients appreciated this and it was imitated by a consulting group among the local physicians.[186]

A similar development took place in Mashhad. During the first years (early 1920s), Dr. Hoffman and Dr. Lichtwardt encouraged Iranian doctors to join them in having regular meetings to discuss current medical topics, but it was only in 1928 that for the first time they expressed an interest to do so. This happened mainly because of the superintendent of the Pahlavi (Shrine) hospital. With his encouragement, weekly meetings were held during part of the year, when it was at the American hospital under the presidency of the American physicians, if it was at the Pahlavi hospital then under his. Most Iranian doctors attended regularly, and the discussions were valuable. In these meeting the American physicians used clinical material and

---

184. RG91-19-9, Resht Medical Report 1919-20.
185. RG91-19-9, Resht Medical Report 1923-24.
186. RG91-19-9, Resht Medical Report 1924-25

occasionally showed still-films.[187] During the winter of 1929-30, these weekly meetings for doctors were held at the American hospital. The American physicians showed unusual cases, specimens removed at operations, while TB cases were presented by them and a few by outside doctors. The American physicians also cooperated with the Health Department and local physicians in giving a series of health lectures and still films in the Public Library in one of the city parks. While they prepared the material and operated the lantern, 10 of the 12 talks were given by Iranian doctors. Dr. Lichtwardt also gave a series of simple talks for new army recruits at the request of the GCO Army of the East. The meetings for doctors stopped in the spring of 1930 due to their work load.[188] Because there were European trained doctors in Mashhad, the missionary doctors didn't make house calls. Nevertheless, they were called out frequently for consultation with Persian doctors, which they tried to do as much as possible in the late afternoon so as not to interfere with the normal schedule. However, house calls might come at any time of the day and night.[189]

Because of the difficulty of effectively treating patients, the Mashhad staff began placing emphasis on preventive care in 1928 and thereafter. They submitted that the objective of medicine should not only be diagnosis and treatment but also be prevention. In that year the two physicians began a program of medical education. "We have now two stereopticon projectors, with a growing library of still-films, covering a variety of subjects, and have made great use of the 'magic lanterns', throughout the year." In the winter of 1928-29, Dr. Hoffman gave two courses on hygiene in the school building. "Later the governor and the superintendent of education asked us to co-operate in planning for a series of public lectures of hygiene and health subjects." In the spring of 1929, weekly meetings were held in the Nader Shah garden and the large lecture room of the public library. It

187. RG 91-20-2, Mashad Medical Report 1929.

188. RG 91-20-2, Mashad Medical Report 1929-1930.

189. RG 91-20-2, Mashad Medical Report 1930-1931: Presbyterian Church 1926, pp. 206, 217; RG 231-1-6, Hoffman, Pioneering in Meshed, pp. 57-59.

was always very crowded and many were even standing outside. Most talks were given by local Iranian doctors, although the US physicians supplied most of the material and showed still-films weekly.[190] Also, in the following years the US physicians gave public health lectures, illustrated by stereopticon, at the local Shah Reza High school, where about 500 students gathered for the talks.[191] In the winter of 1935-36, the public health lectures were held bi-monthly to a high school's boys club; attendance was some 60 students. Patients were given health literature in the form of printed folders on diseases, while physicians emphasized the need for continued treatment. "We gave mimeographed sheets of information and instruction to the many suffering from trachoma, malaria, syphilis, tuberculous glands, intestinal worms, diarrhea, favus, etc. and we had evidence that they were being read and treasured." In 1936 and thereafter, the local Health Department also was putting out pamphlets and posters.[192] Similar activities took place in Rasht. In 1933-34, Dr. Frame and Dr. Brinkman produced a number of lantern talks using film slides and collections of pictures, which they gave in the hospital waiting room on Thursday evening and in Lahejan. The topics were: Pasteur and the Cause of Disease; Trudeau and the Cure of TB; How disease is spread; How to prevent disease; General personal hygiene; and Malaria.[193]

In Tehran, already in 1898, part of the year clinics were held once per week to which doctors in the city and students of the Shah's College were invited and they gladly came.[194] It is not known whether these collegial clinics were continued, but good relations existed among the American and Western Iranian trained doctors. This led to the creation of the Medical Society probably in 1931. It consisted of a small select group of Iranian physicians, who met twice per month at the American hospital. Anyone could suggest an interesting case to

---

190. RG 91-20-2, Mashad Medical Report 1929.

191. RG 91-20-2, Mashad Medical Report 1931-1932.

192. RG 91-20-2, Mashad Medical Report 1935-1936; RG 231-1-6, Hoffman, Pioneering in Meshed, p. 82-93, 128 (with details).

193. RG 91-19-7, Resht Medical Report 1933-1934; Ta'eb 1384, p. 49.

194. Presbyterian Church 1899, pp. 187-88.

discuss. In 1933, the Tehran Medical Society was infused with new life under Dr. Habib Adle. Initially, there were a dozen members: the two American missionary physicians, the British Legation doctor, the other nine were Iranians, all leaders in their profession. One was the leading X-ray specialist, trained in Paris (Dr. Habib Adle), a second was a good general and genitourinary surgeon, lately national chief of health department; one had recently returned from the US (Dr. Abu'l-Hasan Bakhtiar), where he had been in practice in New York, and had now become the chief of the government hospital for women. The others were mostly teachers at the Medical College. Between these physicians, friendly relations existed, whom they also saw when asked for consultations. After the British doctor had left (presumably Dr. Cyril Elgood, who left Iran in 1931), the two US doctors were the only foreigners and the Medical Society didn't intend to include more. Thereafter, there were 16 members, many young Iranians fresh from medical schools in Europe. The Society focused on clinical work and as of 1934 wanted to publish a small medical journal in Persian. In the winter of 1933-34, much time was spent on professional organization and medical defense. Dr. Hoffman (who was on loan from Mashhad) found it very interesting to sit in on fierce discussions how to get rid of foreign doctors and their competition. The two American doctors were very flattered, when told that they were not considered foreigners.[195] Dr. McDowell and Dr. Blair were members of the Tehran Medical Society.[196]

A similar Medical Society was also created in Mashhad. The changed attitude and good relations created by the earlier discussion group and professional meetings and presentations were sustained by a series of outside developments, such as: less fanaticism, modernization and arrival of a well-trained Armenian doctor, who had fled from Russia. Also, the number of local medical leaders was only

195. RG 231-1-5, Hoffman/Tehran to Dr. McClanahan/Cairo (31/07/1932); RG 231-1-2, Report Medical Work Teheran 1934.

196. RG 91-19-11-1, Report Medical Work Teheran 1936; Idem, Report of Medical Work Teheran 1937-1938; RG 231-1-2, Rolla Hoffman, no date (probably 1938).

about 12 (Iranian doctors with modern medical training were: Dr. Ziai from AU Beirut, Dr. Moezed from the Jesuit University in Beirut, Dr. Eftekhari from Germany), which made developing contacts easier. Most important was an emergency operation on one of these doctors (strangulated hernia). As a result of the good relations, Iranian doctors referred patients to the Christian hospital. When in 1935, Dr. Cochran came from Urumiyeh, where the government had closed the mission station, his arrival led to the founding of the Mashad Medical Society, which met twice per month to discuss medical subjects. Another interesting contact was that with the city architect, who came to the American doctors, since he wanted to study the design of their hospital, because it was a compact and conveniently arranged building, hence more economical to operate than others.[197]

In 1935-36, the Mashhad Medical Society, which was established in the US hospital, continued to meet monthly. As in the preceding years, the US physicians presented cases of interest at each meeting; often using films from the Shah Reza hospital and discuss the interpretation of films and the usefulness of X-rays. In 1936, it was decided to meet at the Shah Reza hospital during 1936-37, while one of its doctors was elected as chair. These meetings led to a further improvement of the attitude toward each other; its members sent patients for surgery or diagnosis to the Christian hospital. The great event was the medical conference of the Presbyterian Iran Mission in March 1936 with representatives from all six American missionary hospitals. One evening, a dinner and discussion with the Mashhad medical society was held. The conference apart from praise for the Mashhad missionary doctors also made suggestions for improvements.[198] Prof. Hammerschlag, a German gynecologist and superintendent of the Shah Reza hospital attended the meetings of the Medical Society and he was elected president. He had the meetings transferred to the Shah Reza hospital, where the Society met every month. He knew little Persian, yet insisted on remaining president, so the Society faded away. Some lost interest, but others joined and brought new life, and 1937 was the best year yet for the

---

197. RG 91-20-2, Mashad Medical Report 1934-1935.
198. RG 91-20-2, Mashad Medical Report 1935-1936.

Society, according to Dr. Hoffman. The missionary doctors conducted one meeting on the topic of 'blood pressure.'[199] The medical society continued to meet monthly at the Shah Reza hospital. The general tone was improving and several meetings were worthwhile. Also, the spirit of better ethics and cooperation that the society promoted continued. Most members referred their patients to the Christian hospital for lab exams and surgery, while the American physicians refused to make house calls, except when asked by an Iranian doctor for consultation. This also saved them a lot of time, as house calls were time-consuming.[200] The good spirit of cooperation continued due to the monthly meetings of the medical society. Iranian doctors sent more referrals for surgery and made more use of the Christian hospital's lab for diagnosis, while the American doctors sent more patients to the Shrine hospital for X-rays. Again, these exchanges were an opportunity for increased friendship and mutual help in a shared profession with a common goal.[201]

---

199. RG 91-20-2, Mashad Medical Report 1936-1937; RG 231-1-6, Hoffman, Pioneering in Meshed, p. 123.

200. RG 91-20-2, Mashad Medical Report 1937-1938.

201. RG 91-20-2, Mashad Medical Report 1938-39; Idem, RG 91-20-2, Mashad Medical Report 1940-1941.

V

QAL`EH-YE MEHRAB KHAN: THE FIRST LEPROSARIUM IN IRAN

Before discussing the establishment and functioning of the first real leprosarium in Iran, a brief explanation is given of the pathology of leprosy, the various names are listed under which it was known in Persian, and the earliest archeological evidence of its occurrence is presented. Also, societal behavior in Imperial Iran towards lepers is highlighted, while reference is made to the earliest medical descriptions of leprosy in Persian. Little is known about the occurrence of leprosy in Iran over the centuries, as evidenced by the lack of knowledge about its prevalence among medical practitioners and institutions in Iran, even as late as the 1920s. Although segregated villages with lepers existed prior to 1926, it was only as of then that the Mehrab Khan village became the first true Iranian leprosarium, when regular institutional medical treatment was offered by American missionary physicians. The funding agencies, medical personnel and treatment, the living environment of lepers and their numbers in Mehrab Khan are discussed as well as how its population size and status changed over time, and how it was transformed into a structural component of public medical care. Finally and briefly, the establishment and functioning of two other Iranian leprosaria is discussed as well as the slow but sure disappearance of the disease in Iran.

The Disease

Leprosy, also known as Hansen's disease, is an infection caused by bacteria called *Mycobacterium leprae*. These bacteria grow very slowly and it may take up to 20 years to develop signs of the infection. The disease can affect the nerves, skin, eyes, and lining of the nose (nasal mucosa) and may cause the affected areas to lose the ability to sense touch and pain, which can lead to injuries, as well as eventually the loss of toes and fingers as well as saddle-nose deformity. Usually, the affected skin changes color and either becomes lighter or darker, often dry or flaky, with loss of feeling, or reddish due to inflammation of the skin.[1] According to Browne, lepromatous leprosy, the most severe and most infectious type, was the form of significance in the past, while Dols submitted that tuberculoid leprosy, the least damaging and the least infectious type, which does not show clinical signs of the disease, were certainly known in the past.

Leprosy, a term derived from the Greek term 'lepros', which means 'scaly.' In Persian many words exist to denote leprosy. One may distinguish a three-fold division, viz. one group of words that refers to the disfiguring destructive nature of the disease, the other to the change in color of the skin due to the disease, and the third a more generic type of terminology. In group one finds: جذم *jadhm* and جذام *jodham*, Arabic words meaning, 'amputating, lopping, and mutilating.' Its Persian counterparts are خوره *khvareh, khvureh* and کلی *koli,* i.e., 'anything that eats or corrodes.' In group two one finds words that denote white leprosy or morphew, either malignant or not, such as: برص *baraṣ*, the malignant white species of leprosy; بهق *bahaq* or بهك *bahak,* (distinct from *baraṣ*); بیستگی *bistegi,* پیس *pis*, پیسگی *pisegi,* سرچپ *sarchap,* شوره *shureh*. In group one there are تن قره: *tan qara,* black leprosy as well as لری *larri,* and لوری *luri*, both meaning 'leprosy.' *Jodham* (جذام) has gradually substituted the other terms since the earliest centuries of the Islamic period in Iran and is still the common term for leprosy in use in Persian.[2] A hyperbolic way of referring to the disease is the term *ʿellat-e `areza suda'i* (علة عارضا سوداي), meaning a 'scorbutic affliction.'[3] Some of the above terms have other meanings, such as *khureh*, which also means

1. CDC website (accessed 2 July 2018).
2. *Loghatnameh-ye Dehkhoda*; Matin 1388, p. 643; Schlimmer 1970, p. 228; Zambaco Pacha 1924, p. 570; Wolff 1860-61, p. 286. According to Polak 1863, p. 175, the term *pis* was used by Turkish speakers.
3. Brydges-Jones 1976, p. 78.

'shanker'.[4] Its use to denote leprosy probably is due to the fact that traditional physicians often did not make a distinction between the two afflictions. According to Zambaco Pacha, the tubercular form of leprosy was most prevalent and often mistaken for syphilis and treated as such. Likewise, psoriasiform leprosy was treated as if it were common psoriasis with purifying agents and various pomades.[5]

Earliest Literary Evidence

Leprosy is an ancient disease known since at least 2000 BCE. There are literary references to leprosy in India and China from the first millennium BCE as well as in Egypt from around 1500 BCE.[6] Likewise the Avesta mentions leprosy. The Avestan term for leper (*paesa-*) is related to the term *vitərəto.tano*, meaning "whose body is isolated', suggesting that isolation of lepers was practiced. Greek authors such as Herodotus (b. 485 BCE) report that those affected by leprosy or *leuke* (a skin disease like leprosy) stayed outside the towns and avoided contact with non-lepers. This social exclusion is confirmed by Ctesias of Cnidus (a 5th century BCE physician) who reports that Persians, like others in Antiquity, considered lepers to be pariahs. He used the term *pisagas* to refer to lepers, which is the Greek rendering of the Old Persian term *pesag*, or leper. Iranians considered the affliction the result of divine punishment, having offended the Sun, possibly meaning Mithra, or the Babylonian Sun or Moon-god. According to Yasht 14.48, believers who don't lie to Mithra and sacrifice to Verethragna will receive protection against leprosy and other plagues. Yasht 5.92-93 states that lepers could not receive the libations offered to Anahita, the goddess of 'health giving.'[7] Videvdad (9.33-35) prescribes

---

4. Schlimmer 1970, p. 123.
5. Zambaco Pacha 1924, p. 570. The Persian terms used for white leprosy probably mostly referred to non-leprous skin diseases, Polak 1865, vol. 2, pp. 307-08.
6. Griffith, 1895, Book I, hymns XXIII and XXIV; Aufderheide et al. 1998, p. 148; McLeod at al. 1981; Bryan 1930, pp. 88-94.
7. Coloru 2017, pp. 65-66; see also Modi 1911; Idem, 1917, p. 281.

for men and women in state of uncleanliness isolation in a building called *armeshtgah* or 'house of seclusion.'

> He shall sit down there in the place of infirmity, inside the house, apart from the other worshippers of Mazda. He shall not go to the fire, nor near the water, nor near the earth, nor near the cow, nor near the trees, nor near the faithful, either man or woman. Thus shall he continue until three nights have passed. When the three nights have passed, he shall wash his body, he shall wash his clothes with *gomez* and water to make them clean.[8]

There is not only literary evidence, but also in art. Three small masks recently found in the remains of the Tepeh Hasanlu, dating back to the 1st millennium BCE, may be considered as the first visual instance of the effect of leprosy on Iranian art. Of one of three masks "the nose is deformed which is quite compatible with the impact of leprosy on the nose cartilage tissue and deformity. Furthermore, the mask has empty sockets."[9]

EARLIEST MEDICAL EVIDENCE.

Despite the literary evidence, Dols maintains that 'There is no persuasive evidence that true leprosy occurred in ancient Egypt, Mesopotamia, or Persia before the time of Alexander the Great."[10] However, the literary evidence for the early prevalence if leprosy is borne out by recent paleo-pathological studies of ancient skeletal remains. The earliest corporate evidence of leprosy is from Balathlal (Rajastan-India) in skeletal remains from the second millennium BCE. This finding is further confirmed by skeletal evidence from the Harappa site in Pakistan. These findings seem to support the hypothesis that leprosy migrated from Africa to Mesopotamia and India in the third millennium

---

8. Coloru 2017, pp. 65-66.
9. Moghadas 2015, pp. 1162-63.
10. Brown and Simcock 2012; Dols 1979.

BCE.[11] Further osteo-archaeological evidence of leprosy is from first millennium CE from the Ustyurt Plateau, Uzbekistan.[12] A Ptolemaic Period cemetery in the Dakhleh Oasis in Egypt contained the skeletons of four adult males of European type of the second century BCE. Dzierzykray-Rogalski diagnosed leprosy on the features of facies leprosa and has suggested that these Europeans in a predominantly negroid burial ground possibly represented lepers segregated from the Ptolemaic capital because of their disease.[13] In addition, DNA taken from skeletal remains of a man dated 10-50 CE, in a tomb next to the Old City of Jerusalem showed the presence of leprosy.[14] Adequate clinical descriptions of lepromatous leprosy did appear during this period, the best perhaps by Aretaeus of Cappadocia, a contemporary of Galen in the second century CE. In Sasanid Iran, according to Christian hagiography, Christians healed royals of afflictions such as leprosy through miracles.[15]

The first Iranian physician who described leprosy was `Ali b. Rabban Tabari (838-70 CE), the author of *Ferdows al-Hekmat*. Thereafter, `Ali b. `Abbas Majusi Ahvazi (10th century CE) described the clinical manifestations of leprosy in his book entitled *Tebb Maleki*. Ibn Sina (980–1037 CE) also discussed the clinical findings of leprosy in his *Canon of Medicine* and was the first to describe the saddle-nose deformity, typical for leprosy, since its first known description in the 3rd century BCE Chinese text *Feng zhen shi*.[16] Later, Esma`il Jorjani (1040-1136 CE), in his *Dhakhireh-ye Khvarazmshahi* described the various stages in the development of the destructive and contagious nature of leprosy.[17]

---

11. Robbins et al. 2009; Robbins at al. 2013.
12. Blau 2005.
13. Dzierzykray-Rogalski 1980.
14. Anonymous 2009; Spigelman 2001; Matheson et al. 2009.
15. Coloru 2017, p. 70.
16. Najmabadi 1353, pp. 316-20, 460, 591; Matin 1388, pp. 642-53.
17. Matin 1388, p. 643.

LEPROSY IN THE QAJAR PERIOD (1794 – 1925).

Not much is known about the prevalence and geographical distribution of leprosy in Iran from the year 1,000 until the Qajar period. The occasional mention of the disease is found, such as in 1590, when, according to Teixeira, Arabs in the Persian Gulf area were much afflicted by leprosy.[18] However, such mention of leprosy during this intervening period is rare.[19] Although we know more about leprosy during the Qajar era still the information for that period is not overwhelming either. Most 19th century authors who report on the disease during this period had little experience with the disease, both in terms of the number of patients seen and the parts of the country visited. Sometimes mistaken for, but not related to leprosy, was vitiligo or *baras*.[20] Alphos (*pis* or *baras*) was an endemic disorder, also sometimes mistaken for leprosy, about which little was known at that time.[21] Likewise, sphacelus, described as a dry gangrene, occurred in some towns, and it was feared as much as leprosy.[22] European trained physicians sometimes did not recognize the disease either. In 1854, Dr. Bock, the Russian Legation's physician, amputated part of the knuckles of a patient from the Khamseh, as he did not suspect leprosy.[23]

The general opinion of nineteenth century European physicians and travelers was that leprosy mainly occurred in N.W. Iran. According to Ussher, "The whole of north-west Persia would seem to be afflicted with this frightful scourge of humanity."[24] De Gobineau encountered

18. Teixeira 1991, p. 228.
19. Elgood 1951 and Najmabadi 1353 don't mention it at during this time period. The same holds for the entry *jodham* by Matin 1388 in the *Dar al-Ma`aref Bozorg Eslami* and by Dols in the *Encyclopedia of Islam.*
20. Polak 1865, vol. 2, p. 307.
21. Schlimmer 1970, pp. 28-31, 365-66 (q.v. melas); Polak 1863, pp. 178-79.
22. Polak 1863, p. 179.
23. Polak 1863, p. 177.
24. Ussher 1865, p. 652.

deformed leprous beggars at Miyaneh.[25] In 1906, Azerbaijan was reported to be the most afflicted province, although the same report stated that leprosy was endemic in Iran.[26] According to Polak, leprosy (*jodham*; *pis*) was mainly concentrated in the Khamseh province with its center at Zenjan, and in the districts of Khalkhal and Qaradagh. He had never heard of a case south of Qazvin.[27] Häntzsche concurred, for he submitted that leprosy occurred in endemic form among certain families in the higher parts of Iraq-e Ajam, Azerbaijan, and Qaradagh.[28] Hirsch reported cases of leprosy in Iraq-e Ajami, Kohestan near Baluchistan and Azerbaijan.[29] In 1908, Loew wrote that the disease in particular occurred in NW Iran (Tabriz, Qazvin area).[30] Feistmantel reported that there were also loci in the NE, East and South, in particular among pearl fishers. Klingmüller, citing Abol-Ghassem Khan, went even further and reported that leprosy was not widespread in Iran and only isolated cases occurred in the North-West and the South.[31] In Fars leprosy was seldom seen.[32]

This shows how little was known even about the areas where the disease mostly occurred. Dr. Johan Louis Schlimmer, practiced in Talesh and Rasht from 1849-52 treating, among others, lepers. Dr. Schlimmer described a case of a leprosy patient referred to him, who was cured after ten months.[33] However, according to Häntzsche, leprosy was rarely seen in Caspian provinces.[34] Contrariwise, Dr. Christides,

---

25. de Gobineau 1923, vol. 2, p. 259.
26. Römer 1906, p. 146.
27. Polak 1865, vol. 2, pp. 305-07, vol. 1, pp. 311-12; Idem 1863, pp. 175-76; Schlimmer 1970, pp. 228-254. Polak also tried to treat the illness and showed a case to his medical students in the Dar ol-Fonun. *Vaqaye`-ye Ettefaqiyeh*, vol. 2, p. 1235 (no. 193, 19 Moharram 1271/ March 8, 1856).
28. Häntzsche 1863, p. 181.
29. Klingmüller 1930, p. 50.
30. Loew 1908, p. 701.
31. Klingmüller 1930, p. 50.
32. IOR/L/PS/20/7, p. 88; Adamec 1989, vol. 3, p. 693 (Shiraz).
33. Schlimmer 1970, p. 306.
34. Häntzsche 1863, pp. 181-82; Fraser 1826, p. 200. In 1920 and

who had worked for many years in Rasht, reported that in that town, mainly among the poor, many lepers were seen, who allegedly mostly came from Azerbaijan and Kurdistan.[35] In 1886, Dr. Vaume reported that leprosy not only occurred in Gilan, but also in Mazandaran, Talesh and Khamseh/Zanjan, as well as in Kurdistan, which until then had been unknown.[36] Leprosy was allegedly "especially prevalent among the Kurds, lepers are not segregated, although leper settlements are found in a number of places."[37] Leprosy also occurred in Khuzestan[38] as well as in Bushehr, where the medical staff of the British dispensary was very pro-active in treating lepers.[39]

The above demonstrates that even the medical community in Iran, including the in 1904 reestablished Sanitary Council, was rather ignorant about the incidence and geographical prevalence of leprosy in Iran, although it was the Council's task to deal with all aspects of public health of the country and advise the government what action needed to be taken. However, the Council had a rather patchy notion of the occurrence of leprosy in Iran. This is evident from a session of the Sanitary Counsel in February 1911, when this medical supervisory body was not even aware that the government of Iran had drawn up regulations dealing with leprosy. During this session, "Persian members present described the regulations made by the Persian Government for the isolation and feeding of the unfortunates." The same session further demonstrated the total lack of knowledge about leprosy in Iran, for the Council "decided to request the Government to see

---

thereafter, leprosy was seen more common than usual in Rasht. RG 91-19-9, "History of Resht Station," p. 2; Idem, Resht Medical Report 1930, p. 3; Resht Medical Report 1931, p. 2. Polak reports that in 1858, at the orders of the Minister, one of his students was sent to Zanjan to treat leprosy patients there, accordance with instructions given. Polak 1859, p. 140.

35. Zambaco Pacha 1924, p. 569.

36. Vaume 1886, p. 160.

37. Anonymous 1902, p. 46.

38. IOR/L/MIL/17/15/8, p. 42.

39. Administration Report 1908, p. 12.

that the regulations were carried out, and to collect information on the question of leprosy in Persia generally."[40] This not only shows the ignorance about the occurrence of the disease in Iran, but also what to do about it. Because, when in September 1912, a center of leprosy was discovered in Bibianlu (Astara district) by the medical officer, the Council "decided to instruct him to take him whatever measures of isolation were possible at once,"[41] rather than refer him to the government regulations. Because of the outbreak of WW I the intended assessment of the incidence of leprosy in Iran did not happen. According to Dr. Neligan, a former member of the Sanitary Council, the main endemic foci of leprosy in Iran were Khorasan, Azarbaijan, Gilan, Kermanshah, and Kurdistan, thus ignoring the Khamseh province and the Persian Gulf littoral. He added that lepers were not allowed to enter towns and that in Khorasan and Azarbaijan officials encouraged lepers to live in their own settlements.[42]

Despite the incomplete and imperfect knowledge about the disease and its sufferers there was a beginning of both medical and official government interest in dealing with the disease and caring for those afflicted by it. In 1862, Dr. Schlimmer wrote a book on dermatological disorders, including leprosy, entitled 'Beauty of the Human Bodies' (*Zinat al-Abdan*), while in 1874 he published his lessons on leprosy taught at the Dar ol-Fonun in his *Terminologie*.[43] `Abdol-Hoseyn Khan Zonuzi Filsof al-Dowleh (1866-1942) was the first Qajar era physician to write a treatise on leprosy.[44] He submitted that leprosy was not widespread in Iran and only isolated cases occurred in the North-West and the South.[45]

According to Häntzsche, in Iran there was no therapy for the disease. He treated leprosy with Sublimat internally with some weak

---

40. IOR/L/PS/10/284, Neligan to Walter Townley, 03/02/1914.
41. IOR/L/PS/10/284, Neligan to Walter Townley, 04/11/1914.
42. Neligan 1926, part II, pp. 694.
43. Schlimmer 1970, pp. 238-55.
44. Monzavi 1348, vol. 5, p. 3398; 30. Azizi and Bahadori 2011, p. 426.
45. Klingmüller 1930, p. 50.

results, but patients left fearing they would lose their affliction and thus their justification for alms. Schlimmer had good results with Jodkali int.[46] A traditional medicine in the Tabriz region was to drink large quantities of fermented goat milk.[47] A Zand courtier was advised to daily to swallow a certain quantity of china-ware broken fine, of which he died.[48] Other traditional medicines used for leprosy included turnip, *hashishu'l-baraṣ,* bucks-horn plantain, *sangisboyeh,* cinquefoil, *rijlu'l-ghurab,* crows-foot, and *sharabi kadar,* a decoction gained from this tree, which was believed to be useful against leprosy and other diseases of the skin.[49]

THE NUMBER OF LEPERS

In 1908, according to Dr. Loew, there were not more than 100-200 lepers in Iran and this number was diminishing.[50] In 1923, Abol-Ghassem Khan held the same opinion, when he reported that leprosy was not widespread in Iran and that in the two preceding years only one new case had been reported, although he admitted that possibly unreported cases had been treated in hospitals.[51] In 1932, the Director of the Public Health Administration (*Sehhiyeh-e koll-e mamlekati*), established in 1926, reported that lepers were scattered in various parts of Iran, but were mostly found in Khorasan, Mazandaran, Azerbaijan, Qazvin, and Kurdistan. He added that a leper colony was established near Mashhad and one leper house outside the port city of Bushehr. The official number of registered leper patients was 400; however, the Director believed that the actual number was much higher.[52] In 1936, Dr. Lichtwardt estimated that the number of lepers in Iran was

46. Häntzsche 1863, pp. 182-83.
47. Vinkhuijzen 1868, p. 188.
48. Brydges-Jones 1976, p. 436 note.
49. *Loghatnameh-e Dehkhoda*; see also Matin 1388, p. 643 (bloodletting, diet, etc.).
50. Loew 1908, p. 701.
51. Klingmüller 1930, p. 50.
52. Rusta'i 1382, vol. 1, p. 473.

between 500 to 1,000 sufferers.[53] In the 1940s, leprosy was reported not to be very prevalent and to occur in Khorasan, Azerbaijan, Gilan, Kermanshah and Ardalan.[54]

Segregation of Lepers

Although Iranians didn't believe that leprosy was contagious, they nevertheless feared it.[55] Therefore, as soon as somebody showed signs of leprosy he or she was expelled from the community as they were held to be 'unclean.'[56] Wilson reported that when a woman was banned from the village her family wanted to depart with her. The village owner, who was a traditional physician, did not want to lose the benefit of having such a hard-working family in his village and "offered to give her a medicine that would kill or cure her in eight days. His intention was to poison her."[57] Usually the expelled person had to go to a leper village situated on a caravan route, which consisted of dilapidated mud huts with holes instead of windows and a door. The local governor was supposed to give them some flour and butter, and in years of need the Shah sent them some sacks of flour. However, these gifts usually did not reach them and therefore, dressed in rags; they lived by begging from passing caravans and family.[58] Lepers were banned from coming into the cities and, e.g., they were rarely seen in Tehran.[59]

---

53. Mashad Medical Report 1935-1936.
54. Government of Great Britain 1945, p. 421.
55. Häntzsche 1863, p. 182; Zambaco Pacha 1924, p. 570. On the belief in contagion, see Floor 2018, pp. 47-48.
56. Loew 1908, p. 701; Wilson 1896, pp. 271-72
57. Wilson 1896, pp. 271-72.
58. Loew 1908, p. 701; Polak 1863, p. 176; Idem 1865, vol. 1, pp. 311-12; vol. 2, p. 305; Wilson 1895, p. 140; de Gobineau 1923, vol. 2, p. 259 (deformed beggars at Miyaneh); Watelin 1921, p. 6 (near Alulak); Häntzsche 1863, p. 183; Loew 1908, p. 701; Feuvrier 1900, p. 120; Lycklama 1872, vol. 4, p. 30; Brugsch, 1886, p. 170.
59. Polak 1863, p. 176. The governor of Gilan once expelled lepers from Rasht who had come suddenly from Ardabil. Häntzsche 1863, pp. 183.

A different view was offered by Dr. Christides, who had worked for many years in Rasht. He reported that in Tehran and Tabriz lepers lived among the population and mixed freely with them. In Gilan lepers walked in the streets and bazaars asking for alms. However, Iranians were not afraid to be contaminated by them and even ate with them from the same plate. Because Iranians did not believe in contagion they even employed leprous servants. The same lack of segregation held for the public baths. Here lepers mingled with others in the basin, the water of which was changed only once per month. He concluded that in Iran there was neither prophylaxis, segregation, nor disinfection for leprosy or for any other disease, thus, according to Zambaco Pacha, presenting the optimal case for its propagation.[60] This view, which totally differed from all other sources and actual practice, must have been due to Dr. Christides having mistaken *baras* and other dermatological conditions for leprosy (see above).

The reality was that it was not uncommon for lepers to live together in rural communities near an urban center. In 1853, Dr. Polak saw at about one km from Zanjan and Miyaneh where he saw some 60 leprous men, women and children, who lived in a few huts.[61] In 1854, he wrote that there were whole villages that were home to lepers. They lived segregated from the rest of the community; usually one km from the city and food was brought to their small huts. When strangers passed they came begging, but were unable to use their voice due to the nodes in their throat.[62] In 1885, Dr. Vaume visited a leper village of 20 huts, housing 45 lepers from four surrounding villages, at almost 2 km from Sanandaj.[63] A number of villages north of Tehran were exclusively inhabited by lepers, according to Dr. Verrier.[64] In Qaradagh in the 1850s, there were said to be well maintained villages for them.[65] In 1895, Rev. Wilson reported that "There is a village of them about

60. Zambaco Pacha 1924, pp. 569-70.
61. Polak 1853, p. 510.
62. Polak 1855, p. 270.
63. Vaume 1886, p. 159.
64. Zambaco Pacha 1924, p. 567.
65. Häntzsche 1863, p. 183.

six miles from Tabriz. Their hamlet is called Payon, or the 'Village of the Sick,' and there are about five hundred of them, little, if at all, segregated."[66] It was allegedly the only leper village in Iran at that time. In the late 1850s, `Aziz Khan Sardar, then governor of Tabriz, ordered to assemble all the lepers from Azerbaijan at one location. He assigned a piece of land to them, "furnished them with oxen and farming implements, and established them as a separate community. At first they were given charity, month by month from the public treasury. If it was delayed beyond the regular time they came trooping down to the city. Now, on the contrary, it is said that they pay taxes to the government."[67] According to Dr. Mary Bradford, that village still existed in 1906, for she reported that "About 10 miles from Tabriz there is a village where all the lepers from the northern province of Persia are supposed to be sent, though no one sees to it that all go there." The government gave them wheat each year to the value of $400. Everything else they had to beg. Eight people lived together in a windowless 10 x 12 yards room. It had a smoke hole and a door of 4 feet high and 2 feet wide. The village had no bath and in the summer the villagers bathed in a nearby salty river throwing modesty to the wind. In 1906, the Rev. F.N. Jessup collected money for the lepers in the village and brought them supplies that each year, foreigners in Tabriz as well as Iranians, both Armenians and Moslems, gave to the American missionaries.[68] In early 1912, the German ambassador in Tehran informed the Sanitary Council that Mrs. Wanneman, the wife of the American missionary physician in Tabriz, did much for the lepers in Tabriz and the German society had given £50 for the amelioration of the lepers' lot,[69] which suggests that either the leper colony did not exist any longer or that lepers in that village were still rather neglected.

66. Wilson 1895, pp. 140-41; Cochran 1899, p. 105.

67. Wilson 1895, pp. 140-41; Neligan 1926, part II, pp. 693; Brugsch 1886, vol. 1, p. 179.

68. Bradford 1906, p. 502.

69. IOR/L/PS/10/284, Neligan to Walter Townley, 03/02/1914.

Although by the 1930s, the segregation of lepers was not considered necessary anymore by the international medical community, not only the government of Iran, but many other governments, such as that of Great Britain, still maintained this measure as the guiding principle of their medical policy towards lepers. Concerning its Persian Gulf protectorates, Great Britain went even so far to consider returning Iranian lepers to their country. When in 1942 Bahrain wanted to start a leper colony, the British adviser to the Sheikh did not want to care and feed non-Bahrainis there.[70] Because he had heard that there was a leper colony at Rezaieh he proposed to send Iranian lepers in Bahrain to Rezaieh. "But before the question of sending Persian lepers there from Bahrain can be taken up with the Persian Government, further information is necessary. The question of whether they contracted leprosy in Persia or Bahrain is also important." Therefore, he asked the British Political Agent in Bahrain, "how many you want to return to Persia, where are they from, where did they contract it."[71]

Despite this continued government policy of segregation, in actual practice little was done by the government of Iran to effectively control the spread of lepers. Only in Khorasan (Mehrab Khan) and Azerbaijan (Babi Baghi) advanced cases were segregated in villages, where they cultivated land and received a wheat allowance from the government.[72] Were these villages just places where lepers were forced to live or were they institutions where they were medically cared for and looked after? Here, I will only consider the case of Mehrab Khan.

THE FIRST REAL LEPROSARIUM NEAR MASHHAD.

THE EARLY BEGINNINGS

In 1884 or 1885, a leper village, the *Jodham-khaneh-ye Mehrab Khan* (Mehrab Khan Leper House) was established in the old Qal`eh-ye Mehrab Khan, 3 km north-east of Mashhad. The village was named

---

70. IOR/R/15/2/1297, Adviser to Political Agent, 21/03/1942.

71. IOR/R/15/2/1297, Adviser to the Govt. of Bahrain to Political Agent, 12/09/1942.

72. Government of Great Britain 1945, p. 421.

after Mehrab Khan Qajar, who was governor of Mashhad (1603-10) and Merv (1610-13), because, when he died in 1614, he bequeathed some landed property north-east of Mashhad to the charitable foundation (Astan-e Qods Razavi Organization) that manages the Shrine of Imam Reza.[73] Prior to the establishment of this leper village, lepers lived unencumbered in rags and misery in Mashhad among its inhabitants and begged in the streets of Mashhad as well as near the Shrine. Given the contagious nature of the disease, or so it was believed, and to provide comfort to the sufferers of leprosy, in 1884, the governor and Custodian of the Shrine, Mirza `Abdol-Vahhab Asaf al-Dowleh (1301-03/1884-86) decided to concentrate all lepers in the dwellings of the Mehhrab Khan fort and ban them from entering the city.[74] He allocated an annual budget of 500 *tuman*s for each leper. Thereafter they continued to be taken care of by the Shrine, which gave the 80 or so inmates an allowance of bread, a small money pittance and odds and ends of clothing.[75] However, there existed some doubt whether the Shrine money really was used to help the lepers. On 27 April 1914, the newspaper *Now Bahar* wrote: what happened with the Zargandeh *vaqf* property designated to assist the lepers? If it still exists, why are they begging freely in the streets? On 9 June 1914, the Shrine Custodian, Morteza Qoli Khan Tabataba'i replied that there was no particular Shrine property allocated to help lepers. In 1896, Sadr al-Mamalek had decided to assign some of the *vaqf* funds of the *Dar al-Shafa* to be used for the lepers, who lived in the Qal`eh-ye Mehrab Khan. At that time, the village had 40 to 60 inhabitants, but in 1914 there were more than 160 of them. Although care for the lepers was the city's responsibility, the Shrine gave 1,000 *tuman*s in cash and 100 *kharvar* of wheat annually to the lepers in Mehrab Khan. Due to negligence, some of the lepers were indeed engaged in begging on the Quchan and Qahqaheh road, but the Shrine had asked

---

73. Nasiri 2008, pp. 241, 246; Mehrab Khan built a mosque in Mashhad in the Darvazeh-ye Nowghan quarter, which mosque still exists. Adhari-Khakestar 1395, p. 80.

74. Mo'tamen 1348, p. 411; Adhari-Khakestar 1395, p. 80.

75. RG 231-1-6, p. 67.

the governor to detain them. Also, the Shrine was ready to make a permanent allocation from the Zargandeh property to assist lepers, on condition that lepers were reallocated to Mehrab Khan. The Shrine had spent money to build many dwellings, a special bath-house, and a water reservoir and Tabataba'i believed that those buildings were better than those elsewhere.[76]

Because nothing was really done to change the situation of the lepers, in 1921, the Sanitary Council of Khorasan decided that all lepers had to be removed from the city of Mashhad to Qal`eh-ye Kalat or some other location. Also, amenities such as water supply and a bath-house had to be readied for them there. On 20 August 1921, the city council under Col. Mohammad Taqi Pesiyan also decided that lepers had to be gathered at one location. He sent some of the lepers treated in the *Dar al-Shafa* of Mashhad to one of the farms belonging to Shrine to be taken care of there.[77] However, all these plans failed to materialize due to lack of funds and, in November 1923, when part of the Shrine funds did not reach the lepers in Mehrab Khan, some of them returned to Mashhad and congregated around the Shrine and sought asylum there. The newspaper *Mehr-e Monir* wrote that their presence was a danger to the pilgrims and public health and accused the Shrine authorities of negligence in their duties.[78] The Mehrab Khan village consisted of dirty, one room huts without windows at that time.[79]

The above shows that the general public considered lepers a threat to public health and that official care of lepers was not a sustained affair, but only incidental in nature, but also that a leper community continued to exist at Mehrab Khan, be it that many still lived and begged in Mashhad for their living. Because there was no medical treatment of the inhabitants of this village until 1926, it is only as of that year that this village may be referred to as a leprosarium, i.e., an institution to treat people suffering from leprosy.

---

76. Adhari-Khakestar 1395, pp. 81-82.
77. Nezam al-Saltaneh 1361, vol. 2, p. 366.
78. Adhari-Khakestar 1395, p. 82.
79. Klingmüller 1930, p. 50.

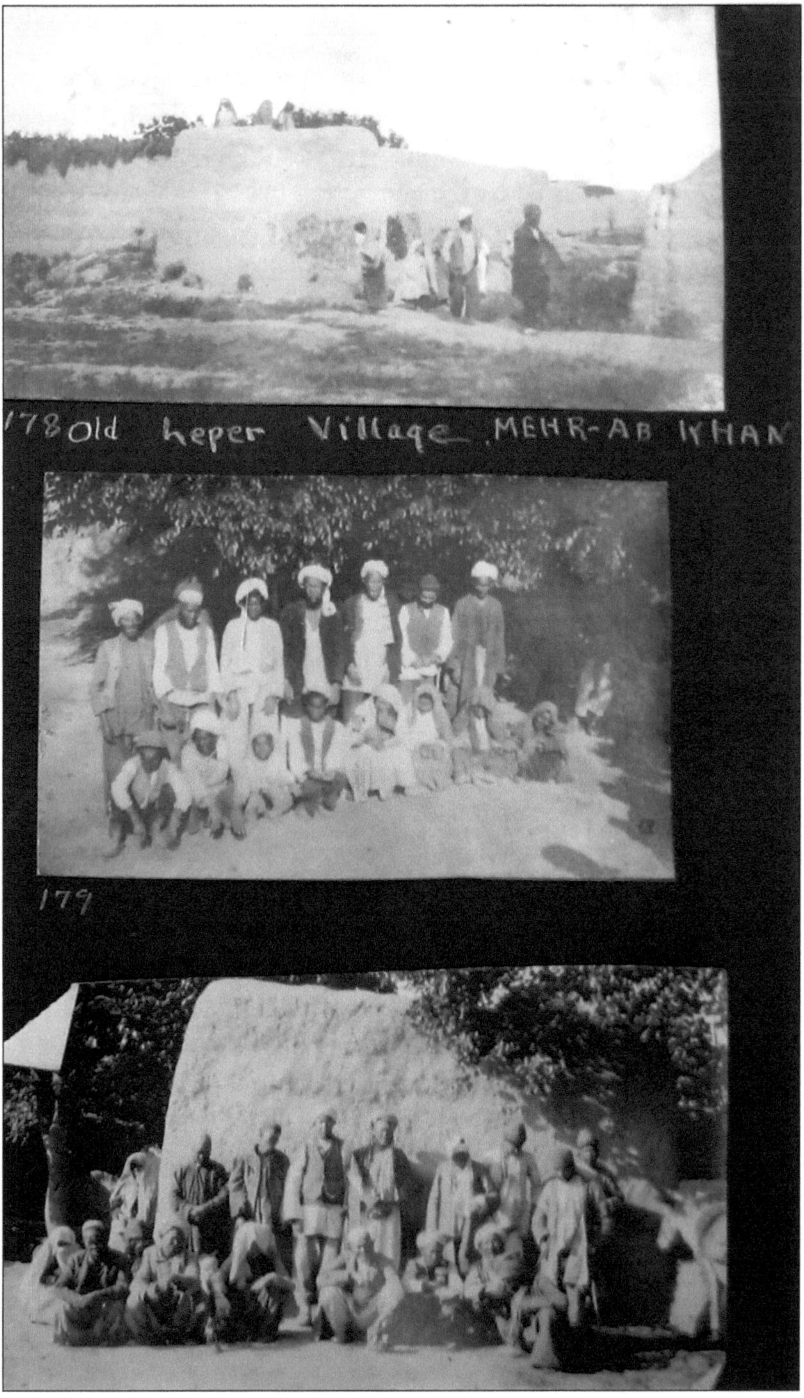

Mehrab Khan, the old leper village and some of its inhabitants, late 1920s

CONSTRUCTION AND FUNDING OF THE LEPROSARIUM.

For in 1926, Dr. Hartman A. Lichtwardt, a physician of the American Presbyterian Missionary Hospital who had begun working in Mashhad as of March 1920, began making visits to the village of Mehrab Khan.[80] He was spurred by the conviction that "if diagnosed early this disease may be cured when thoroughly and adequately treated and in more chronic cases the ravages of the disease may be arrested, so that lepers may return to their villages."[81] Dr. Lichtwardt's work for the lepers stimulated great interest among the leading citizens of Mashhad and prodded the authorities to take action. The governor of Khorasan, Mehdi Vosuq al-Saltaneh Dadvar and several citizens of Mashhad organized an Anti-Leprosy Society, which met under the presidency of Mohammad Vali Khan Asadi, the deputy-chairman of the Astan-e Qods Organization. On 6 October 1926, the board of this Society met and decided to make improvements in Mehrab Khan and to construct a new building. The next day the chief of Public Works and the chief city architect went to Mehrab Khan to select the building site, such that it both in summer and winter it had a sunny side. Thereafter the design of the buildings was finalized. Hajj Sayyed Hadi Khadem together with Mr. Nazem, the city's architect (*me`mar*) was appointed as the supervisor of the works. The Society raised money to erect a new building and dwellings, whose construction was realized in 18 months' time, when they were dedicated with much ceremony. The new building had 29 rooms, built on two sides with an open square, each with a window and door and also a fireplace. According to Adhari-Khakestar, the new building measured 80 x 80 *dhar`* and had 128 rooms. Reza Shah and his wife headed the list of donors with 1,000 *tuman*s each and together with other gifts a total of 4,300 *tuman*s were received (see Table 11). People in Mashhad were encouraged to give clothes and cash to the leper colony, and

80. RG 231-1-6, p. 67. Adhari-Khakestar 1395, p. 90 mentions that prior to Dr. Lichtwardt's regular visits Dr. Stoker of the British Consulate-General in Mashhad did so, but not with what frequency and over what period.

81. RG 91-20-2, Mashad Medical Report 1929-30, p. 39.

lepers were then banned from begging in Mashhad. In 1929, people in Mashhad gave 380 *tumans* and two *qrans*, among the donors were Drs. Hofmann and Lichtwardt of the American Christian Hospital, who donated 12 beds, sofas and couches to the leprosarium. The American Mission to Lepers[82] initially gave $700/year to the American Christian Hospital for this work, and Persians gave 6 times more.[83] Despite local support to help lepers and the fact that there were doctors with training in modern medicine in Mashhad, who daily attended part of the sufferers from diverse diseases, only the American missionary doctors were willing to spend time on the lepers.[84]

Table 12: List of major donors for the construction of buildings at Mehrab Khan 1928

No.	Name	Amount in rials	No.	Name	Amount in rials
1	Reza Shah	10,000	13.	Sadr al-Tojjar Bozorg-niya	500
2.	The queen	1,000	14.	Mirza Hasan Sar-keshik	200
3.	Cdr. of the Army of the East	1,000	15.	Mas`ud Na'eb al-towliyeh	250
4.	Mirza Nazer 2 x	130	16.	Shoja` al-Dowleh 2 x	500
5.	Sheikh al-Ra'is Afsar	200	17.	Rokn al-Tojjar	100

82. An American Christian charity organization that aims to eradicate leprosy and was founded in 1906.

83. RG 231-1-6, p. 67; Adhari-Khakestar 1395, pp. 83-84, 89-90. According to Mo'tamen 1348, p. 412, the original building measured 80 x 80 meters and had 38 rooms in which the lepers lived. In the middle of its circumference was the kitchen. The small hospital was located in the south side of the building and had a courtyard for healthy family members.

84. RG 91-20-2, Mashad Medical Report 1932-1933, p. 5.

No.	Name	Amount in rials	No.	Name	Amount in rials
6.	Motavalli mosque	200	18.	Yusef Khan Hazarah	250
7.	Sar kashik-e avval	300	19.	Hajj Behnud Khan	100
8.	Hajj Ra'is-e Daftar	250	20.	Major Lewis, treasury manager	100
9.	Sardar Mokarram	200	21.	Amir Showkat al-Molk	100
10.	Salar Mo'ayyad	250	22.	Zabet-e ketabkhaneh	20
11.	Mo`in al-Sal-taneh	500	23.	Hajj Khabir Razavi	500
12.	The late Hajj Gholamreza Sabzavari	500	24.	Two anonymous Ameri-cans	200

Source: Adhari-Khakestar 1395, p. 92. According to RG 231-1-6, the queen also gave 10,000 rials.

In addition to the expenditures made by the Anti-Leprosy League in 1929, the following contributions were made by: the American Mission to Lepers 1350 rials; the Girls school in Rasht: 81 rials; the Christians in Isfahan 155 rials, or a total of 1586 rials. Moreover, in the fall of 1928, Iranian and American women gave 120 woolen shirts. Christians in Mashhad gave at Christmas food to the lepers on that day.[85]

85. Adhari-Khakestar 1395, p. 91.

Table 13: Income and expenditures of the Anti-Leprosy Association in 1929

Income in *qrans*		Expenditures in rials	
111494, 5	in cash	2128,75	office, paper, mail, seal
1386,6	value of in kind income	43474,95	for the construction of the new building
46822,7	contribution Shrine	204,8	treatment building *(darmangah)*
11586	contribution Americans	55777,30	clothes, bathhouse, medicine, nursing
826,65	contribution *Shir va Khorshid-e Sorkh*	9570,5	Cash in hand
11149,45	Total	11149,45	Total

Source: Adhari-Khakestar 1395, p. 91.

OCCASIONAL IRREGULAR FUNDING NO OBSTACLE

In 1929 the Shrine under Asadi gave to each leper: 10 *sir* of bread/p.p./day; for children half of that. To each leper 5 *qran*s per month was given for food. Each month, 15.5 *man* of oil for lighting the rooms. Per day 30 *shahi*s as fee for the bath-house; its water was always warm. To transport bread daily to the leprosarium 30 *shahi*s was paid.[86] In that year, the lepers also received things in kind such as meat, rice, oil, mash, beans, and sugar from the American team. The Shrine made *pustin*s and clothes during two years available, all of which had a positive impact on their welfare.[87] Sometimes the American missionaries gave winter clothes and charcoal, above to what the Shrine supplied.[88] This situation was quite an improvement compared to the one prior to 1926, when the lepers at Mehrab Khan lived in ruins, were hungry and had no medicine, as Asadi, the deputy-Custodian of the Shrine wrote in 1944, when he reported on the major improvements made at the leprosarium and in the condition of its inhabitants.[89]

Despite the Shrine's commitment to Mehrab Khan, it sometimes happened that payments by the Shrine were late. The money eventually was paid, but on several occasions the Shrine authorities had to be reminded to make their contribution. Adhari-Khakestar blames this on the constrained budget situation of the Shrine, to the fact that the allocation only was designated for the needs of Khorasan and that with the growth of the number of lepers coming to Mehrab Khan from outside the province the allocation did not and could not suffice. For example, 130 new lepers arrived in 1930, who had come from as far as Kermanshah and Kurdistan. Therefore, the Shrine had to construct a new building to house 23 of them. Also, in 1943 the Health Department transferred a number of lepers from Zanjan and elsewhere to

86. Adhari-Khakestar 1395, p. 85; for a list of other payments made by the Shrine in 1929 to help the lepers at Mehrab Khan, see Idem, pp. 86-87.

87. Adhari-Khakestar 1395, p. 90.

88. RG 91-20-2, Mashad Medical Report 1932-1933, p. 5.

89. Adhari-Khakestar 1395, p. 87.

Mehrab Khan.[90] Although it is true that most of the lepers were not from Khorasan, this was the reality from the very beginning, when the leper village of Mehrab Khan had been created in 1884. The reason was simple; the lepers were Shiites who came to Mashhad to seek healing at Imam Reza's Shrine, an attraction that was touted by the Shrine authorities themselves. After all, Imam Reza was the healer par excellence and throughout history miraculous healings had been ascribed to his powers.[91] In fact, in 1929, Mehrab Khan received 56 additional lepers due to the activities of the Anti-Leprosy Society that tried to attract lepers from all over the country, among whom were many Barbaris (Afghan Hazaras).[92] In short, the Shrine authorities not only had a moral, but also a religious and institutional obligation to help lepers and other people afflicted with a disease. Therefore, it was not surprising that Afghans pilgrims who often came to the Shrine to find a cure there were told by Shrine officials to go to Mehrab Khan for treatment. The Shrine guardian and the governor-general of Khorasan also suggested that people give gifts to the lepers in time of illness, wedding or death in the family.[93] Therefore, many believers bequeathed assets to the Shrine to explicitly help that group of people. For example, one third of the *vaqf* of the Fazak property left by Hajj Mirza `Abdol-Karim, known as Hakim Radkani, in 1917 was to be used for poor, the sick and the lepers. As a result, the Shrine committed to give each leper one *charak* of bread/day and 5 *qran*s/month, which was regularly paid thanks to Hakim Radkani, but, unfortunately, later the *vaqf* manager was sentenced in court and the property transferred.[94]

This budget uncertainty sometimes led to non-delivery or late delivery of the allowance to the Mehrab Khan lepers. On 3 May

90. Adhari-Khakestar 1395, pp. 87-88.

91. Kaempfer 2018, p. 92.

92. Adhari-Khakestar 1395, p. 90. Also, government officials sent lepers to the leprosarium. On 27 April 1935 the mayor of Mashhad had two lepers detained who were begging in the city and sent them to the leprosarium. Adhari-Khakestar 1395, p. 92.

93. RG 91-20-2, Mashad Medical Report 1935-1936, p. 6.

94. Adhari-Khakestar 1395, pp. 81, 89.

1928, about 40 lepers gathered in the garden of the Custodianship to demand their allowance over the last 8 months. Dr. Lichtwardt offered to construct with his own funds two rooms where leper patients could relax, if the Shrine gave its permission.[95] Dr. Lichtwardt wrote on 1 December 1932 to the deputy Custodian that the Shrine funds had not arrived as yet. In case there was no budget could he see his way and allocate some funds of the *Shir va Khorshid-e Sorkh* Society to Mehrab Khan?[96]

Despite these problems they did not have a negative impact on the work in Mehrab Khan as they were incidental; in fact they are not even mentioned in the official reports by Dr. Lichtwardt or his colleagues. Moreover, as to the arrangements to help the lepers at Mehrab Khan, Dr. Lichtwardt wrote: "This work has been an excellent example of co-operation, international and inter-religious." The Presbyterians provided physicians, the American Mission for Lepers funds, the British Empire Leprosy Relief Association certain medicines; land and bread by the Shrine, funds for building and hosting the lepers by the local 'Anti-Leprosy Society, "which is organized and run by Iranians, and to which Reza Shah and his wife gave money." Moreover, the work was supported by the deputy-Custodian of the Shrine who "is most loyal in his co-operation and most sincere in his friendship."[97]

The cooperation between the Shrine and the American missionaries continued to be very positive, as both parties were clearly interested to work for the benefit of the leprosy sufferers. On 9 December 1928, Dr. Lichtwardt sent the deputy Custodian a letter asking the Shrine and the Anti-Leprosy Society to help protect the lepers against the cold and also to remove snow and other obstacles from the road to Mehrab Khan to make access easier to leprosarium.[98] In 1932, Dr. Lichtwardt reported that the Shrine "continues to provide a bread ration of one and a half pounds daily per adult, as well as an allowance of

95. Adhari-Khakestar 1395, p. 89.
96. Adhari-Khakestar 1395, p. 88.
97. RG 91-20-2, Mashad Medical Report 1929-30, pp. 40-41.
98. Adhari-Khakestar 1395, p. 250 doc 10. The extra help was given in the form of *pustin*s, see Idem, p. 90.

five rials (18 c.) per month, per adult, for the purchase of 'extras.' They also provide some fuel, some kerosene and some soap. We assume the responsibility for the medical treatment, and have also provided some food, some clothing and some wool which they have to knit into socks and scarves."[99] In 1936, Dr. Hoffman reported that the Shrine regularly supplied the lepers of Mehrab Khan with bread, occasionally with meat, kerosene, a simple cooking allowance and this year quilts and 10 bedsteads for the small hospital. The Shrine also agreed to increase the allowance of 60 lepers who were totally and permanently helpless. The Shrine Treasurer said: "Well, what else can we do, when you people take such an interest in our poor lepers."[100] Even when the Sacred Shrine organization had become a government department in 1937, it continued to send supplies of food, kerosene and occasionally clothing and bedding to the whole colony and cooperated in making a nice garden of the yard for the healthy children, and granting them a special allowance for food and fuel.[101] This positive attitude continued in the years thereafter. The Shrine continued to work well with the American Christian Hospital and paid many cost of the leprosarium.[102]

Nevertheless there was some dissatisfaction among the lepers at the end of the 1930s about the height of the Shrine's contribution and the manner in which it was made available. In 1938 and 1939, a group of lepers of Mehrab Khan wrote a petition to the *Majles* asking for an increase in their allowance. They also complained that during 6 months of the year the water of the bath-house was not heated and consequently, they had to wash themselves with cold water. Further, that the supervisor (*mobasher*), who had been there for 14 years, be replaced as he was not as caring as before, and they asked for the appointment of an intermediary between them and the bakery and the bathhouse. Furthermore, they requested that the *Majles* appoint an

---

99. RG 91-20-2, Mashad Medical Report 1931-32, p. 17 (on p. 7 a photo of Dr. Lichtwardt examining a leprous patient).

100. RG 91-20-2, Mashad Medical Report 1935-1936, p. 5.

101. RG 91-20-2, Mashad Medical Report 1937-1938, pp. 2-3.

102. RG 91-20-2, Mashad Medical Report 1938-39, p. 1.

observer who discretely would check whether their demands would be implemented and that they would be properly treated. Finally, they asked for a letter from the *Majles* that stipulated the duties of those who worked at Mehrab Khan. The petitioners drew attention to the fact that they already had made these requests several times.[103] Despite these complaints, during the difficult war years when everything was scarce and expensive, the Treasurer of the Shrine, who was formally in charge of the leprosarium, continued to be most cooperative and supplied food, fuel, some clothing and a small financial allowance, and, in 1946, appointed a more efficient caretaker.[104] In 1949, the Shrine allocated 440,000 rials for the lepers.[105]

Despite the fact that Mehrab Khan Leprosarium had been functioning since 1884, 90% of Mashahdis had never heard about it, according the newspaper *Tus* on 14 February 1946. The newspaper wanted to correct this ignorance among the public and wrote that most of the about 130 lepers were Barbaris and Azeris. Before 1926 their situation was not good, but since then the Shrine and the American hospital had worked together to improve their situation. In the past, the lepers only received one warm meal per week, now every day the kitchen prepared food and their bread was baked from good wheat, prepared in the Shah Reza hospital and daily brought to them. According to the Shrine officials in the past it happened that people gave a sheep for the lepers, but the last years this did not happen, and this may have been one of the reasons that the article was written.[106] The local press did not always have the same appreciation for the Shrine's work during this difficult time. On 5 January 1942, the newspaper *Azadi* wrote that, since a few days lepers were seen in Mashhad begging. Had they fled from the leprosarium or had they come from elsewhere? It was said that those in Mehrab Khan were working in the surrounding villages. If true, woe on those people. It

---

103. Adhari-Khakestar 1395, p. 242, doc. 4 (17 Ordibehesht 1317 rec.)

104. RG 91-20-2, Mashad Medical Report 1942-1943, p. 2; Idem, Mashad Medical Report 1945-1946, p. 3.

105. Adhari-Khakestar 1395, p. 89.

106. Adhari-Khakestar 1395, p. 95.

was hoped that the Shrine or the Health department would take steps immediately in the interest of the common weal.[107]

Role of Government

Although the Iranian government did nothing to address the problem of leprosy sufferers, hospitals were required by law to report cases of leprosy, which the missionaries did, hoping the government finally would take action.[108] This changed in 1936, when the Health Department financed the construction of new rooms in Mehrab Khan. These rooms were completed and occupied in 1936. The direct involvement of the Health Department had to do with the fact that government health officers sent about 20 lepers to Mehrab Khan. Therefore, these patients were not supported by the Shrine, so that their support came from the government, which was less than that from the Shrine.[109] In 1937, Dr. Falati (sic; ?), head of the National Health Department, visited Mehrab Khan and was favorably impressed and endorsed immediately several of the recommendations of the American physicians for its improvement and gave 12,000 rials and increased its annual budget.[110] Although I have not found further information about government activities and its funding of Mehrab Khan patients, a fact is that there continued to be Shrine and Government supported patients at Mehrab Khan. In 1942 there were 136 lepers in Mehrab Khan and 130 in May 1944, of which 59 were paid for by the Shrine and the other 71 by the Health Department. In August 1944 there were 127 lepers, of which 57 supported by the Shrine and 70 by the Health Department.[111]

---

107. Adhari-Khakestar 1395, p. 94.
108. RG 91-20-2, Mashad Medical Report 1931-32, p. 17; RG 91-19-9, Resht Medical Report 1930, p. 3; Idem, Resht Medical Report 1931, p. 2.
109. RG 91-20-2, Mashad Medical Report 1935-1936, p. 5.
110. RG 91-20-2, Mashad Medical Report 1936-1937, p. 4.
111. Adhari-Khakestar 1395, p. 94.

OTHER SUPPORTERS

The British Empire Leprosy Relief Association continued to supply Alepol, although it is not known until when. The American Mission to Lepers (AML) continued to pay $1,000/year to buy medicine, food, dressings, etc. In 1932, AML also shipped a large amount of woolen scarves, wristlets, bandages, and gauze, all really needed. These supplies were prepared by women of several churches.[112] In 1935, the AML increased its funding to Mehrab Khan and each leper received a good mattress, a pair of mittens, two pairs of socks, a pair of shoes (made of old tires and very serviceable) and those most in need of them sheepskins, besides a small monthly allowance.[113] The grant by the AML supported the hospital and clinic and also some money was left for overcoats for most and shoes for many. At X-mass special gifts of sugar, tea, woolen socks and mittens were made to the whole colony; the same happened at Easter.[114] In 1940, AML reducing its funding of Mehrab Khan, but due to a better rate of exchange more money became available for the lepers, which made it possible to supply them with more shoes and better food.[115] AML funds continued to support the activities of the American physician to provide the lepers at Mehrab Khan with clothing, sometimes food, and medical care.[116]

Apart from institutional support, Mehrab Khan also received help from individuals. In 1938, with help of the foreign community the American missionaries could buy shoes for all of them. There also was a gift of a rice dinner by an Iranian doctor, while the women of the church in Mashhad sewed clothes for women that were given at X-mass time.[117] In 1942, aside from gifts of shoes, dark glasses, and overcoats from local friends the missionaries gave them special rice

---

112. RG 91-20-2, Mashad Medical Report 1931-32, p. 17.
113. RG 91-20-2, Mashad Medical Report 1935-1936, p. 5.
114. RG 91-20-2, Mashad Medical Report 1937-1938, p. 3.
115. RG 91-20-2, Mashad Medical Report 1939-40, p. 3.
116. RG 91-20-2, Mashad Medical Report 1940-1941, p. 2.
117. RG 91-20-2, Mashad Medical Report 1938-39, p. 2.

dinners. The women of the church sowed dresses for the leper women.[118] In the fall of 1944, the missionaries realized that the clothes of the lepers were in tatters as they had forgotten the usual gifts of overcoats, due to the terrible high cost of cloth. Mr. Irwin helped and the 140 inhabitants each got a good sheepskin coat (*pustin*).[119] In 1945, the missionaries gave *pustin*s to all those who had not received them the previous year, and everybody received shoes and the women new dresses; they also spread the gospel.[120]

Composition and Number of Lepers at Mehrab Khan

Many of the lepers in Mehrab Khan village, who had been driven from their villages, came from all over Iran and Afghanistan.[121] According to the American missionaries, who treated them, "None of the lepers were true Persians," i.e. Persian speakers. In fact, "about half were Turks from W. Iran, the rest Mongolians, about 20 were not lepers, but had other disfiguring diseases." The so-called Mongolians were Afghan subjects, also in this case, not 'real' Afghans, but Barbaris, the Khorasani name for the Shiite Hazaras of Afghanistan.[122]

The erection of the new leper hostel in 1928 was one of the most important reasons for the improvement of the lepers' condition. "They now live on dry, light, clean rooms, better than then average homes of 80% of the Persians." These living conditions improved their general health and resistance to disease. Also, the amount and quality of the food had improved somewhat, although it was still insufficient. Moreover, more and better clothes were given and a regular though

118. RG 91-20-2, Mashad Medical Report 1942-1943, p. 2

119. RG 91-20-2, Mashad Medical Report 1944-45, p. 2.

120. RG 91-20-2, Mashad Medical Report 1945-1946, p. 2.

121. Of the 60 arrivals in 1934, 25 were from Afghanistan. Mashad Medical Report 1934-1935, p. 3.

122. RG 231-1-6, pp. 67-68; RG 91-20-2, Mashad Medical Report 1928-29, p. 2; Lichtwardt 1934, pp. 75-76; Mo'tamen 1348, p. 412; Adhari-Khakestar 1395, pp. 80, 90-91.

small allowance of fuel enabled the lepers to better tolerate the long cold winters, although the condition inside their homes was still far from comfortable, according to Dr. Lichtwardt.[123] He was not the only one to think so, because living conditions in the leper village had improved, such that "it is occasionally necessary to turn away non-leprous malingerers who seek admission to the village."[124] Because of this interest of non-lepers to become a member of the Mehrab Khan Village population, the Shrine official in charge of the lepers required an official diagnosis before he would admit newcomers to the Home. Among them "are malingerers, who singe off their eyebrows or irritate their skin sores."[125]

In 1926, the number of lepers in the village amounted to sixty and thereafter their number grew. According to Adhari-Khakestar, on 12 Mehr 1307 (4 October 1928), the day of the creation of the Anti-Leprosy Society, the leprosarium had twenty-five men, thirty-two women, and six children, a total of eighty-six persons. Later, new arrivals amounted to forty-four men, six women, and five children, a total of fifty-six, or a total of 117 lepers. In March 1929, Dr. Lichtwardt reported that there were 118 lepers and during that year 39 new ones arrived. Also, 11 were dismissed as cured and 9 died. According to Dr. Lichtwardt, most lepers came voluntarily after having heard that leprosy sufferers were housed and medically treated in Mashhad. Many came on foot from as far as Tabriz and Van, begging their way. A few were sent by Western and Iranian physicians. Barbaris came from Afghanistan traveling 40 days or more. Their number was 140 in 1934, which included 60 new arrivals. However, 25-30 lepers died each year, who were replaced by new cases. In 1934 there were 60 new arrivals and 30 deaths, so that there was a net increase of 30 in that year. In 1936, the leper colony had grown to 200, of whom 184 were lepers. Thereafter, there was an unexplained drop in the number of inhabitants of the leper colony, for in 1939 this number had decreased

123. RG 91-20-2, Mashad Medical Report 1929-30, pp. 41-42.

124. Presbyterian Church 1930, p. 187.

125. RG 231-1-6, p. 67.

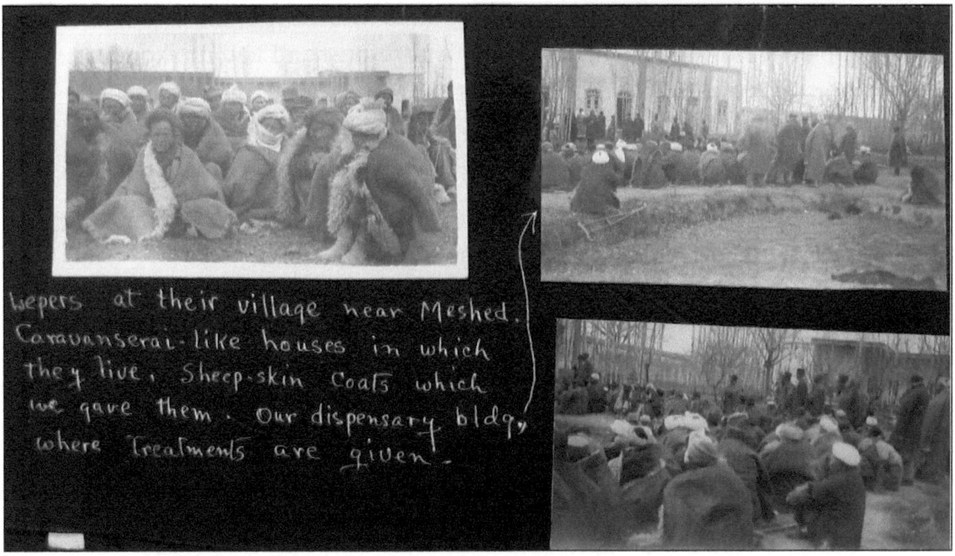
Lepers at their village near Meshed.
Caravanserai-like houses in which
they live. Sheep-skin coats which
we gave them. Our dispensary bldg,
where treatments are given.

Lepers dressed in *pustins* – in the background the dispensary where treatment was given

to 120 lepers. In 1945, the leper village had 140 members.[126] It were not only the better living conditions that drew more lepers to Mehrab Khan, but so was the certainty of regular and sustained medical treatment, which gave rise to great optimism among the leprosy sufferers. One leper said: "For years we had been living in squalid holes like unwanted wild animals, with no one caring whether we died. Now in clean light rooms, we live in comfort, our sores are cleansed, our pains are relieved, our disease is cured."[127]

A related issue to control the influx of non-leprous persons in Mehrab Khan was the presence of some healthy women, who lived with their leprous husbands. In the fall of 1934, `Ala al-Soltan, the deputy-Custodian and Dr. Lichtwardt decided that in case of death

---

126. Adhari-Khakestar 1395, pp. 84, 90; RG 91-20-2, Mashad Medical Report 1932-1933, p. 4; Idem, Mashad Medical Report 1929-30, p. 39; Idem, Mashad Medical Report 1934-1935, p. 3; Idem, Mashad Medical Report 1935-1936, p. 5; Idem, Mashad Medical Report 1938-39, p. 1; Idem, Mashad Medical Report 1944-45, p. 2.

127. RG 91-20-2, Mashad Medical Report 1929-30, p. 39.

or divorce the healthy person had to leave the leprosarium. It so happened that two healthy women, whose husband had died or had divorced her, married in secret to leprous men in the village, which was not allowed and, therefore, they were expelled; to remain with their wives, the leprous husbands left Mehrab Khan village.[128]

In 1936, the American missionaries reported that no new Afghan lepers were arriving at Mehrab Khan, because it was reported that Iran barred their coming across the border. The Americans worried about their fate, because these Afghan lepers were "cast off by their relatives and driven out of their villages, and are penniless."[129] This was the result of official government policy. The governor-general of Khorasan was worried about lepers walking freely around and pressed the Shrine to take steps that lepers stayed in the leprosarium. He also suggested giving them a piece of land so that they might farm, while he informed the Shrine that the police had orders to send lepers back immediately. Also, orders were given to the Customs officials and border governors not to allow Afghan lepers entry into Iran. The deputy-Custodian replied that the lepers of Mehrab Khan had been given their allowance regularly, even though the budget was tight, bread, clothes and fuel etc. was assured to them.[130]

MEDICAL TREATMENT

Initially, Dr. Lichtwardt visited the village of Mehrab Khan bi-weekly on Saturday afternoon in a droshky, accompanied by some dressers, the American Hospital's druggist and Ms Reynolds, the evangelist. With

---

128. Adhari-Khakestar 1395, p. 92. Art. 1123 of the new Iranian civil allowed a man to cancel the marriage "in case his wife had black leprosy (*juzam*) and leprosy (*baras*)." IOR/L/PS/12/3416. The expulsion of the two women very much upset the community of lepers, because in 1938 and 1939 they requested an allowance for these two healthy women. Adhari-Khakestar 1395, p. 242, doc. 4 (17 Ordibehesht 1317 rec.)

129. RG 91-20-2, Mashad Medical Report 1936-1937, p. 4.

130. Adhari-Khakestar 1395, p. 93.

his team he gave the patients injections of the traditional chaulmoogra oil, dressed their mainly foul ulcers as well as gave other treatments and necessary medicines. Ms Reynolds talked with the women, gave them wool yarn, taught them knitting socks and mittens and told Bible stories.[131] Already in 1927, Dr. Lichtwardt made weekly visits, enabled by an increased grant of $1,000 from the American Mission to Lepers. However, as of 1929 he and his team made visits twice a week hoping that this more intensive treatment might be more effective. The work pattern remained the same; injections were given, wounds dressed, and medical treatment as needed. During the first 18 months that Dr. Lichtwardt treated lepers he gave them increasing doses of esters of chaulmoogra oil, intramuscularly, with satisfactory results, although in larger doses the injections occasionally caused much discomfort and produced local abscesses. For a second period of 18 months he used Alepol in the recommended 3% and 1% solutions, intramuscularly and intravenously, with less annoyance to the patients and with as good therapeutic results. Because in increased doses it caused discomfort, and therefore, in 1929, he gave Alepol in 6% and 2% solutions to certain lepers and found that some tolerated this more concentrated solution quite well, but that it caused higher temperature and an increase in nodules in others. In such cases he returned to the 3% and 1% solutions. In 64% of the cases there was definite improvement, but only three cases were cured. Improvement meant, healing of ulcers, except of the nose and throat and "all those who have bacteriological evidence of such ulcers are still liable to disseminate the disease." There was a definite improvement with younger patients, with old chronic cases the treatment prevented the worsening of the situation. Those who were not cured were relieved, because their living conditions were better than in a normal Iranian village. Unfortunately, most cases in Mehrab Khan were so chronic that longer treatment was needed to achieve a complete cure. Most patients had diagnosed their disease before they came here, so they must have had it for a long time already. The death rate in 1309

131. RG 91-20-2, Mashad Medical Report 1930-31, p. 6; Idem, Mashad Medical Report 1936-1937, p. 5.

(1929-30) was 19% due to pneumonia, nephritis and dysentery, which are diseases difficult to treat in patients weakened by leprosy and other ailments, for many patients also suffered from malaria, syphilis etc. Moreover, all of them had insufficient food intake. "In spite of their inadequate food-ration of only one and a half pounds of daily bread, plus five *krans* (50 ¢) per month to buy 'extra; many are quite plump and well nourished."

Table 14: Statistics concerning the medical situation of lepers in Mehrab Khan 1929-30

Leper men and boys receiving regular treatment now	92
Leper women and girls now receiving regular treatment	14
Leper men (hopeless burnt-out cases) not receiving treatment	15
Leper women (hopeless burnt-out cases) not receiving treatment	11
Untainted children of lepers still living in village	8
Total number people still living in village	140

Number of lepers, men and women who have died in past 4 years	
(19% of all treated)	29
Lepers who have left village improved, not entirely cured	16
Lepers who have left village cured 92% of all treated)	3
Total under observation in past four years	188
Total number of lepers receiving treatment part four years	154
Lepers who have become worse under treatment, 3%	5
Lepers who have remained same as when treatment started, 12%	18
Lepers who have shown definite improvement under treatment, 64%	99
Population of leper village when our work started in 1926	
(95 to 100 in 1922 or [19]24)	81
New lepers admitted in past four years	101
Children born to lepers	6

To give the lepers a sense of normalcy and of self-esteem the Americans encouraged the lepers to work in the fields when they were able to. As a result, they were more cheery than the average non-lepers in a Persian village. They had nicer garden plots than in most Persian villages. There were of course quarrels among them, but they also had happy times, and sometimes a traveling minstrel came to entertain them, and they enjoyed singing and chanting. Ms Reynolds during her weekly visits worked with the women in the village. She usually organized her knitting, reading from the Bible and other activities outside under the trees, but when it rained, everybody moved into the village mosque, which the Americans found amazing, as 'infidels' usually were not allowed in Shiite mosques. Also, the lepers kept their rooms fairly clean, which meant that the allocation of funds for cleaners in 1929 had either been canceled or they did not work or come any longer. To stimulate cleanliness, "Large religious pictures from Sunday School picture rolls are given to lepers as rewards for keeping their rooms neat and clean, and they are very anxious to secure them and to tack them on their bare wall."[132]

In 1931, Dr. Lichtwardt continued his weekly visits treating some 120 out of 150 living in the village with injections; also additional medication was given, as needed, as well as dressing of their many ulcers. Most patients showed slow improvement; "several have been cured entirely and will soon return to their villages, and three who were clinically and bacteriologically cured had already gone." Almost every week one new leper applied for admission; some in 1931 were children from the Afghan border and others had the disease in an advanced stage and had little hope of cure. When in March 1932, Dr. Lichtwardt was away for three weeks, on his return, lepers begged for treatment, "stating that their pains, ulcers, and swellings had become much worse in even this short interval without treatment." [133]

Dr. Lichtwardt distinguished two types of groups among his leprous patients. Class I of 28 were those without visible signs of the disease; they were well and Alepol worked well with them; over

---

132. RG 91-20-2, Mashad Medical Report 1929-30, pp. 42-44; Idem, Mashad Medical Report 1928-29, p. 6; Idem, Mashad Medical Report 1938-39, p. 5. On alepol, see Bhandari 1932 and Dikshit 1932. For the treatment with chaumogra oil and treatment in general, see Klingmüller 1930, pp. 676-743. For the 1929 budget allocation for female cleaners, see Adhari-Khakestar 1395, p. 86 (item 6).

133. RG 91-20-2, Mashad Medical Report 1931-32, p. 16.

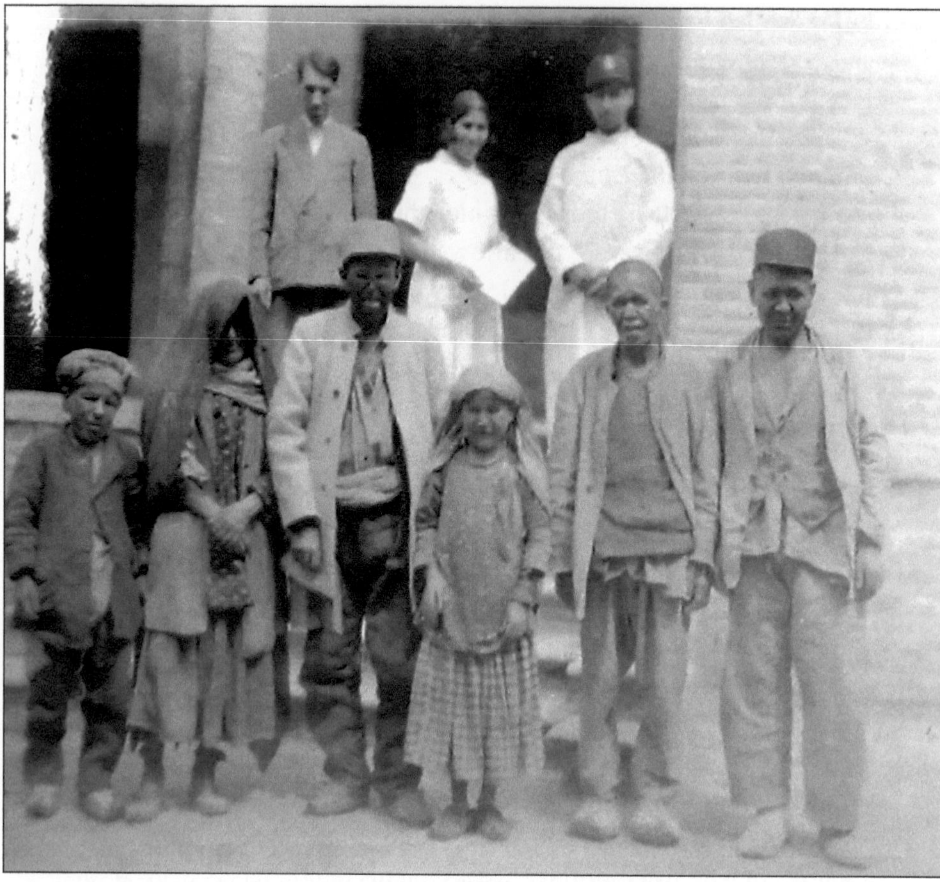

Above and opposite: Lepers in Mehrab Khan and a typical windowless dwelling

dosages sometimes did harm. Class II of 64 were in the active stage; for them he used intravenous injections of Chaulmoogra oil, for Alepol often stirred up a leprous reaction and made them worse. Class II included the old, burnt-out cases with gnarled stumps of fingers and toes. "Specific treatment here merely discredits the treatment; so we merely dress ulcers and try to relieve their aches and pains, malaria and coughs."[134] Sometimes, Dr. Lichtwardt made extra visits, such "as at Christmas and to operate on several poor sufferers." At the weekly

134. RG 91-20-2, Mashad Medical Report 1932-1933, p. 4.

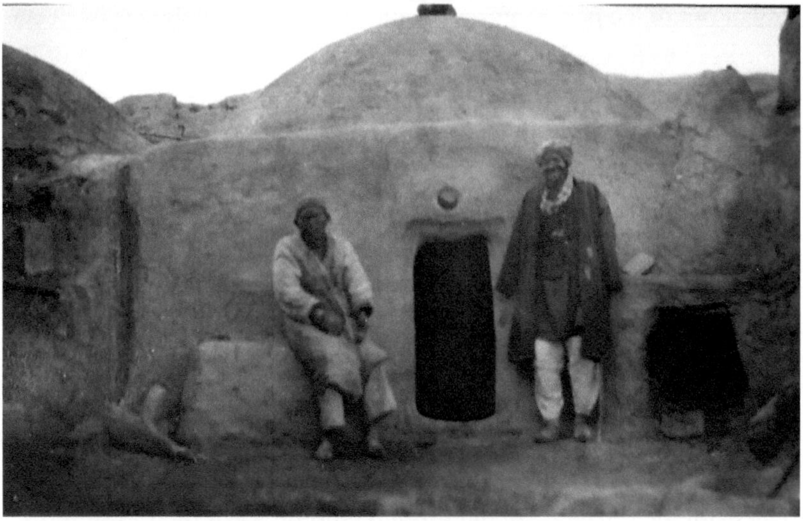

visits one bread was given to each who came for the injection; which did the trick, "for they need little stimulus beyond the vague hope of improvement, especially since the injections are sometimes painful." Sometimes the Americans gave winter clothes and charcoal, above to what the Shrine supplied.[135]

New Buildings

In 1931, five new rooms were added, three of which for treatment and examination of patients; one was used as a store-room, and one where Ms Reynolds told her Bible stories to the women and children, and taught them to knit and sing simple hymns. "A gramaphone [sic] and records have been given to the lepers this year and they enjoy it very much. This new building has enabled us to release three large rooms for the use of new lepers that have arrived. A new, high veranda has been built, extending along one half of the leper rooms."[136] By 1935, the leper colony had grown to 200, of whom 184 were lepers. This required the construction of new rooms, which were erected by the Health Department. These rooms were completed and occupied in

135. RG 91-20-2, Mashad Medical Report 1932-1933, p. 4.

136. RG 91-20-2, Mashad Medical Report 1931-32, p. 17.

1936. Four of the new rooms were allocated to the American physicians to be used as a small 9-bed hospital for comfort and treatment of the patients. The rooms were screened for flies.[137] Mrs. Helen Hoffman, the wife of Dr. Hoffman and a nurse herself, worked hard in the fall of 1936 to get three rooms fixed up for the use as an hospital at the village. Although the rooms were built by the Health Department, the American missionaries plastered, fixed them up and furnished them with funds from AML. Ten old bedsteads were given by the Shah Reza hospital, which had to be repaired. In January 1937, the three wards, with three beds each, were opened and as of then the sickest were taken care of in clean beds and fed warm food and milk.[138] In 1937-38, Mrs. Hoffman supervised the cleaning, plastering and repairs of the six rooms in the children's ward for which she obtained 3,000 rials from local friends in the foreign colony. As of then the children lived with such of their parents who were infectious.[139]

CHANGE OF STAFF – NOT OF TREATMENT

In 1934, Dr. Lichtwardt, who had started the program of medical treatment at Mehrab Khan was transferred to the American Christian Hospital in Hamadan. His work was continued by Dr. Hoffman, who had worked in Mashhad since 1915 and was the head of the American Christian Hospital there. He was assisted by Dr. Adelaide Kibbe, who in April 1935 went of furlough. Her place was filled by Dr. Cochran, who came from Urumiyeh, where the government had closed the American mission station. These changes interfered with the treatment schedule, if there was only one physician at the hospital. After Dr. Kibbe's return in 1936, one doctor's day/week was given again to the lepers. To make life for the lepers more meaningful, boost their morale, and reduce their own workload, the American physicians had

137. RG 91-20-2, Mashad Medical Report 1935-1936, p. 5; RG 231-1-2, Hoffman to Mother, 04/10/1936.

138. RG 91-20-2, Mashad Medical Report 1936-1937, pp. 3-4; Mashad Medical Report 1935-1936, p. 5.

139. Mashad Medical Report 1937-1938, p. 3.

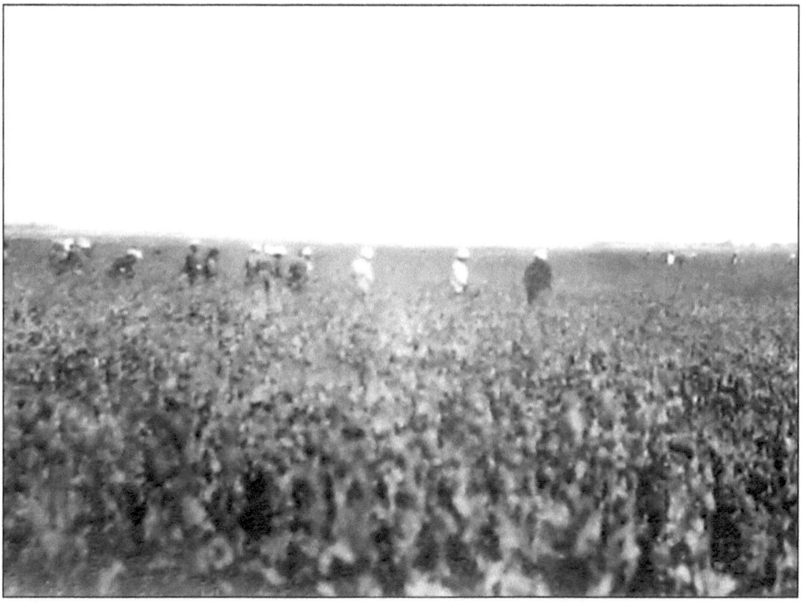

Lepers picking opium near Mehrab Khan village

begun training interested male leprosy patients as nurses. As a result, by 1936, more and more dressings and injections were done by these leper nurses, who also took care of the nursing in the small hospital. Here they daily dressed ulcers and gave medicines to relieve fever and pain. Consequently, the ailing lepers were being cared for better than ever before.[140] One of the two American physicians in Mashhad continued with weekly visits accompanied by three helpers. There were also additional visits by Naderi, their male nurse, to see to it that the four lepers that they employed as nurses dressed the many sores and took care of the patients in the little hospital there. To save money, gauze and bandages were washed and re-sterilized as long as they held together.[141] In addition to the four male nurses, the Americans also employed two women as washerwomen. To make the mullah of the village stop begging from them, the Americans employed him as keeper of the record cards of the lepers, which had the desired effect.

140. RG 91-20-2, Mashad Medical Report 1935-1936, p. 5.
141. RG 91-20-2, Mashad Medical Report 1936-1937, p. 3.

In addition, they arranged work for some 25-30 able bodied ones in the opium fields as day laborer and other farming jobs nearby.[142]

As of 1937, Dr. Cochran made the weekly visit with Naderi, and three helpers to Mehrab Khan. The village mullah handed out the record cards, the doctor checked the patients and prescribed for each one of them, one assistant supervised the injections given by leper nurses, while another supervised the dressing of ulcers and the third dispensed the medicines prescribed for fevers, aches and pains. The nine beds were always occupied, a near 100% occupancy, more than in any other hospital. The worst cases lay there screened from flies, were looked after and given hot food, milk and curds by the four leper nurses. Two leper women did the cooking and washing, one nurse was always on night duty. The four nurses also did "the daily dressings of the many painful sores, always worse in winter because the lepers burn their numb fingers and toes in the scanty fires trying to get warm, and give the injections." In addition, after the doctor's visit, Naderi later came twice per week to Mehrab Khan on his bike to direct the nursing.[143] The beds in Mehrab Khan's small hospital were always occupied by the worst cases. Therefore, in the fall of 1938, three beds were added for female patients. Even then the 12 beds were occupied by the most sick and helpless in the group of 120 lepers throughout the year.[144] As of 1944, the weekly visits were reduced because of lack of time. One hospital worker went there three times per week, while 3-4 went there once/week for special treatments. Dr. Hoffman could go there only once/month as he was the only physician in the Mashhad hospital. By that time, the little hospital had 15 beds,

142. RG 91-20-2, Mashad Medical Report 1936-1937, p.4. It is interesting that in 1942 the work on farms was decried by a local newspaper as "woe betide' the villagers, who employed lepers, see Adhari-Khakestar, p. 94. The village mullah probably was called `Aziz Khan and was himself a sufferer of leprosy. Mo'tamen 1348, p. 411, note.

143. RG 91-20-2, Mashad Medical Report 1937-1938, p. 2.

144. RG 91-20-2, Mashad Medical Report 1938-39, p. 2; Idem, Mashad Medical Report 1939-40, p. 3; Idem, Mashad Medical Report 1940-1941, p. 2; Idem, Mashad Medical Report 1944-45, p. 2.

which usually were all filled. It was repaired under supervision of Mrs. Hoffman, and, according to Dr. Hoffman, "It is one of the best hospitals in the region."[145] After Dr. Hoffman left in 1948, Dr. Cochran was responsible for both the hospital and leprosarium. When in 1949 the number of lepers had grown Dr. Cochran requested the Shrine to build new rooms. "At the moment the beds of the hospital of the leprosarium are currently occupied by almost 15 blind lepers, so that there is no place for the other lepers. It is requested to construct two rooms for the hospital."[146]

Between 1943 and 1954, 38 buildings were constructed for the cured lepers and their families. The additional building erected in 1953 and 1954 by the Shrine measured 80 x 70 meters. At its north side it had 14 rooms for the lepers, and at the south side, which was also the entrance, there were rooms for staff. In 1955, to the south-east a bath-house was constructed with 12 shower stalls, 12 water taps for clothes washing, which was out of use by 1968. By 1955, the number of lepers at the Mehrab Khan Leper House reached 312. In 1957, the supervision of Mehrab Khan was transferred from the Shrine to the Ministry of Health (*Vezarat-e Behdari*) and gradually the old buildings were destroyed.[147] It is not known when the Americans stopped working in Mehrab Khan, their reports for the period after 1948 have not been preserved. According to Mo'taman, they still provided support to the leprosarium in the mid-1960s, when the Presbyterian missionaries ended their work in Iran. One thing is clear that around 1960, some French nurses started working at Mehrab Khan. The praiseworthy work of Mary Gabriel Kurot (Corot?), sister Zhaleh, and sister Rahebeh, who came to Mashhad via the WHO, is mentioned in particular. They lived next to the leprosarium. When they stopped working there is not known. In the mid-1960s, i.e. after the American hospital had closed, the Department of Health funded

145. RG 91-20-2, Mashad Medical Report 1945-46, p. 2; Mashad Medical Report 1942-43, p. 2; Mashad Medical Report 1944-45, p. 2.

146. Adhari-Khakestar 1395, p. 89.

147. Azizi and Bahadori 2011, p. 428; Mo'tamen 1348, pp. 412-13. Mo'tamen's text is copied in 'Ataradi 1371, vol. 2, pp. 511-13.

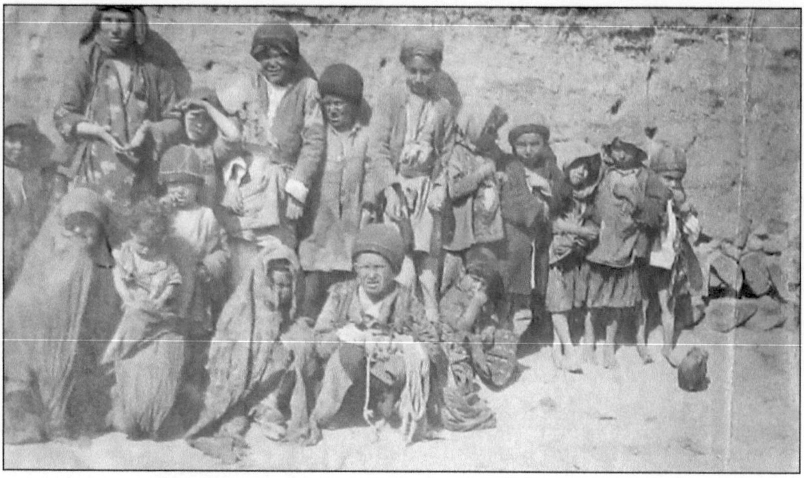

Above and opposite: Lepers in Mehrab Khan

the visits of an Iranian physician.[148] In 1958, a new asylum with 130 rooms was constructed and the eight hectares of land of the Mehrab Khan Leprosarium was enclosed by a fence. At that time, it was the best equipped leprosarium in Iran. This was because its budget was subsidized by a grant from the Shrine, which in 1962 amounted to 20 rials/day per patient. Also, a nursery had been established by the Lepers Aid Association of Mashhad where the 50 children of the by then more than 500 leprosy patients were looked after. In 1962, it was proposed to build a large hospital for the treatment of leprosy in Mashhad.[149] Finally, the Ministry of Health officials dissolved the Mehrab Khan Leprosarium and on its site constructed the Hashemi-nezhad Hospital, located in northeast of Mashhad, which as of 1982 is affiliated with the Mashhad University of Medical Sciences.[150] According to Ataredi, the leprosarium was moved to a village near Bojnord.[151]

148. Adhari-Khakestar 1395, p. 96.

149. Iran Almanac 1963, p. 379. According to Mo'tamen 1348, p. 413 the Shrine paid the Health Department 50,000 rials/month for its work at Mehrab Khan in 1957.

150. Azizi and Bahadori 2011, p. 428.

151. 'Ataradi 1371, vol. 2, p. 513.

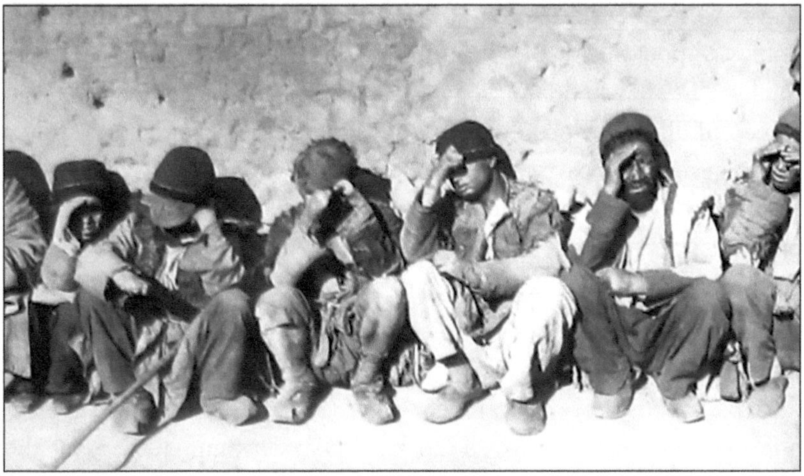

Other Leprosaria

In those provinces where there was no leprosarium, which meant most of Iran, there was no Iranian institutional support for lepers and hardly any medical care, private or public. The only incidental medical care that was available to lepers came from American and European medical institutions, either missionary or government supported. Of the latter, the British dispensary in Bushehr is an excellent example, which treated all kinds of diseases, including that of leprosy. The most modern methods and treatments were introduced as soon as these became available. For example, in 1908, with some pride, the Political Agent in Bushehr reported the "Successful treatment of leprosy cases by means of the new Nastine treatment inaugurated by Professor Deycke Pasha."[152] The Nastin treatment was continued and 1910 "ten patients were treated with encouraging results."[153] Elsewhere, such as in Rasht, Dr. Frame of the American Christian Hospital treated lepers. For those that had no proper housing and were out of town, Frame advised them to go to Mashhad or Tabriz, which each had a leprosarium with the facilities to treat them. However, because most

152. Administration Report 1908, p. 12; Das 1911; Anonymous 1909.
153. Administration Report 1910, p. 20.

lepers were poor and had no money to travel, they returned to their homes without treatment. Government institutions were of no use, even though "The newly organized health department wants to make a clean sweep of all health problems but has neither the organization, funds nor experience to carry out their program immediately."[154] Although in modern treatment of leprosy segregation was not necessary or even desirable there was nevertheless a need for a refuge for leprosy sufferers. However, the situation of such refuges did not look bright.

By 1920, three leper colonies were reported to exist in Iran; one at Mashhad (Mehrab Khan), another at Khalkhal, and a third one at Arpadarrehsi (آرپا درەسی), near Ahar (Azerbaijan).[155] However, it appears that there also was a leper colony near Senneh, perhaps the one visited by Dr. Vaume.[156] There also seems to have been one in the village of Savudluq in the mountainous district of Vanyar (W. Azerbaijan), situated on the road between Tabriz and Ahar. Coming down from their heights the leprous villagers engaged in banditry, attacking travelers, who out of fear for contact with the leprous bandits fled leaving their possessions. This situation lasted till the end of the 1920s and thereafter the Savudluq lepers were moved to Baba Baghi.[157]

Whereas in the early 1920s there were at least 3 to 5 leper colonies in Iran (see above), some 25 years later the Ministry of Health of Iran only operated two leprosaria with about 400 patients in the provinces.[158] It is not clear whether the village of Pāyon was discontinued or developed into a leprosarium. In 1921, it was decided to designate the village of Baba Baghi (بابا باغی) as the location where all lepers from Azerbaijan had to be concentrated. The village was located around 15 km N.W. from Tabriz; in the 19th century the Baba Baghi village had been a royal hunting lodge. However, it was impossible to realize this plan at that time until ten years later, when again it was

154. RG 91-19-9, Resht Medical Report 1930, p. 3.

155. Gilmour 1924, p. 30; see also Polak 1865, vol. 1, p. 132 (leper colonies in Azerbaijan, Khamseh, and Khalkhal).

156. Rasooli and Allen 1958, pp. 22-23.

157. https://fa.wikipedia.org/wiki/بابا_باغی [accessed 15 June 2018]

158. Andrews 1950, pp. 2.

decided to house there all lepers there from North, West and N.W Iran. However, due to lack of funds and other means it was impossible to prepare the village to house leprosy patients. Two years later, in 1933, the Municipality of Tabriz bought the village for 600 *tuman*s and took steps to make the necessary preparations to receive the future leper inhabitants. In that same year, 75 hectares of Baba Baghi lands were transferred to the Public Health Administration and thus, a beginning was made with the Baba Baghi leper village.[159] Because the village was surrounded by a 3-meters high wall it looked like an army barracks. At first, 40 mud (*kahgelli*) rooms were built; thereafter the village was gradually expanded and lepers from different parts of Iran settled in Baba Baghi. The first group of patients who came to the Baba Baghi Leprosarium were the lepers from Arpadarrehsi of whom there were seventy-five. In the beginning, the neighboring villagers supported these lepers with donations.[160]

Because no regular medical treatment was offered at Baba Baghi it was not as yet a real leprosarium. However, the government of Iran wanted to improve the way in which it dealt with leprosy. To that end Dr. Brown of the WHO visited Iran in 1956, who assessed the leprosy situation in the country. Following his visit, the Ministry of Health decided to launch a large-scale leprosy treatment campaign, because there were reportedly some 12,000 lepers under treatment in Iran. The majority of the patients was located in Azerbaijan, Kurdistan, Khuzestan, Lorestan, Tavalesh, Gilan, Torkmansahra, Zabol, Bandar Abbas and Mashhad. There also were a few in Tehran. Many of them lived and were treated in the two leper colonies Baba Baghi and Mehrab Khan. In Tehran, lepers were treated in a special ward at the Loghman al-Dowleh Adham hospital. Despite the government's intention to improve medical services at the two leprosaria, no Iranian physician or nurse wanted to work in the two leper villages. Their refusal led to great controversy and caused much national uproar. Finally, two French nuns offered to help the lepers in Baba Baghi, who were later joined by four Frenchmen, who worked there for several years. Among

---

159. https://www.mehrnews.com/news/1018043/ [accessed 15 June 2018].

160. https://fa.wikipedia.org/wiki/بابا_باغی [accessed 15 June 2018].

them was Dr. Alphonse David, who trained his Iranian successors. In 1962, there were 530 patients in the 100-room Baba Baghi leper colony and its annual budget was 6 million rials/year.[161]

Despite the establishment in 1957 of the "Society for the Support of Lepers" in Tabriz to help the lepers of the Baba Baghi Leprosarium,[162] living conditions there were very unfavorable. In 1962, their neglected suffering was highlighted by the documentary "The House is Black" (*Khaneh Siyah Ast*) made by Forugh Farrokhzad (1935-67), a poet and film director.[163] Because the government of Iran erected new medical buildings in Baba Baghi, as well as improved living conditions and the medical treatment of its inhabitants it received assistance from the WHO, so that in 1963 the first batch of medicines for the 600 patients reached Baba Baghi. In the 1970s and thereafter the situation gradually improved under the leadership of Dr. Mohammad Hoseyn Mobayen, who had started his professional career at the Baba Baghi Leprosarium in 1962. One year later he became its director, which he remained until 1988. Under his direction the 3-meter wall around the village was taken down, new facilities were constructed and medical care of the lepers was put on a sound scientific foundation. After the Revolution of 1978 further improvements were made to the village (piped drinking water, baths, gas, electricity, asphalt road, etc.). Some 80 medical and administrative staff live in the village as well as about 470 patients of whom 80% with their family. Most patients engaged in agriculture and animal husbandry. The Baba Baghi Leprosarium is now affiliated with the Tabriz University of Medical Sciences.[164]

In 1961, a third leprosarium was added, the *Behkadeh Raji*, now renamed as *Behkadeh-ye Razavi*, which was established near Birjand, due to the efforts the Health Minister of the time, Dr. `Abdol-Hoseyn Raji (1902-72) and the active support of Farah Diba, the queen of

161. Iran Almanac 1963, pp. 378-79.

162. Azizi and Bahadori 2011, p. 427.

163. Matin 1388, p. 645.

164. https://fa.wikipedia.org/wiki/بابا_باغی [accessed 15 June 2018]; http://www.bartarinha.ir/fa/news/90156/ [accessed 15 June 2018]; http://www.hamshahrionline.ir/details/304736 [accessed 15 June 2018].

Iran. The Razavi Leprosy Rehabilitation Center was the first modern, economically self-sufficient leprosarium in Iran complete with a hospital, school, bathhouse, cinema and all administrative services and other modern amenities. In this modern village, the lepers were treated, in accordance with the recommendations of the WHO. In 1968, the government of Iran began a systematic fight against leprosy. It allocated more medical staff, several leprosies were built (Siyahqol, Kolbar, Reza Khan, Basri) and a number of special clinics were established. At that time, the Mehrab Khan leprosarium had 700 lepers and the Baba Baghi leprosarium housed 573 lepers, while some 232 leprosy patients were treated by other clinics and mobile teams in rural areas.[165] In 1960, 900 lepers and their 180 healthy children lived in the *Behkadeh Raji*. By 1977, 400 houses and several educational, professional training and entertainment centers, as well as six villages near the *Behkadeh Raji* were erected by French and German charity foundations. For a number of years it was supervised by the 'Society for Help to the Lepers in Iran'. In 1980, the name of the society changed to the 'Organization for Fighting against Leprosy', which was supervised by the Ministry of Health. Finally, in the 1980's this rehabilitation center was dissolved and patients who were cured and their families were transferred to the buildings near the asylum.[166]

Table 15: New cases of lepers by sex and age for the stated year (1960-2008)

Year	Sex			Age	
	Both sexes	Male	Female	14 years and under	15 years and over
1340/1960-61	123	-	-	-	-
1350/1971-72	320	-	-	-	-
1351/1972-73	375	-	-	-	-
1370/1990-91	191	132	59	37	154
1375/1976-77	112	69	43	13	99

165. Iran Almanac 1970, p. 496; Matin 1388, p. 645; Pahlavi 2005, p. 143. For leprosy related medical education and research in Iran, see Azizi and Bahador 2011, pp. 428-29.

166. Aziz and Bahadori 2011, p. 428.

Year	Sex			Age	
1380/2001-02	96	44	52	3	93
1383/2004-05	93	64	29	0	93
1384/2005-06	89	48	41	5	84
1385/2006-07	71	39	32	0	71
1386/2007-08	37	22	15	1	36
1387/2008-09	38	24	14	0	38

Source: Iran Almanac 1974, p. 407; Iran Statistical Yearbook 1387 (2008-09), Table 16.16, p. 719.

Since 1364/1985, the number of leprosy patients in Iran has dropped (see Table 13). Therefore, the prospects of the elimination of leprosy in Iran look good, because since 1996 its prevalence was less than one case per 10,000 persons. In 2016, its prevalence was 0.003 per 10,000 persons and the rate of new cases was 0.22 per 100,000 people. In 2016, only 15 new cases were reported, of which 11 were Iranian.[167] Let's hope that these are the last sufferers of leprosy in Iran and that its chapter of leprosaria may be closed.

---

167. http://tb-lep.behdasht.gov.ir/Leprosy_Situation_In_Iran_World.aspx (accessed 14 June 2018).

BIBLIOGRAPHY

ARCHIVES

PRESBYTERIAN HISTORICAL SOCIETY, PHILADELPHIA (USA).

DOWLATABAD – MALAYER

RG 280-1-10, Medical Reports (Mary Zoeckler) 1914-1949.
Report of Medical Work Daulatabad 1924-1925
Report of Medical Work Daulatabad 1928-1929
Report of Daulatabad Medical Work 1938-1939
Report of Daulatabad Medical Work 1939-1940
Report of Daulatabad Medical Work 1940-1941
Report of Daulatabad Medical Work 1941-1942

HAMADAN

RG 91-19-27, Hamadan Hospital 1927-1956
Hamadan Medical Report 1933
Hamadan Medical Report 1934
Medical Report Hamadan Station 1935
Healing in the Home of Avicenna 1936
Hamadan Medical Report 1937
Report on Medical Work Hamadan 1937-1938
Christian Healing in Hamadan 1939
Healing in Hamadan 1940
Hamadan Hospital 1945-1946

RG 280-1-10, Medical Reports (Mary Zoeckler) 1914-1949. M. A. Zoeckler,
Report of the Women's Medical Work Hamadan 1914
Report of Medical Work Hamadan 1920-21

KERMANSHAH

RG 91-19-30, Kermanshah Hospital 1927-47
Report Westminster Hospital 1933
Report of Westminster Hospital 1933-1934
The Westminster Hospital Annual Report 1934-35[mimeo pamphlet]

Kermanshah Medical Report 1937
Annual Report Westminster Hospital Kermanshah 1938
Annual Report Westminster Hospital Kermanshah 1938-39
The Westminster Hospital Bulletin. vol. 2/1. October 1939
Report Westminster Hospital Kermanshah 1940
Annual Report Westminster Hospital Kermanshah 1944-45
Social and Education Project – Kermanshah 1944-45

MASHHAD

RG 91-20-2, Mashad Hospital 1925-1948.
Mashad Medical Report 1928-29
Mashad Medical Report 1929-30
Mashad Medical Report 1930-31
Mashad Medical Report 1931-32
Mashad Medical Report 1932-33
Mashad Medical Report 1933-34
Mashad Medical Report 1934-35
Mashad Medical Report 1935-36
Mashad Medical Report 1936-37
Mashad Medical Report 1937-38
Mashad Medical Report 1938-39
Mashad Medical Report 1939-40
Mashad Medical Report 1940-41
Mashad Medical Report 1941-42
Mashad Medical Report 1942-43
Mashad Medical Report 1944-45
Mashad Medical Report 1945-46

RG 231-1-2, Rolla Hoffman Correspondence 1910-1919
NN [Hoffman] to Friends, Meshed, March 1918
Hoffman to Mother, 04/10/1936
Hoffman to N.N., no date (probably 1938).

RG 231-1-5, Rolla Hoffman Correspondence 1930-1949
Memo Medical Needs Rasht Hospital undated, probably 1948.

RG 231-1-6.
Rolla Edwards Hoffman, *Pioneering in Meshed, the Holy City of Iran. Saga of a Medical Missionary*. Duarte, California, 1969 (typescript).
Annual Report of the Medical Work at Meshed, Persia. The American Hospital. For the year ending June 30, 1929.
The American Christian Hospital, M, Iran, 31st Annual Report, 1945-1946

Rasht

RG 91-19-9, Resht Medical Reports 1918-1944.
- "History of Resht Station."
- Report Medical Work 1919-20
- Medical Report Resht 1921-22
- Resht Medical Report 1923-24
- Resht Medical Report 1928-29
- Resht Medical Report 1930
- Resht Medical Report 1931
- Resht Medical Report 1932
- Resht Medical Report 1933
- Resht Medical Work 1934
- Report of Resht Medical Work 1934-35
- Medical Report Resht 1935-36
- Resht Medical Report 1936-37
- Resht Hospital Report 1937-38
- Resht Hospital Report 1938-39
- Resht Hospital Report 1939-40
- Resht Hospital Report 1940-1941
- Medical Report Resht Hospital 1941- 1942
- Resht Hospital Report 1943
- Resht Hospital Report 1944
- Resht Hospital Report1944-45

RG 91-20-8 - Resht Hospital ?-1957
- Frame/Rasht to Speer/NY 17/02/1931
- Resht Hospital Social Service Center 1942-43
- Resht Hospital Social Service Center 1944-45

Tabriz

RG 161.3.51, Institutions- Christian Hospital, Tabriz 1956, 1958-1964
- Arnold Schneider M.D. Tabriz. Kirkwood Hospital. Questionnaire for the Medical Office, 1958, Tabriz, 17/01/1959.
- Arnold Schneider (Tabriz) to Stevenson and Sundberg (N.Y.), 04/08/1958,
- Drs. Wallstrom M.D. Questionnaire for the Medical Office 1958 , Resht, 26/12/1958
- Gloria Simpson, Nurses education
- Christian Hospital Tabriz Report 1962-1963
- N.N. to Stevens (N.Y.), 07/14/1964
- Memo Sundberg to Stevenson and McGilvray, 06/12/1964

TEHRAN

RG 91-19-11-1: Tehran Medical Work-reports 1922-52

Notes on medical work of Teheran station Jan. 1922
S. W. McD. Historical Sketch of Teheran Medical Work
Teheran Hospital Report 1928
Report of the Medical Work Teheran 1931-1932
Report of Teheran Hospital 1933
Report of Tehran Medical Work 1934-1935
Report of Teheran Hospital 1936
Report Teheran American Hospital 1937
Report Medical Work Teheran 1937-1938
Report American Hospital Teheran 1940-1941
Teheran Medical Report 1941-1942

RG 91-19-17: Medical Committees Reports 1938-41

Jane Payne, Health Center for Children
Memo Bussdicker-Blair, 14 May 1938
Circular letter concerning the Health Center, 11 November 1938.

RG 231-1-2, Rolla Hoffman, no date.

Report of Medical Work Teheran Station 1934.

RG 231-1-5, Rolla Hoffman, Correspondance 1930-1949

Gifford [?] to Allen/Wysham, Tehran 17/08/1936, Government Nurses' School Project
Hoffman/Tehran to Dr. McClanahan/Cairo (31/07/1932).

URUMIYEH

RG 91-20-7: Rezaieh Hospital 1926-31

Report of Mission Medical Work in Urumia. Nov. 1922-1923
Report Jessie Lee Ellis. [1925?]
Famous Urumia Hospital to be rebuilt - memo
Ellis to Williamson, charge d'affaire Tehran 30/09/1930
Cochran Memorial Hospital Report 1933
Last annual report of the Cochran Memorial Hospital, Rezaieh 1934

BRITISH LIBRARY, INDIA OFFICE (IOR), LONDON (UK).

IOR/L/PS/10/284, File 2612/1912 Pt 2 'Persia. Tehran Sanitary Council',

IOR/L/PS/12/3416, Coll. 28/20 'Persia Judicial. Civil, Commercial + Penal Code, and various laws.'

IOR/L/MIL/17/15/8, 'Military Report on Southern Persia'.

IOR/L/MIL/17/15/10/1, *Military Report on S. W. Persia*, 4 vols. Simla, 1909.

IOR/L/PS/20/7, 'Report on Fars by Captain A T Wilson, Indian Political Department',

IOR/R/15/2/1297, 'File 6/78 Necessity to start leper settlement at Bahrain'

Websites

http://tb-lep.behdasht.gov.ir/Leprosy_Situation_In_Iran_World.aspx (accessed 14 June 2018).

https://fa.wikipedia.org/wiki/بابا باغی [accessed 15 June 2018];

http://www.bartarinha.ir/fa/news/90156/ [accessed 15 June 2018]; http://www.hamshahrionline.ir/details/304736 [accessed 15 June 2018].

Iranicaonline.org is the online version of the *Encyclopedia Iranica*.

Books and Articles

Abbasi-Dezfouli, A.; Daneshvar-Kakhi, A; Arab M.; Javaherzadeh M.; Shadmehr M.B.; Abbasi S.; Nournbala, A.A. 2014. "Development of Thoracic Surgery in Iran," in Azizi ed. 2014, pp. 201-04.

Adamec, Ludwig 1989. *Historical Gazetteer of Iran*. 4 vols. Graz: Akademische Verlag.

Adamiyat, Fereydun 1348/1969. *Amir Kabir*. Tehran: Khvarezmi.

Adhari-Khakestar, GholamReza 1395/2016. *Tarikh-e Pezeshki-ye Novin-e Mashhad*. Tehran: Daneshgah-e Azadi-ye Eslami.

Administration Report = *Administration Report on the Persian Gulf Political Residency for the year (1873 to 1940)* in Government of India. *The Persian Gulf Administration Reports 1873-1947*, 10 vols., Gerrards Cross, Archives Editions, 1986.

Amanat, Abbas 1998. "E`tezad al-Saltana, `Aliqoli Mirza," iranicaonline.org.

Algar, Hamed 1969. *Religion and State in Iran 1785-1906. The role of the Ulama in the Qajar Period.* Berkeley: UCLA Press.

Andrews, Justin M. 1950. "Planning a malarial control program for Iran." *CDC Bulletin, Malaria Control in Iran*, July, pp. 1-24.

Anonymous 1902, "Leprosy in Persia," *All Nations, an illustrated missionary magazine* vol. 2, January, p. 46.

Idem 1909, "Nastin treatment of leprosy according to Prof. Dr. Deycke." For unsuccessful treatment results with nastin, see "The treatment of leprosy with nastin," JAMA 13 November, pp. 1646-47.

Idem 1911. "Traveling in Persia," *Bulletin of Pharmacy*, vol. 25, p. 425.

Idem 1918. "Notes on Current Topics," *The Moslem World*, vol. 8, p. 303.

Idem 1922, "Encouraging contrasts in Persia," *The Missionary Review*, vol. 45 (February), p. 146.

Idem 1924. «Current Topics», *The Moslem World* 14, p. 182.

Idem 1954. *Auguste Rollier, M.D. (1954).The British Medical Journal* 2: (4897): 1169-1170.

Idem 2009. "DNA of Jesus-Era Shrouded Man in Jerusalem Reveals Earliest Case of Leprosy," *Science Daily,* 16 December.

Arasteh, A. Reza 1970. *Education and Social Awakening in Iran*. Leiden: Brill.

Ardakani, Hoseyn Mahbubi 1368/1989. *Tarikh-e Mo'assesat-e Tamaddoni-ye Jadid dar Iran.* 3 vols. Tehran: Daneshgah-e Tehran.

Arjah, Akram- Hadiyan, Farideh- Soltanifar, Sadiqeh- and Chehrekhand, Zahrah eds. 1371/1992. *Ketabshenasi-e Nosakh-e Khatti-ye Pezeshki-ye Iran* (Tehran: Ketabkhhaneh-ye Melli.

`Ataradi, Azizollah 1371/1992. *Tarikh-e Astan-e Qods-e Razavi.* 2 vols. Tehran: Utared.

Aubin, Eugène 1908. *La Perse d'aujourd'hui.* Paris: Armand Colin.

Aufderheide, A. C.; Rodriguez-Martin, C. & Langsjoen, O. 1998. *The Cambridge Encyclopedia of Human Paleopathology.* Cambridge; CUP.

Azizi, Hossein Mohammad and Azizi, Farzaneh 2010. "Government Sponsored Iranian Medical Students Abroad (1811-1935)," *Iranian Studies* 43/3, pp. 349-63.

Azizi, M.H. 2014 a, "In Memory of the Late Professor Charles Oberling, the First Dean of Modern Medicine at Dar Al-Fonun," in Azizi, Mohammad Hussein ed. *A Collection of Essays on the History of Medicine in Iran.* Tehran: Academy of Medical Sciences, 2014, pp. 291-94.

Idem 2014 b. "The Biography of Dr. Abol Hassen Bakhtiar (1872-1971)," in Mohammad Hussein ed. *A Collection of Essays on the History of Medicine in Iran.* Tehran: Academy of Medical Sciences, 2014, pp. 295-97

Azizi Mohammad Hussein ed. 2014. *A Collection of Essays on the History of Medicine in Iran.* Tehran: Academy of Medical Sciences.

Azizi, Mohammad Hossein and Bahadori, Moslem 2011. "A History of Leprosy in Iran during the 19th and 20th Centuries," *Archives of Iranian Medicine* November, pp. 425-30.

___, 2014. "A Brief History of Tuberculosis in Iran during the 19th and 20th Centuries," in Azizi ed. 2014, pp. 355-64.

Azizi, Mohammad-Hossein; Bahadori, Moslem; Raees-Jalali, Ghanbar-Ali 2014. "In commemoration of Haj Mohammad Nemazee (1895-1972): The Founder of Nemazee Hospital in Shiraz," in Mohammad-Hossein Azizi ed. *A Collection of Essays on the History of Medicine in Iran.* Tehran, 2014, pp. 239-43.

Bahadori M. 2014. "A Historical Review of Pathology in Iran," in Azizi M. H. ed. 2014, pp. 143-50.

Baladiyyeh-ye Tehran (Servis-e Ma`aref va Ehsa'iyeh va Nashriyat) 1310/1931. *Dovvomin Salnameh-ye Ehsa'iyeh-ye Shahr-e Tehran.* Tehran.

Bamdad, Mehdi 1356. *Tarikh-e Rejal-e Iran qorun-e 12-13-14.* 6 vols. Tehran: Zavvar.

Bhandari, Amdba Datt 1932. "Alepol in the treatment of leprosy," *The Indian Medical Gazette* May, pp. 244-46.

Billings, F. T. 1957. "Dr. Auguste Rollier." *Transactions of the American Clinical and Climatological Association* 68: 52-53.

Blau S, Yagodin V. 2005. Osteoarchaeological evidence for leprosy from western central Asia. *Am J Physical Anthropol* 126, pp. 150-58.

Bradford, Mary E. M.D. 1906. "Something of Persian Lepers," *The Assembly Herald* vol. 12/1, January. pp. 502-03.

Brown, Simon and Simcock, David C. 2012. "Leprosy in Mesopotamia," *Research on History of Medicine* Nov. 1(4), pp. 147-56.

Brugsch, Heinrich 1863. *Reise der K.Preussischen Gesandtschaft nach Persien 1860 und 1861.* Leipzig: Hinrichs.

___, 1886. *Im Lande der Sonne. Wanderungen in Persien.* Berlin.

Bryan, C.P. 1930. *The papyrus Eberus.* London: Geoffrey Bless.

Brydges-Jones, Harford 1976. *An Account of the Transactions of His Majesty's Mission to the Court of Persia in the Years 1807-11*. Tehran: Imperial Organization for Social Services.

CARE 1961. *Resume of Current or Recently Completed Technical Assistance Programs Of Private American Agencies In Iran prepared for STUDY GROUP ON TECHNICAL ASSISTANCE IRAN of the American Council of Voluntary Agencies for Foreign Service February 1, 1961 prepared by The American Council in cooperation with the Program Research Department of CARE, the Cooperative for American Relief Everywhere*. n.p.

Chaqueri, C. ed. 1978. *The Condition of the Working Class*. Florence: Mazdak.

Clarke, H.T. 1837. "Sketches on the State of Medical Knowledge in Persia," *London Medical and Surgical Journal* 2, pp. 707-10.

Cochran, James P. 1899. "Treatment of the Sick and Insane in Persia," *The American Journal of Insanity* 56, pp.105-07.

Coloru, Omar 2017. "Ancient Persia and silent disability," in Chr. Laes ed., *Disability in Antiquity*, London and New York, Routledge, pp. 61-74.

Curzon, G.N. 1892. *Persia and the Persian Question*. 2 vols. London.

Daniel, Rabbi Mooshie G. 1901. *Modern Persia*. Toronto: The Carswell Co.

Daniel, T.M. 2006. "The History of Tuberculosis," *Respiratory Medicine* 2006 Nov;100 (11):1862-70.

Das, P. 1911. "Leprosy and Nastin." *The Indian Medical Gazette*, *46*(11), pp. 421–422.

de Gobineau, A. 1923. *Trois Ans en Asie (de 1855 A 1858)* 2 vols. Paris, Bernard Grasset.

Dikshit, B. B. 1932. "Alepol in leprosy," *The Indian Medical Gazette* January, pp. 7-12.

DCR (Diplomatic and Consular Reports) no. 3189, "Trade of Kermanshah and District for the year 1903-04" by Consular Agent H.L. Rabino. London: HMSO, 1904.

Dodge, Bayard 1958. *The American University of Beirut- A Brief History*. Beirut: Khayat.

Dols, M. 1979. "Leprosy in Medieval Arabic Literature," *Journal of the History of Medicine and Allied Sciences*, Volume XXXIV, Issue 3, 1 July, Pages 314–333.

Dowlatabadi, Yahya 1336/1957. *Hayat-e Yahya*. 4 vols. Tehran: Mosavvar.

Dzierzykray-Rogalski T. 1980. "Paleopathology of the Ptolemaic inhabitants of Dakhleh Oasis (Egypt)," *Journal of Human Evolution* 9(1) January, pp. 71-74.

Iran Almanac 1963, 1970. Tehran: Echo of Iran.

Ebrahimnejad, Hormoz. "Introduction de la médecine européenne en Iran au XIXe siècle," *Sciences Sociales et Santé* 16/4 (décembre 1998), pp. 69-96.

Idem 2000, Theory and Practice in Nineteenth-Century Persian Medicine: Intellectual and Institutional Reforms," *History of Science* 38, pp. 171-78.

Idem 2002, "Religion and Medicine in Iran: from Relationship to Dissocation," *History of Science* 40, pp. 91-112.

Idem 2014. *Medecine in Iran. Profession, Practice, and Politics, 1800-1925*. New York: Palgrave-MacMillan.

Ehtesham al-Saltaneh 1366/1987. *Khaterat*. ed. Sayyed Mohammad Mehdi Musavi. Tehran: Zavvar.

Eilers, Wilhelm 1979. *Die Al, ein persisches Kindbettgespenst*. Munich: Bayerischen Akademie der Wissenschaften.

Ekhtiar, Maryam Dorreh 1994. *The Dar al-Funun: Educational Reform and Cultural Development in Qajar Iran*. unpublished thesis, New York University.

Elgood, Cyril 1951. *A Medical History of Persia and the Eastern Caliphate. The Development of Persian and Arabic Medical Sciences from the Earliest Times until the Year A.D. 1932*. Cambridge: CUP.

Encyclopedia Iranica 1989, "Bongah-e hemayat-e madaran o kudakan," iranicaonline.org.

E`temad al-Saltaneh, Mohammad Hasan Khan 1345/1967. *Ruznameh-ye Khaterat*. ed. Iraj Afshar. Tehran: Amir Kabir.

`Eyn al-Saltaneh, Qahraman Mirza Salur. 1376/1997. *Ruznameh-ye Khaterat*. 10 vols. eds. Mas`ud Salur and Iraj Afshar. Tehran: Asatir.

Farahmandfar, Amir Qoli 1384. "Tolu`-e pezeshki-ye modern va ta'sis-e daneshkadeh dar Shiraz," in Sadeq Homayuni ed. *Yaran-e yekshanbeh*. Shiraz: Novid, pp. 117-28 (with the text of the agreement).

Ferrel, Jno. A. 1914. *The Rural School and Hookworm Disease*. Washington DC: GPO.

Feuvrier, Dr. 1900. *Trois Ans à la Cour de Perse*. Paris: F. Juven.

Firth, Stanley J. 1927. "Treatment of ringworm by thallium acetate," *The British Medical Journal* 18 July, p. 1097.

Floor, Willem 2004. *Public Health in Iran*. Washington DC: MAGE.

Idem 2011. *Labor and Industry in Iran 1850-1941*. Washington DC: MAGE.

Idem 2012. "Hospitals in Safavid and Qajar Iran: an enquiry into their number, growth and importance," in Fabrizio Speziale ed. *Hospitals in Iran and India 1500-1950s*. Leiden: Brill, pp. 37-116.

Idem 2018. *Studies in the History of Medicine of Iran*. Washington DC: MAGE.

Fraser, James Baillie 1826. *Travels and Adventures in The Persian Provinces on the Southern Banks of The Caspian Sea*. London: Longman.

Garrison, Fielding H. 1933. "Persian Medicine and Medicine in Persia," *Bulletin of the Institute of the History of Medicine. The Johns Hospkins University*, Vol. 1, No. 4 (May, 1933), pp. 129-153.

Ghorban, Zabih 1989. *Medical Education in Shiraz, A Personal Memoir*. N.p.

Gilmour, John 1924. *Rapport sur la situation sanitaire de la Perse*. Geneva, Société des Nations.

Good, Byron J. 1981. "The Transformation of Health Care in Modern Iranian History," in Michael E. Bonine and Nikki Keddie eds. *Modern Iran. The Dialectics of Continuity and Change*. Albany: State University of New York Press, pp. 59-82.

Government of Great Britain 1945. *Geographical Handbook Series – Persia*. n.p.

Government of France 1914, *Rapports Commerciaux des agents diplomatiques et consulaires de France* – Année 1914 no. 1079 Perse. Paris.

Government of Iran n.d. A, *Modhakerat-e Majles, Dowreh-ye Dovvom-e Taqniniyeh*. 3 vols. Tehran: Majles.

Government of Iran n.d. B, *Majmu`eh-ye Qavanin ... dar chahar dowreh-ye taqniniyyeh*. Tehran: Majles.

Government of Iran 1317/1938. Rahahan-e sarasar-e Iran. Tehran: Vezarat-e Toruq.

Griffith, Ralph T.H. 1895. *Hymns of the Atharva Veda*. Benares, E.J. Lazarus & Co.

Griscom, Mary W. 1921. "A medical motor trip through Persia," *Asia. The American Magazine on the Orient* March, pp. 233-40.

Grothe, Hugo 1911. *Zur Natur und Wirtschaft von Vorderasien. I. Persien*. Halle: Gebauer-Schwetschke.

Gurney, John and Nabavi, Negin 1993. "Dar al-Fonun," iranicaonline.org.

Hajbaghery. Adib M and M. Salsali. A model for empowerment of nursing in Iran. *BMC Health Serv Res*. 2005; 5(1):24. Published 2005 Mar 16. doi:10.1186/1472-6963-5-24.

Hamed, Mohammad Sadeq and Habibi, Manuchehr 1376/1997. *Tarikh-e San`at-e Barq dar Iran*. Tehran.

Häntzsche, J.C. 1863. "Lepra in Persien," *Virchows Archiv für pathologische Anatomie und Physiologie* 27, pp. 180-83.

Hasanbegi, Mohammad Reza 1377/1998. *Tehran-e Qadim*. Tehran: Mansuri.

Hedayat, Mohammad. 1344/1965. *Khatarat va Khaterat*. Tehran: Zavvar.

Hedayat, Rezaqoli Khan 1338-39/1959-60. *Tarikh-e Rowzat al-Safa*. 10 vols. Tehran: Khayyam.

Ingram, John T. 1932. "Thallium acetate in the treatment of ringworm of the scalp," *The British Medical Journal* (2 January), pp. 8-10.

Iran Almanac 1963. Tehran: Echo of Iran.

Jorjani, Esma`il 1380/2002. *Dhakhireh-ye Khvarazmshahi*. Moharreri MohammadReza ed. 3 vols. Tehran: Farhangestan-e `olum-e pezeshki.

Jozani, Niloufar 1994. *La Beauté Menacée*. Paris-Tehran: IFRI.

Kaempfer, Engelbert 2018. *Exotic Attractions in Persia: 1684-1688*. Washington DC: MAGE.

Karamati, Yunos and EIr 1999. "Faculties of the University of Tehran. v. Faculty of Medicine." Iranicaonline.org.

Khakestar, Gholamreza Adhari 1395/2016. *Tarikh-e Pezeshki-ye Novin-e Mashhad*. Mashhad: Daneshgah-e Azad-e Eslami.

Klingmüller, Victor 1930. *Die Lepra*. Berlin: Springer.

Lichtwardt, Hartman A. 1934. "Leprosy in Afghanistan: a preliminary assessment," *International Journal of Leprosy* vol. 2/1, pp. 75-76.

Loew, Dr. 1908. "Zur Lepra in Persian," *Deutsche medizinische Wochenschrift*, Volume 34/1, 1908, pp. 701-02.

Loghatnameh-ye Dehkhoda.

Lycklama à Nijeholt, T.M 1875. *Voyage en Russie, au Caucase et en Perse*. 4 vols. Paris-Amsterdam: Aethus Bertrand - C. L. van Langenhuysen.

Mahdavi, Shireen 2009, "Kofri, Mohammad Kermanshahi," iranicaonline.org.

Malekzadeh, Elham 1392. *Mo'assesat-e Kheyriyeh-ye Refahi – Behdashti dar Dowreh-ye Reza Shah*. Tehran: Tarikh-e Iran

Idem 1394. *Seyr-e Takvin va Tatavvor-e Herfeh-ye Mama'i dar `Asr-e Qajar va Pahlavi*. Tehran: Pazhuheshgah-e `Olum-e Ensani.

Matheson C.D., Vernon K.K., Lahti A. et al. 2009. Molecular exploration of the first-century Tomb of the Shroud in Akeldama, Jerusalem. *PLoS ONE* 4: e8319.

Matin, Peyman. "Jodham," *Dar al-Ma`aref Bozorg Eslami* vol. 17, pp. 639-45.

McLeod, Katrina C. D.; Robin D. S. Yates June 1981. "Forms of Ch'in Law: An Annotated Translation of The Feng-chen shih". *Harvard Journal of Asiatic Studies*. 41 (1), pp. 111–163.

Modi, Jivanji Jemshedji 1911, "Leprosy, an old Iranian view of it. The legend suggesting cow-urine as its supposed preventive," *Anthropological Papers* Part III. Bombay: British India Press, pp. 93-118.

Idem, 1917, "Ancient Palipatura," in *Asiatic Papers* II, Bombay: The Times Press, pp. 211-86.

Moghadas, Abdorreza Naser 2015. "First Visual Evidence of Leprosy in the Continental Shelf of Iran," *Iran J Public Health*. Aug; 44(8): 1162–1163.

Morton, Rosalie Slaughter. 1940. *A Doctor's Holiday in Iran.* New York: Funk & Wagnalls.

Mostowfi, Abdollah 1343. *Sharh-e Zendegani-ye Man ya Tarikh-e Ejtema`i va Edari-ye Dowreh-ye Qajariyeh.* 3 vols. Tehran: Zavvar.

Mo'tamen, `Ali 1348/1969. *Rahnama ya Tarikh va Towsif Darbar-e Velayatmadar-e Razavi.* Tehran.

Najmabadi, Mahmud 1353/1974. *Tarikh-e tebb dar Iran pas az Eslam.* Tehran: Daneshgah.

Idem 1354/1975, "Tebb-e Dar al-fonun va kotub-e darsi-ye an," in Qodratollah Rowshani Za`faranlu ed., *Amir Kabir va Dar al-Fonun.* Tehran, pp. 202-37.

Idem 1364/1985. *A Bibliography of Printed Books in Persian on Medicine and Allied Subjects.* Tehran.

Nasiri, Mirza Naqi 2008. *Titles & Emoluments in Safavid Iran.* translated and annotated by Willem Floor. Washington DC: MAGE.

Neligan, A.R. 1926. "Public Health in Persia. 1914-24," *The Lancet* Part I; Part II-March 27, pp. 690-94; Part III-April 3, pp. 742-44.

Nezam al-Saltaneh 1361. *Khaterat va asnad-e Hoseyn Qoli Khan Nezam al-Saltaneh Mafi.* 2 vols. ed. Mansureh Nezam Mafi, Sirus Sa`dvandiyan and Hamid Rampisheh. Tehran: Nashr-e Now.

Overseas Consultants, Inc. 1949. *Report on the Seven Year Development Plan for the Plan Organization of the Imperial Government of Iran.* 5 vols. New York.

Pahlavi, Farah 2005. *An Enduring Love. My Life with the Shah.* New York: Miramax.

Paidar, Parvin 1995. *Women and the Political Process in twenty-century Iran.* Cambridge: CUP.

Piemontese, Angelo Michele, "The Statutes of the Qajar Orders of Knighthood," *East and West* 19/3-4, 1969, pp. 431-73.

Idem 1984. "Gli Ufficiali Italiani al servizio della Persia nel XIX secolo," in: G. Borsa and Brocchieri P. Beonio. *Garibaldi, Mazzini et il Risorgimento nel Risveglio dell'Asia e dell'Africa.* Milan: Francio Angeli, 1984, pp. 65-130.

Polak, J. E. 1852. "Briefe aus Persien," *Wiener medizinische Wochenschrift* vol. 2, pp. 742-43, 789-90.

Idem 1853. "Briefe aus Persien," *Wiener medizinische Wochenschrift.* vol. 3, pp. 219-21, 509-10.

Idem 1854. "Briefe aus Persien," *Wiener medizinische Wochenschrift.* vol. 4, pp. 59-60, 396-97.

Idem 1855. "Briefe aus Persien," *Wiener medizinische Wochenschrift.* vol. 5, pp. 269-70.

Idem 1859 a. "Briefe aus Persien," *Wiener medizinische Wochenschrift.* vol. 9, p. 765.

Idem 1859 b. "Medicinische Briefe aus Persien (17/11/1858)," *Zeitschrift der k.k. Gesellschaft der Aerzte zu Wien* vol. 15, pp. 138-40.

Idem 1860, "Ueber 158 Stein-Operationen ausgefuehrt in Persien," *Zeitschrift der K.K. Gesellschaft der Aertze zu Wien,* vol. 15, pp. 694-99.

Idem 1862. "Die medizinische Schule und Spitäler in Teheran," *Zeitschrift der k.k. Gesellschaft der Aerzte zu Wien* vol. 12, pp. 235-36, 249-51.

Idem 1863. "Lepra in Persien," *Virchows Archiv für pathologische Anatomie und Physiologie* 27, pp. 175-80.

Idem 1865. *Persien, das Land und seine Bewohner,* 2 vols. Leipzig.

Political Diaries = *Political Diaries of the Persian Gulf* 1904-1947, 17 vols. n.p. Archive Editions, 1990.

Presbyterian Church 1876, The Thirty-Ninth Annual Report of the Board of Foreign Missions. New York.

Presbyterian Church 1877. The Fortieth Annual Report of the Board of Foreign Missions. New York.

Presbyterian Church 1883, The Forty-Sixth Annual Report of the Board of Foreign Missions. New York.

Presbyterian Church 1884, The Forty-Seventh Annual Report of the Board of Foreign Missions. New York.

Presbyterian Church 1886, The Forty-Ninth Annual Report of the Board of Foreign Missions. New York.

Presbyterian Church 1887, Seventeenth Annual Report of Board of Home Missions. New York.

Presbyterian Church 1888. Eighteenth Annual Report of Board of Home Missions. New York.

Presbyterian Church 1889, Nineteenth Annual Report of Board of Home Missions. New York.

Presbyterian Church 1890. Twentieth Annual Report of Board of Home Missions. New York.

Presbyterian Church 1891. Twenty-First Annual Report of Board of Home Missions. New York.

Presbyterian Church 1892. Twenty-Second Annual Report of Board of Home Missions. New York.

Presbyterian Church 1893. Twenty-Third Annual Report of Board of Home Missions. New York.

Presbyterian Church 1894, Twenty-Fourth Annual Report of Board of Home Missions. New York.

Presbyterian Church 1895. Twenty-Fifth Annual Report of Board of Home Missions. New York.

Presbyterian Church 1896. Ninety Fourth Annual Report. Board of Home Missions. New York.

Presbyterian Church 1897. Ninety Fifth Annual Report. Board of Home Missions. New York.

Presbyterian Church 1898. Ninety Sixth Annual Report. Board of Home Missions. New York.

Presbyterian Church 1899. Ninety Seventh Annual Report. Board of Home Missions. New York.

Presbyterian Church 1901. Ninety Ninth Annual Report. Board of Home Missions. New York.

Presbyterian Church 1902. One Hundred and First Annual Report. Board of Home Missions. New York.

Presbyterian Church 1904. *Hundred and Second Annual Report of the Board of Home Missions of the Presbyterian Church in the U.S.A*. New York.

Presbyterian Church 1905. One Hundred and Third Annual Report. Board of Home Missions. New York.

Presbyterian Church 1906. One Hundred and Fourth Annual Report. Board of Home Missions. New York.

Presbyterian Church 1907. One Hundred and Fifth Annual Report. Board of Home Missions. New York.

Presbyterian Church 1908. *Reports of the Missionary and Benevolent Boards and Committees to the General Assembly of the Presbyterian Church in the USA*. New York.

Presbyterian Church 1909. One Hundred and Seventh Annual Report. Board of Home Missions. New York.

Presbyterian Church 1910. One Hundred and Eighth Annual Report. Board of Home Missions. New York.

Presbyterian Church 1911. One Hundred Ninth Annual Report. Board of Home Missions. New York.

Presbyterian Church 1912. One Hundred Tenth Annual Report. Board of Home Missions. New York.

Presbyterian Church 1913. One Hundred Eleventh Annual Report. Board of Home Missions. New York.

Presbyterian Church 1914. One Hundred Twelfth Annual Report. Board of Home Missions. New York.

Presbyterian Church 1915. *One Hundred Thirteenth Annual Report of the Board of Home Missions*, Reports of the Missionary and Benevolent Boards and Committees to the General Assembly.

Presbyterian Church 1919. *One Hundred Seventeenth Annual Report of the Home Missions of the Presbyterian Church of the U.S.A.*

Presbyterian Church 1919-20. *Annual Report, By Presbyterian Church in the U.S.A. Board of Foreign Missions*, Volumes 82-83, 1919-20, p. 265-266.

Presbyterian Church 1920. One Hundred Eighteenth Annual Report. Board of Home Missions. New York.

Presbyterian Church 1920. *The Eighty-third Annual Report of the Board of Foreign Missions of the Presbyterian Church in the U.S.A.*, 1920.

Presbyterian Church 1921. *The Eighty-fourth Annual Report of the Board of Foreign Missions of the Presbyterian Church in the U.S.A.*

Presbyterian Church 1922 a. *The Eighty-fifth Annual Report of the Board of Foreign Missions of the Presbyterian Church in the U.S.A.*, 1922.

Presbyterian Church 1922 b. *The Presbyterian Hospital Bulletin*. Chicago, Ill. January 1922, no. 48.

Presbyterian Church 1928 a. Annual Meeting Actions of the East Persia Mission of the Presbyterian Church in the USA. Daulatabad, August 1-10, 1928.

Presbyterian Church 1928 b. Minutes to the General Assembly of Presbyterian Church in the USA, Third Series-Volume VIII-1928, Part II. Philadelphia, July.

Presbyterian Church 1930. *Seventh Annual Report of the Board of National Missions of the Presbyterian Church in the USA*. New York.

Presbyterian Church 1932. Minutes to the General Assembly of Presbyterian Church in the USA, Third Series-Volume XI-1932, Part II. Philadelphia, July.

Rahnama-ye Daneshkadeh-ye pezeshki, daru-sazi, dandan-pezeshki. 1333/1954. Tehran: Daneshgah.

Rasooli, Jay M. and Allen, Cady H. 1958. *The Life Story of Dr. Sa'eed of Iran* (Grand Rapids: Grand Rapids International Publications.

Rastegar Dr. 1312/1933. "Hefz al-Sehheh-ye `Omumi-ye Atfal," *Salnameh-ye Pars*, part 2, pp. 80-96.

Reza'i, Maryam 1398/2019. "Goft o gu ba Safiyeh, qabeleh'i dar Jarquyeh-ye Esfahan," *Zan-e Emruz* 6/25, pp. 87-92.

Rice, Clara 1923. *Persian Women and Their Ways*. London: Seeley, Service & Co.

Robbins, Gwen; Tripathy, V. Mushrif; Misra, V. N.; Mohanty, R. K.; Shinde, V. S.; Gray, Kelsey M.; Schug, Malcolm D. 2009. "Ancient Skeletal Evidence for Leprosy in India (2000 B.C.)". *PLOS ONE*. 4: e5669.

Robbins Schug, G. Blevins, K. Elaine; Cox, Brett; Gray, Kelsey; Mushrif-Tripathy, Veena December 2013. "Infection, Disease, and Biosocial Process at the End of the Indus Civilization," *PLOS ONE*. 0084814: e84814.

Römer, R. 1906. "Le Lèpre," *Bulletin de l'Académie royale de médecine de Belgique*, vol. 20, pp. 99-165.

Rusta'i, Mohsen 1382. *Tarikh-e Tebb va Tebabat dar Iran*, 2 vols. Tehran: Asnad-e Melli.

Ruznameh-ye Dowlat-e `Aliyeh-ye Iran 1370-72/1991-93. 2 vols. Tehran: Ketabkhaneh-ye Melli (reprint).

Sadeq, Isa 1340/1961. *Yadegar-e `Omr*. 3 vols. Tehran: Amir Kabir.

Sadid al-Saltaneh Kebabi, Mohammad `Ali 1342/1963, *Bandar `Abbas va Khalij-e Fars*. Tehran: Amir Kabir.

Sajjadi, Sadegh 1994. "Dentistry," iranicaonline.org.

Salnameh-ye Pars 1308/1929. Tehran: Jahed.

Sani` al-Dowleh, Mohammad Hasan Khan 1295-97/1878-81. *Mer'at al-Boldan*. 4 vols. Tehran (lithograph).

Idem 1296/1879. *Ketab al-Ma'ather va'l-Athar*. Tehran (lithograph).

Idem 1300/1883. *Montazam-e Naseri*. 3 vols. Tehran (lithograph).

Sardari-Niya, Samad 1382/2003, *Dar al-Fonun-e Tabriz*. Tabriz: Neda-ye Shams .

Schlimmer, Joh. L. 1970. *Terminologie Medico-Pharmaceutique*. Tehran: Daneshgah.

Sepehr, `Abdol-Hoseyn 1368/1889. *Mer'at al-Vaqaye`-ye Mozaffari va Yaddashtha-ye Malek al-Mo'arrekhin* ed. `Abdol-Hoseyn Nava'i. Tehran: Zarrin.

Shahri, Ja`far 1368/1989. *Tarikh-e ejtema`i -Tehran dar qarn-e sizdahom*, 6 vols. Tehran: Farhang-Rasa.

Shanks, S. Cochrane M.B. B. Ch. 1931. "Correspondence", *The British Medical Journal* (16 January), p. 121.

Slaby, Helmut 1982. *Bindenschild und Sonnenlöwe. Die Geschichte der österreichisch-iranischen Beziehungen bis zur Gegenwart*. Graz: Akademische Druck u. Verlagsanstalt.

Shteglova, O.P. 1975. *Katalog litografirovannykh Knig na persidskom yazyke v sobranii LO IV AN SSSR*. 2 vols. Moscow: Nauka.

Soltani, Mohammad `Ali 1370/1991. *Joghrafiya-ye Tarikhi va Tarikh-e Mofassal-e Kermanshahan*. 3 vols. Tehran.

Spigelman M, Donoghue H.D. 2001. "Unusual pathological condition in the lower extremities of a skeleton from ancient Israel." *Am J Physical Anthropol* 114, pp. 92-93.

Stamp, Dr. 1922. "What do teeth do?" *`Alam-e Nesvan* 2 (November), pp. 6-10.

Sureshjani, Salem Hoseynzadeh 1395/2006. *Tarikh-e Dar al-Shifa-ye Astan-e Qods-e Razavi az dowreh-ye Safavi ta Payan-e dowreh-ye Qajariyeh*. Tehran: Daneshgah-e Azad-e Eslami.

Ta`eb, Hasan 1384/2005. *Bimarestanha-ye Rasht az mashruteh ta 1357*. Rasht: Iliya.

Tarbiyat 1377/1998. 3 vols. Tehran, Ketabkhaneh-ye Melli.

Teixeira Pedro 1991. *The Travels of Pedro Teixeira with his "Kings of Harmuz"*. Nendeln - Liechtenstein: Kraus Reprint.

UNESCO 1963. *Iran-Shahr: a survey of Iran's land, people, culture, government and economy*. 2 vols. Tehran: University.

UNESCO 1343/1964. Komisiyun-e Melli-e Yunesko-Iran. *Iranshahr*, no. 22, Tehran.

US Army 1963. *Area Handbook for Iran*, Washington DC.

US Government 1956. *United States Operations in Iran, Hearings of the Subcommittee on Government Operations pf the House of Representatives*. Washington DC: GPO.

Ussher, John 1865. *A Journey from London to Persepolis*. London: Hurst and Blackett.

Vaqaye`-ye Ettefaqiyeh 1373-74/1994-95. 4 vols. Tehran: Ketabkhaneh- Melli.

Vaume, Dr. 1866. "La lèpre dans le Kurdistan Persan," *Bulletin de la Société d'Anthropologie de Lyon* 5, pp. 158-62.

Vessal K, Rad. S., Alizadeh A., Jalal-Shokouhi, J. 2014. "Development of Radiology in Iran," in Azizi ed. 2014, pp. 157-64.

Vinkhuijzen, H.J. 1868. *De melaatschheid: vooral met betrekking tot hare oorzaken en verhouding in de maatschappij*. the Hague: van Cleef.

Warne, William E. 1956. *Mission For Peace. Point 4 in Iran*. Indianapolis/New York: Bobbs-Merrill.

Watelin, Louis-Charles 1921. *La Perse Immobile*. Paris: Chapelot.

Waterfield, Robin E. 1973. *Christians in Persia - Assyrians, Armenians, Roman Catholics and Protestants*. London: George Allen & Unwin.

Wells, R. P. 1878, *A Year in Persia. A discourse in memory of Mrs. Hattie Lyman Stocking*. Holeyoke, Mass.: Transcript Steam Book and Job Printing House.

Williams, Molly 1994. *The Rich Persian Tapestry of My Persian Years*. Bendigo: Keith Cole.

Wilson, S.G. 1895. *Persian Life and Customs*. New York: Fleming. H. Revell.

Idem 1896. *Persia*: *Western Mission*. Philadelphia: Presbyterian Board of Publication.

Wishard, John G. 1908. *Twenty Years in Persia*. New York: Fleming H. Revell.

Wolff, Joseph 1860-61. *Travels and Adventures of the Rev. Joseph Wolff*. London: Saunders, Otley and Co.

Yaghma'i, E. "Madraseh-ye Dar al-Fonun," *Yaghma* 23, 1349/1970-71, pp. 233-38, 361-66, and 423-26.

Zambaco Pacha, Démétrius Alexandre 1924. *La lèpre a travers les siècles et les contrées*. Paris: Masson & Cie.

INDEX

C

D

E

F

G

N

O

P

T

U

V

W

X

Y

Z

www.ingramcontent.com/pod-product-compliance
Ingram Content Group UK Ltd.
Pitfield, Milton Keynes, MK11 3LW, UK
UKHW041844031026
15587UKWH00003B/1008

9 781949 445237